YOGA NIDRA
THE ART OF TRANSFORMATIONAL SLEEP

*Restore your health, reshape your life
and change your destiny.*

by Kamini Desai, PhD
Inspired by the Teachings of Yogi Amrit Desai

First Lotus Press Edition 2017
ISBN: 978-0-9406-7639-8

Library of Congress Number: 2016441639

Published by:

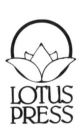

Lotus Press
P.O. Box 325
Twin Lakes, WI 53181 USA
800-824-6396 (toll free order phone)
262-889-8561 (office phone)
262-889-2461 (office fax)
www.lotuspress.com (website)
lotuspress@lotuspress.com (email)

Printed In USA

This book is dedicated to my beloved father and mother, whose love I have come to cherish deeply...my deepest gratitude for all I have learned from you both.

Your teachings have contributed to the lives of thousands of people the world over...and live on through this book.

It is my hope to make such a contribution to humanity.

Yoga Nidra
The Art of Transformational Sleep
Table of Contents

Acknowledgements

I am amazed by the groundswell of support I received that has allowed this book to come to fruition. Thank you, first and foremost, to SuzAnn Gunter for your meticulous, loyal and unwavering support to get this book edited and ready for print. To Lynn Matthews, an outstanding teacher in her own right, who dedicated her valuable time to helping edit this book just because she believes in the value of this method and its healing potential. To Diane and Fred Covan who, out of appreciation for the work, volunteered to help make the book great. To Eric Walrabenstein for your friendship and the keen insights that helped hone these teachings. To the Amrit Yoga Institute and all the teaching staff who carry the essence and teachings of the Amrit Method of Yoga Nidra so beautifully. To my assistant Hamsa, who takes care of me in so many ways.

Finally, to my husband Skuli and my new family, my team, who have brought me more joy and fulfillment than I could ever have imagined.

Foreword

The year was 1972. It was near the beginning of my career as a clinical psychologist and I was working at a hospital-based clinic. The patient was thirteen years old and pregnant for the second time while her maternal grandmother raised her two year-old child. Her mother was a heroin addict; she did not know her own father. She was depressed, anxious and the only thing she looked forward to was the birth of this child. I believed my job was to get her to stop having babies while still a child herself. But she wanted this baby so somebody would love her and it would make her important. She had insight. She knew what she was doing and why she was doing it. This was the first time I clearly saw the limits of psychological insight. Mere insight would not change this girl's lifestyle. Nor has it been enough for thousands of patients who have followed.

Last year, in a social setting, I met a 45-year-old Iraq War veteran. He said he was suffering from Traumatic Brain Injury (TBI) and Post-Traumatic Stress Disorder (PTSD). He reported that he was being treated as an outpatient at a VA Hospital and was taking fifteen different, powerful psychiatric medications to control his numerous symptoms. He was also receiving counseling. I subsequently learned that he committed suicide and joined the ranks of the 23 US Veterans who kill themselves each day.

Different assumptions have underscored the major approaches to psychotherapy, personal change and growth. Psychoanalysis and its many off-shoots are based on the assumption that once the historical antecedents are learned, the patient will understand *why* they are the way they are and will be relieved of their troubling symptoms. This is referred to as "insight." Behavior

Therapy and its derivations assume that changing behavior patterns through learning will result in alleviation of maladaptive behaviors. Cognitive Therapy is based on the belief that by identifying and changing negative, self-defeating thoughts, one will become symptom-free. These and most other psychotherapeutic techniques either ignore or give nodding recognition to the importance of physiological processes in the individual. On the other hand, Yoga Nidra directly addresses, focuses on, and changes habitual physiological reactive patterns. This results in actual change, healing, growth and freedom without the need to go into the story.

In my forty-five years of clinical work with every type of psychological or psychiatric problem at the front-lines of mental health struggles, I have encountered psychotics, schizophrenics, bi-polars, the depressed, traumatized, addicted, neurotic and the "worried well." I have treated children, adolescents, adults and the mature in individual, couples, family and group settings. I have forensically evaluated those accused of murder, white collar and street crime. Although I am not a psychiatrist and do not prescribe psychiatric medication, I have observed their ample use in treatment throughout my career. I have studied various approaches to psychotherapy and human change, ranging from classical Freudian Psychoanalysis to Past-lives Regression Therapy, and everything in between. For at least the past thirty years, I have been impressed with the value of meditation and body-oriented approaches to therapy including massage, yoga and tai chi.

Then, last summer, my wife kidnapped and dragged me to an ashram hidden deep in the Ocala National Forest in Florida to learn Yoga Nidra meditation from a renowned master and his daughter. I was blown away.

The benefits of meditation are well-documented in a wealth of respected scientific literature. I have urged many of my patients to develop a meditation practice and often teach them deep breathing exercises, especially for treating symptoms of anxiety. While a serious and effective meditation practice is difficult to develop and maintain, Yoga Nidra is as easy as—but much more effective than—the breathing techniques I formerly taught. Yogi Amrit Desai perfected the ancient technique of Yoga Nidra to its current level of sophistication. His daughter went on to receive a Doctorate in Psychology and created a ground-breaking curriculum based on his teachings. In this book she integrates her traditional academic learning with Yoga Nidra for a useful guide to the modern applications of this ancient practice.

Traditional meditation requires considerable effort to "empty the mind." Many individuals believe they are incapable of meditation or sitting still. Quieting the mind in that way is difficult because it is antithetical to the actual normal functioning of the brain which is always seeking answers, solving problems, and protecting us from the outside world. Yoga Nidra meditation is easy because it is based on something that the body already knows how to do: go to sleep. Through an ancient and well-designed process, the mind is guided through stages of sleep while the recipient is awake and fully conscious. The process results in the same brain wave changes that occur during deep sleep, although you are aware and awake. It can create the deepest level of meditation achieved by well-practiced Yogis. In this state, various beneficial changes occur. The consequences of stress are reversed. Blood pressure and cortisol levels drop. Heart rate slows and the body begins a process of rejuvenation and healing. The beneficial consequences of entering this state on a regular basis are that the unpleasant symptoms of insomnia, anxiety, depression, addiction and PTSD are reduced.

For example, addicts use the substance to which they are addicted to reduce stress in their lives, including the stress created by the need for more of the substance itself. Removing the addicting substance leaves the individual without the coping mechanism needed to deal with the normal stressors of life. Yoga Nidra both reduces the severity of life's stressors as well as providing a tool upon which the addict can deliberately rely when confronted with the inevitable complications of life.

In this book, Dr. Desai explains how Yoga Nidra can be applied to every aspect of human life. This book not only explains the process, why it works, and what it treats, it also gives an invaluable bonus at the end: exact instructions on how to practice Yoga Nidra and a complete copy of a Yoga Nidra script. So, you can use it for yourself or those you love and, if you're in the mental health business, you can also use it in your clinical work. I conduct Yoga Nidra sessions on a regular basis for my patients and others who don't want to discuss their story but, nevertheless, want relief from the stressors of life. I strongly recommend it.

Frederick L. Covan, PhD

Licensed Psychologist, New York and Florida

Clinical Coordinator of the Adolescent Unit, Harlem Hospital, New York, NY (1972-80); Chief Psychologist of Bellevue Hospital, New York, NY (1980-94); Author of <u>Crazy All The Time: Life, Lessons and Insanity on the Psych Ward of Bellevue Hospital</u> (Simon & Schuster, 1994); Clinical Faculty of the Graduate Schools of New York University, Pace University, Fordham University, Yeshiva University, and St. John's University, New York, NY (1972-94); Currently in Private Practice in Key West, FL, and Clinical Supervisor, U.S. Navy Alcohol and Substance Abuse Program.

Yoga Nidra: The Art of Non-Doing

Yoga Nidra is one of the least known and most under-appreciated practices of Yoga, yet its potential reach is immense. In our modern society, many of us are accustomed to *doing more to get more*. Even when we want to relax, we ask, "How do I *do* that?" Relaxation doesn't happen by *doing* more, yet this is how most of us go about it. Yoga Nidra is not about doing more, it is about doing less. Yoga Nidra is about releasing the struggling and striving to get somewhere. It is the art and practice of doing *nothing* to arrive exactly where you want to be.

It is like floating. Floating is not something you *do*, it is something that *happens* in the absence of *doing*. It is an experience of being held, being carried…but it can only happen when you stop struggling to keep yourself upright. Stop doing and floating *happens*. Stop efforting and sleep happens. When you let go of any doing, everything gets done. This concept is so foreign to the Western mind, we can hardly fathom it.

There is a reason stress is at epidemic levels in the West and I believe this is why: *we don't know how to stop*. Our waking hours have taken over our sleeping hours. Even our sleep and rest is in service of *doing* more, rather than *being* more. We don't sleep to be rested, to revitalize and nourish ourselves, we sleep so we can get up and *do more* the next day. We haven't mastered the art of *non-doing* along with the art of doing. We haven't learned how to relax in action.

What if there was a way we could experience being carried by the waters of life? A way to feel held and supported in the midst of life rather than struggling to keep our head above water? This is exactly what Yoga Nidra is designed to do. Through the practice of Yoga Nidra you learn to relax as deeply as in sleep while awake.

Yoga Nidra is an age-old practice of Yoga described in the ancient texts. It is not new. It is composed of a *series of breath, body and awareness techniques designed to help you move into progressive states of relaxation, of non-doing.* Though it is impossible to achieve relaxation with greater effort, you *can* enter a non-doing state where you are doing nothing and relaxation *happens. The techniques of Yoga Nidra are active techniques that allow access to the non-doing state of being.* The function of the technique is to *do* in such a way that you slip into a state of *non-doing.* So much so, that the experience of the body and mind can disappear completely for a time. The result is a highly regenerative state where the energy normally burned by the mind is fully freed to heal and restore the body. This healing energy of the body, freed from the mind, can also become a spiritual force, unlocking inner guidance, knowing and insight into your true nature.

Yogis state that 45 minutes of Yoga Nidra is as restorative as three hours of sleep. The body needs to let go. It needs to rest. It needs to have profound experiences of *non-doing* so it can regenerate itself. Without this, the body begins to tire. Like a car, it needs maintenance and repair. Keep it in overdrive and it will eventually burn out.

Yoga Nidra is regenerative, but it is more than a nap. *It is a spiritual practice that, through a structured and conscious movement through sleep states, takes you to realms beyond the mind and into the fourth state of consciousness beyond waking, dreaming and deep sleep.* Ancient Yogis knew that a vital, rested and restored body is a necessary first step toward inner awakening. Yoga Nidra is a practice that can be used at many different levels, all of which serve our ultimate potentials as human beings and as evolving souls. It is up to us to determine how far we want to take the practice and for what purpose. Its beauty is that it addresses the entire spectrum from the concrete to the most subtle.

What are the Benefits of Yoga Nidra?

Most people believe that change can only happen in the realm of doing, and that achieving and doing more is the only means to changing one's life. Yet, doing can only take place in the waking state. Change in any other state of consciousness can only be accessed through *non-doing*. Non-doing gives access to change in conscious dream states, deep sleep and in the fourth state beyond waking, dreaming and deep sleep. In Yoga Nidra you are accessing aspects of yourself where your active doing has no access. Its effects are created from *beyond* the mind rather than *through* the mind. Below are some of the benefits of Yoga Nidra that appear from beyond the reach of the logical, analytical, and rational doing mind.

Relaxation, Restoration, Physical Health and Stress Management

Starting at the foundational level, Yoga Nidra brings you to deep states of *non-doing* that help you sleep better, neutralize excess stress and restore profound peace, relaxation and rejuvenation to the body. Yoga Nidra takes you to brainwave states where the organs and systems of the body are nourished and regenerated. Yoga Nidra slows the rate at which you age and keeps you looking younger, longer.

The body is its own healer; it *knows* how to heal itself. However, it needs the right environment to do so. This is what doctors and surgeons do. They don't heal a person; they give the body the best possible environment to heal itself. This is why doctors can never guarantee an outcome; it is all up to the body. What if you could influence your body's capacity to heal itself? In this book, I will show you how Yoga Nidra can free the healing potential of the body to do just that. You will see how Yoga Nidra can be used as an adjunct practice to any mainstream treatment for health or recovery from illness.

I will be surveying numerous studies which show how restoring optimal balance to the body can aid in the prevention and healing of such disparate health challenges as infertility, digestive issues, insomnia, allergies, skin conditions, heart conditions and autoimmune diseases.

Healthy Relationship to Thoughts

Stressful thought patterns influence our health and quality of life. Yoga Nidra allows us to relate differently to our thoughts and redirect the thought patterns of worry, anxiety and fear that affect our ability to enjoy life, our loved ones, and ultimately our health.

At an even deeper level, the practice allows us to create a different relationship to limiting perceptions, beliefs and core programming that unconsciously drive our lives. Consider that we are not tired only because we work hard, we are also tired because of what the mind does. The more we can manage what the mind does, the more energy we will have to live our life.

Detoxification and Integration of Incomplete Experiences

Yoga Nidra allows us to resolve and release incomplete, unprocessed emotions and experiences that came but never left. Sometimes we hold on to overwhelming events that we can't process and we shut down. As a result, these experiences remain stuck and never fully move through us. Yoga Nidra takes us into deep states where we can let go of them. The brakes that normally hold these unfinished experiences in place are lifted, and we begin to rid ourselves of the undigested past. The experiences leave without us ever having to know what they were or where they came from. All we have to do is breathe, relax and let it happen.

Experiencing One's True Nature

Ultimately, all these benefits of Yoga Nidra prepare us for its ultimate purpose: experiencing our true nature, our essence—both kinesthetically and experientially. We may intellectually know that we are more than our mind and body, but how do we experience our essence? It is one thing to say, "I am more than mind and body." It is another to actually *know* our essence with every fiber of our being.

Understanding is only half the solution. Understanding is the map, but the map alone is not enough. We must travel the path as well. Many people may superbly describe the map. They may even write scholarly books. But if they haven't traveled the path itself, the map is ultimately of little use. Combining knowledge with real-life experience is the key.

The beauty of Yoga Nidra practice is that it can serve as a laboratory within which to *practice* the knowledge. Here, the teachings come alive. We have a chance not just to *know* them intellectually, but to *experience* how they work through our own body and mind. This merging of understanding, enhanced and deepened through personal practice, is a potent combination. *The teachings are no longer something to "think" about, they become something we may embody and become.*

The Six Tools of Yoga Nidra

In this book, we will explore each of the Six Tools of Yoga Nidra. These will allow us to optimally attain the benefits we have discussed. The Tools are:

1. Realization
2. Integration
3. Dis-identification
4. Intention
5. Relaxation
6. Restoration

The first Tool, *Realization*, works with the big picture, the ultimate purpose of Yoga Nidra. The remaining Tools speak to the practical, day-to-day benefits to be gained from a Yoga Nidra practice. Most people just want to feel better. They want to be able to sleep, have less stress, and manage their unhelpful habits. Yoga Nidra addresses all of this whether an individual is interested in Self-Realization or not. The Tools of *Integration, Dis-identification, Intention, Relaxation* and *Restoration* allow each person to gain a degree of life mastery. Life mastery grants more peace, more happiness, greater health and self-management. These results can be an end in and of themselves, or they can be a stepping stone to the ultimate Tool of *Realization*. The more quiet and peaceful the mind is and the healthier the body is, the more likely we are to notice that which is beyond it.

The body/mind suffers from identification with limiting patterns known as *samskaras*, the internal aspect of *karma*. This internal aspect of *karma* is made up of thoughts, feelings, experiences and conclusions about our past that we adopted as true. These incomplete experiences and beliefs affect all levels of body and mind. They affect the way we think, feel, and act. They affect the choices we make. If not properly managed, identification with internal *karma* can create undesirable limiting effects. The Tools of Yoga Nidra are designed to help you manage, transcend and neutralize the effects of these limiting patterns.

How This Book is Arranged

This book is divided into three sections. The first section introduces you to the philosophy of Yoga Nidra using the Six Tools of Yoga Nidra as a foundation for *understanding*. The second section *applies* the ancient philosophy of Yoga Nidra to modern maladies including stress, addiction, depression and anxiety. The last section of the book includes suggestions for *practice*, how to set up for Yoga Nidra and a Yoga Nidra script.

This book is not just about Yoga Nidra; it is a handbook for your life. Step by step, it will reveal to you what, up until now, has been running your life. You will see how your patterns of thinking, feeling and acting have been driving and directing your life. You will understand how to use the practice of Yoga Nidra to shape and create the life you want, rather than the one your past has created for you. This book is rich with Yogic insight into the practical, everyday challenges we all face. After reading it, you will have a better understanding of who you are, why you are here and how to make the most of your human journey with the practice of Yoga Nidra.

SECTION ONE

Understanding
The Ancient Secrets
of Yoga Nidra

CHAPTER ONE

Yoga Nidra:
The Art of Transformational Sleep

What is Yoga Nidra?

Yoga Nidra is a little-known ancient meditation technique. It works by taking you to brainwave states similar to those in sleep, where the biology of your body makes it easier to disengage from thoughts. Meditation happens when you are able to disengage from your thoughts and *observe* them rather than believe them. For many, however, seated meditation is challenging and meditation becomes more about the effort of the technique and sitting still, and less about where the technique is supposed to *take us*—to a state of relaxed, spacious awareness. Yoga Nidra is different. The technique itself is composed of a series of body, breath, and awareness techniques designed to effortlessly guide you into a state of complete *non-doing*. You are not practicing *being aware* so much as *resting as awareness itself.* You are resting in a space where thoughts spontaneously come and go without preference or pull toward any one thought. Here, even first-time meditators enter profound states of expanded awareness and deep relaxation.

The secret to Yoga Nidra is that it consciously harnesses the biological function of sleep for a spiritual purpose. Every night when we go to sleep, there is one thing we must do. We must be able to let go of our thoughts. If this does not happen, we will not fall asleep. This is insomnia. The process of sleep happens by dropping into progressively deeper brainwave states. As we enter these brainwave states, the mind slows down and our thoughts naturally begin to move further away from us until we fall asleep. In Yoga Nidra, we enter this process consciously.

The techniques of Yoga Nidra enable the slowing down of our brainwaves and allow us to enter the twilight zone between us and our thoughts.

In this zone, we gain entry to subtle realms where things that seem dense and difficult to change in the waking state become more fluid and easy to shift from the meditative sleep state. As we enter into more fluid states of consciousness, we can easily influence the *visible and manifest* from the *invisible and unmanifest* realm—the pure potentiality from which the visible arises. Making shifts in the waking state is akin to changing the shape of a block of ice. The body, thoughts and all that is visible have already taken a concrete and densified shape. The hammer and chisel of will, discipline and effort are needed here. Making shifts in Yoga Nidra is like making changes to water which quickly and easily assumes the form and direction it is given. This unique element of Yoga Nidra is called *Sankalpa* or *Intention*. The use of *Intention* while in meditation is unique to Yoga Nidra. It is a way to specifically target and shift self-destructive patterns that compromise our health and well-being.

History of Yoga Nidra

The practice of Yoga Nidra is as ancient as the practice of Yoga itself. The first mention of the purpose of Yoga Nidra is in the *Upanishads*, which outline the nature of the universe and Self-Realization. There are eleven principal *Upanishads*. The *Brihadaranyaka Upanishad*, one of the oldest, is estimated to have been composed about 700 BCE, excluding some parts which may have been composed later. *That is almost one thousand years before the birth of Jesus.* Though Ancient Greek philosophy was eventually shadowed by the Dark Ages of Europe, such was not the case in the East. The enormity of accumulated wisdom in the *Upanishads* and other texts has continuously thrived for thousands of years and remains infinitely relevant today. The *Upanishads* sought to answer the question, "What is the single truth, that if known, would solve everything?" This question is the key to solving the riddle of human suffering.

The *Brihadaranyaka Upanishad* includes this verse:

Asatoma Prayer:
asato ma sadagamaya

tamaso ma jyotirgamaya

mrityorma amritam gamaya

-Brihadaranyaka Upanishad-I.iii.28

Lead me from the unreal to the real

Lead me from darkness to light

Lead me from time-bound consciousness (death)

To the timeless state of being (immortality) that I am

As you will come to understand, this verse outlines the ultimate spiritual purpose of both Yoga and Yoga Nidra. You will see this prayer *is* a truth, which if known, could solve everything. Yoga Nidra is a means to do just that.

The *Chandogya Upanishad*, composed around the same time as the *Brihadaranyaka Upanishad*, first discusses the "four states of consciousness" as awake, dream-filled sleep, deep sleep, and beyond deep sleep. Later, the *Mandukya Upanishad*, estimated to have been written in the first or second centuries after the birth of Jesus, describes the four states of consciousness through the sacred syllable, AUM. The sound A relates to the waking state of consciousness, U to the dream state and M to the deep sleep state. The silence that follows represents *turiya*—the state of silent awareness within which all other states of consciousness arise. The purpose of Yoga Nidra is to realize and rest in this *turiya* state. However, although the concept of *turiya* existed, the practice of Yoga Nidra had not yet been born.

Yoga Nidra was first born as a meditation practice 500 - 600 CE, making it over a *thousand years old*. This is around the time when the esoteric teachings of Spirit were brought to the common man. Before then, it was considered holy to renounce all forms that were regarded as mundane—including the body, emotions, sex, money, and householder life. These were seen as obstacles to recognizing one's true nature. Then a new and controversial stream of thought was born. Seekers realized that manifest existence is not separate from consciousness. Rather, it is the visible extension of consciousness. Instead of rejecting forms of human existence such as the body and mind, these forms could serve as *vehicles through which* the formless could be realized. This stream of thought was known as *tantra*. Nowadays, *tantra* has come to be associated primarily with sexual practices, but this perspective is very limited. In reality, any practice that uses the body/mind complex as a vehicle to become Self-Realized is a *Tantric* practice.

This shift in perspective birthed unprecedented access to higher consciousness for the common person occupied with the practicalities of daily subsistence. It opened the door to many new techniques and practices including *asana* (yoga poses), *mantra* (chanting of sacred syllables), *mudra* (hand gestures which open up energy channels) and *yantras* (visualization of geometric forms). Yoga Nidra is one of these practices born as a means to guide a practitioner from the three states in which the body exists (waking, dreaming and deep sleep) into *turiya*—awareness of existence beyond the body.

The *Mahanirvana Tantra*, written in the Seventeenth Century, describes the technique of *nyasa*—placing attention and visualization combined with seed sounds on various energy points in the body. This is the basis of the 61-Point Yoga Nidra Technique that is still used hundreds of years later.

CHAPTER TWO

Yoga Nidra: The Secret Door to Freedom
The First Tool of Yoga Nidra: *Realization*

Yoga Nidra allows us to kinesthetically experience the Self beyond body and mind.

Here, we simply rest as the space through which all experiences come and go.

The more we rest as who we are, the less we are at the effect of what is passing through.

We can be at peace and steady in the midst of external and internal disturbance.

Yoga Nidra consists of a set of tools. If we know the purpose of the tools we are using and what we are trying to build with them, we are much more likely to arrive at the desired result. For example, a hammer is a tool. But that tool can be used in many ways—some helpful, and some not so helpful. However, if we know the purpose of the tool, to build a house for example, we already have some big clues that tell us how to use the tool. It will be obvious that the tool is not to be used to hit other people, but to hit nails. For this reason, it is essential not only to understand the Six Tools of Yoga Nidra, but also to understand what we are trying to build with those Tools. Having a clear picture of the end result shows us *how* to utilize the Tools in the way they were meant to be used. It also helps us know when we have gotten off track and are no longer using the Tools in a helpful way.

For instance, yoga poses are a tool. Yet what are they designed to achieve? A better body? A yoga butt? Or is there more to this 4,000-years-old practice? Knowing what you are trying to build with the tool of yoga poses informs how you approach the poses and what you will get from them. If you know the pose is designed to help you manage not only the body but also create equanimity in the mind, you will know when you are not practicing in a way that moves you toward the purpose of Yoga. You will see that comparison, criticism or excessive body image focus is actually *taking you away* from the original intent of the poses. However, if you do not know what the original intent is, you are less likely to arrive at the desired destination and will be unable to course-correct as needed. When you judge yourself in a yoga pose, that judgment is counter to Yoga's purpose. You could actually be practicing conflict on a yoga mat versus equanimity—in fact, not practicing Yoga at all. This is why it is critical not only to understand the Tools of Yoga Nidra, but for what purpose they are intended.

Without this understanding, the potential under-utilization of Yoga Nidra is great. For many years, Yoga Nidra has been side-lined as a guided relaxation—a spiritual name for a nap. This is because people don't understand what it is really intended to accomplish. Yoga Nidra is so much more than a guided relaxation or a nap. It is a secret door to *liberation*. Without this knowledge, however, one of the most profound practices of Yoga can easily be overlooked in the ego's quest for something more exciting. Using Yoga Nidra as a nap is like using a jet plane to drive to the grocery store. You can do it, but it is a gross under-utilization of its potential. A jet plane can drive, but it is meant to make you fly. Yoga Nidra can help you rest, but it was meant to help you soar. It was meant to liberate you from the suffering that afflicts human existence.

In this chapter, we will explore the purpose of Yoga Nidra. Once we know what we are trying to build with its Tools, the likelihood is great that we will be able to harness the practice to its fullest potential.

The Nature of the Self

The Self has several qualities. It is timeless, eternal and unchanging. It is that which is present before, during and after objects, both subtle and gross, come and go. It is the eternal backdrop of existence—and—it sees. It is the *witness* of all that is passing through it.

Self as Witness

Imagine that you are sitting on top of a hill, surrounded by golden grassed hills on all sides. Down below, you see a road. The road is empty. Far off in the distance, to the right of your vision, you see a car come into your vision, into the center of your vision and then off into the horizon. The car disappears from view.

Can you see that if you are the one seeing the car, it cannot be you? You were there before the car. You were there while the car was there and you were there after the car was gone. You were the one *watching* the car come and go. This is the nature of the eternal Self. It is always there. It is there before things come, while things are there and after they are gone. The eternal Self is *you*—the one who is seeing things come and go. That is why it is called the *witness*.

Let's develop this idea further. Imagine yourself at the age of seven—your body size, your personality, how you were, what you looked like. Now fast forward to a teenager—how you were then, what your personality was like. Now fast forward to the present time. Notice your current body, maybe the wrinkles on your face, your personality. Notice that sometimes you look in mirror and see your body change. Maybe you even ask yourself, "Is that me?"

We said, "If you can see the car, it can't be you." What about the body? Can you see the body? Can you see it change? Are "you" there before the body changes? While it is changing? After it has changed? Consider that if you can see the body change, it can't be you. You are the one *watching* the body change. In fact, you are watching the body change in the same way you watch other bodies change. Some days the body is seen with bags under the eyes, other days not. Some days the body is observed with more weight or less weight. Over time we see the body accumulate more wrinkles and more grey hair. There has to be an *identifier* observing these changes. That means the body cannot be the totality of you. There has to be something greater than the body that is *aware of it*. We could call it *consciousness*. That consciousness is a consistent, eternal thread that watches and observes all things in flux. Consciousness itself is unchanging, but serves as the background behind every changing experience.

Self as Background

Everything that comes, goes. Everything seen, heard, tasted, smelled, felt or thought—lives for a time, then dies. Yet aren't you there before all these things arrive? While they are there? When they leave? *Awareness* identifies the presence and absence of every "thing." You are the one who sees it all come and go, because you are there to identify it. You are the one identifying when an emotion is not present, when it is present and when it is gone. You can say, "I wasn't sad, then I was sad, and now I'm not sad anymore." Just like the *witness* watching the car, you are there to identify changing states. If you are the one *identifying* various gross and subtle objects coming and going, you have to be the unchanging constant within which these objects are coming and going. They cannot be you. *You are not the one who is sad, you are the one who is there before, during and after sadness comes and goes.* See the difference? This small change in perspective has enormous significance, as you will see.

Now, what if we were to remove everything seen, heard, tasted, felt and imagined? Every "thing." What is left? Nothing—right? *No-thing.* This is how Zen defines the Self. *No-thing.* This is why in many traditions it is said that God should not be named or given a form. It *is* the formless itself. To give it a name is to try to capture something in form that is *beyond form itself.*

The formless aspect of the Self has no quality of its own other than its capacity for things to appear in it. It can be understood as space, background, formless capacity for what is. There can be no sound without the backdrop of silence within which the sound arises. Stars only appear in contrast to the background of the night sky. It is only in reference to formless, that forms appear—just as it is only in reference to silence that sound appears. We are not accustomed to paying attention to the space. We are accustomed to focusing on contents. When a thought moves through the mind, we don't pay attention to the silence behind it; we pay attention to the thought itself.

The formless aspect of the Self is where the concept of zero was first born in the East. It is only in reference to nothing that we can have the "something" of numbers. All numbers only appear in reference to nothingness. The concept of zero was at its origin a spiritual one. Even though it was the place from which mathematics were born, mystics would say zero is not something to be known or thought about, but to be experienced. That is exactly where Yoga Nidra takes us—to the experience of zero. That is why my father, Yogi Amrit Desai, the founder of the Integrative Amrit Method of Yoga Nidra, says, "Yoga Nidra takes you to the *Zero Stress Zone.*"

Self as Unconditional Love

The zero background is like a sky of awareness. A sky is simply perfect capacity for whatever is moving through it. It is totally *allowing* of whatever comes and goes through its space. The sky, by its nature, has no preference for clouds over lightning, birds over planes or sun over rain. The sky's nature is to be unconditional capacity for everything to be as it is. Nothing is carved out, separated or labeled as "good" or "bad." The sky does not cleave what it likes from what it doesn't like. That is its nature. From the perspective of the sky-like Self, things simply are. The Self doesn't *try* to be unconditional. It *is* unconditional. Another word for this sky-like spacious allowing is *love*. Not emotional love, but pure, total and unconditional *acceptance*.

I am always struck by those who have near death experiences and come back to report profound experiences of love. The message they return with is that we are wholly, fully and profoundly loved by existence itself in a way we could never imagine. This love is always present, and there is nothing we can do to cause that love to disappear. It is the eternal and unchanging backdrop in which all manifest existence is unfolding. It is said that if we only knew how much we are loved (unconditionally received) we would not suffer the way we do on the human plane of existence.

The nature of the Self then, is not nothingness, but is *love* itself. Everything that has ever taken place—every emotion, every thought, and every experience—has happened in a backdrop of complete, total and unconditional love. Complete, unconditional allowing and acceptance. Imagine a practice that restored our knowledge of this invisible backdrop to accompany our human existence. That is the potential of Yoga Nidra.

Confusing the Container and the Contents

The background, zero-quality of Self renders it very easy not to notice. It is like air. We don't walk around commenting on air or space, even though it is around all the time. We tend to notice the things *in* the space. When someone is speaking or the radio is on, we don't listen to the silence, we listen to the sound. We listen to that which is filling the space, rather than the space itself. Nor do we notice that acceptance *is* the quality of the space that surrounds all our experiences. This, according to Yoga, is where we get caught.

I will share an imperfect metaphor with you, but a useful one nonetheless. Imagine a lobster pot, a huge pot. In truth, the "pot" of awareness has no limits, edges or boundaries, but for now, imagine a pot. The pot, like the sky, is perfect capacity for anything that is put into it. If you put potatoes into the pot, the pot is perfectly allowing of the potatoes. No preference. Completely unconditional. When the potatoes are removed, there is no stain of the potatoes left. The pot is simply total capacity for the next thing—maybe carrots. When carrots fill the container, the pot is total capacity for them.

A frame takes on the qualities of whatever it is framing, but it is perfectly unaffected by what it is framing. In the same way, the container perfectly receives and reflects the qualities of what is in it. If it contains potatoes, the container appears to take on the qualities of potatoes. It is "potatoed." When carrots move through, the container appears to take on the qualities of carrots. It is "carroted." Similarly, sadness and anger are passing experiences which are perfectly contained and allowed. When contained, the container appears to take on those same qualities. When those qualities are present, they are fully felt and received, and when they are gone, the container is left unstained and ready to receive the next experience.

When emotion fills the container, it is fully felt and allowed to be. There is no resistance or fear of what is in the pot. No story about it. It is simply an experience that is present. When the experience comes, it is allowed to come. When it goes, it is allowed to go.

So what is the problem you might ask? Since the container as a background presence doesn't announce itself, we tend to forget its presence and instead notice the contents. Let's say you are cooking spaghetti in a pot. If you lift up the lid, you are not very likely to say, "Nice pot with spaghetti in it." You are more likely to say, "Oh! Spaghetti!" In other words, we tend to notice the contents rather than the container itself.

When we lose awareness of our containerness (the pot), we are subject to become identified with contents. Our perspective changes. Instead of recognizing we are the space through which sadness, anger, and various constellations of experiences are moving, it can appear that we *are* the contents. Just as we only see and experience spaghetti, we only see and experience the sadness, worry or frustration. In forgetfulness of the background, there doesn't appear to be anything greater than the contents. It looks as if that is the totality of who we are. That *is* me. We don't say, "Sadness is moving through the space of awareness that I am." We say, "I am sad." We have become it. *And because we believe ourselves to be it, we are bound by it.*

We no longer experience the sky-like Self which is present before, during and after all experiences come and go. We have lost remembrance of the ground of being. The zero space. The experiences with which we are identified, including the experience of our bodies and minds, become the limit of our existence. The limitless, eternal, unchanging and unconditionally allowing Source becomes limited and locked into identification with the worry, fear and anxiety moving through it. *These changing experiences which constantly gather and dissolve in an unchanging flux appear to have become us. And, bound by this illusion, we suffer.*

This confusion between the container and that which is contained is the *source of suffering*. It is the problem all Yoga practices, including Yoga Nidra, seek to solve. In the *Yoga Sutras of*

Patanjali 2:17, it is said, "The union between the seer and the seen is the source of suffering."

The body/mind is more consistently in the container than anything else. It is present from the moment we wake up until the time we go to sleep at night. Like the spaghetti, every time we look into the container, the body is there. It continues to be in the pot for 80 years or so. It moves like that car through awareness, but very slowly. We see the body grow, we see it flourish, and we see it get old. In truth, we are watching the body/mind just as we watched the car. Unlike the car, the body/mind is rarely ever not there, so it is no wonder we come to identify with the body/mind as the totality of what we are. In fact, one of the few times that the body is not in awareness is when we sleep. This is why Yoga Nidra is such a powerful opportunity. When we enter these sleep-like states consciously, we can experience the container that exists beyond the body.

To clarify one point, Yoga does not say you are not your emotions or the body, but rather that these are *impermanent* aspects of the Self. They will come and go. An emotion, like a wave on an ocean, will live for awhile, will move through the ocean and then dissolve back into the ocean from which it came. The same is true of the body. It will live for a time, move through the container of consciousness, and will die—dissolving back into the consciousness from which it came. Consciousness itself remains eternal.

Once this knowing is established, you will not be subject to the roller coaster of experiences in the same way you are now. Instead of feeling overwhelmed by the waves of thoughts, emotions and experiences that overcome you, you will have a stable and dependable context of stillness and peace within which to experience it all. The contents of life do not disappear, but the *perspective* from which they are experienced changes. You know you can always touch the peaceful stillness that is your eternal nature no matter what is moving through. This knowing radically changes your experience of life. Without this knowing, your happiness is dependent on the contents of the container. You can only be happy when the contents are desirable. Therefore, you have to manage the contents so that you can feel happy for a time. *With* the experiential knowing of your true nature, your peace is *always* available regardless of the contents. This is why many people report that even though nothing about their lives has changed, they simply feel happier and more content as a result of Yoga Nidra practice. The practice is establishing them in the Self, where peace is accessible beyond reliance on circumstances.

Remember the *Asatoma Prayer* first mentioned in the *Brihadaranyaka Upanishad*? It outlined the core question, "What is the single truth that if known, would solve everything?" Read it again based on what you just learned: *"Lead me from the unreal to the real; lead me from darkness to light; lead me from time-bound consciousness (death) to the timeless state of being (immortality)."* This is what the prayer is saying. If you can know the timeless being that you are, you will move from the darkness that comes from falsely assumed limitations, to the truth of the eternal Self. From this place of peace, you can allow all experiences to move through, just as clouds move through a clear blue sky. Yoga Nidra is a tool designed to free us from these assumed limitations and restore our experiential knowledge of the eternal Self. In other words, Yoga Nidra is a tool for *Realization* of our true nature.

How Does Yoga Nidra Solve the Problem of Mis-Identification?

The mechanism by which Yoga Nidra seeks to solve this problem is simple. If you quiet or remove the contents of the container, it is easier to notice the container itself.

This is what is written in Patanjali's *Yoga Sutras*—the first written codification of classical Yoga.

> *1.2 Yoga is the stilling of modifications of mind.*
>
> *1.3 Then the seer abides in his own true nature.*

Imagine a sky background filled with birds, helicopters, planes, bees, and clouds. In that state, are you more likely to notice the stuff in the sky or the sky itself? The stuff—right? Yoga's solution is based on the same principle. The more mindstuff that fills our internal sky of awareness, the more difficult it is to notice our sky-like nature. The quieter it becomes, the less drama, the less weather patterns of the mind, the easier it is to notice what is behind it all. This is what is meant when Patanjali says, "Yoga is the stilling of modifications of mind. Then the seer abides in his own true nature." By removing the clutter that fills the sky of awareness, the sky itself is revealed.

Yoga Nidra is stilling the fluctuations of mind…and abiding as one's true nature…through conscious entry into the sleep state.

Yoga Nidra decreases mental modifications by decreasing the activity of the mind—that with which we are normally identified. As Yoga Nidra takes you toward the conscious sleep state, the electrical activity of the brain slows down and the mind becomes less and less active in order to allow sleep. At some point, the activity of the brainwaves slows down so much that we experience a "gap" of nothingness. No thoughts, no things fill awareness. Here, the only thing left to notice is awareness—the sky-like nature of Self.

Imagine that the mindstuff of our lives is like a movie projected on the screen of awareness. The screen is blank capacity. If the movie is very engaging, with lots of drama, many things happening, lots of ups and downs, we become so involved in the story that it is very hard to notice the screen on which that story is being projected. But the quieter, more calm and peaceful the movie becomes, the more likely we are to notice the screen on which the movie is projected. By calming the movie content of our lives, by becoming internally more still, more calm, and more peaceful, we quiet our movies. The more we can do this, the more likely we are to notice the screen itself—*our true nature.*

Each time we enter Yoga Nidra, we shift our perspective. The movie is temporarily calmed or even stopped. In the deepest states, the only thing left is the screen itself. Here, we come to identify with and rest as the screen more and more. The more we rest as the screen, the less we are affected by what is projected onto it. We can simply allow "the screen"—our true nature—to be.

Each time we emerge from Yoga Nidra and the movie of our lives begins again, we are less engaged by the drama. In other words, the more we begin to rest back as capacity, the less we are affected and dragged around by the contents.

This is what *Realization* is: noticing and resting as the container *that you are* rather than identifying with the contents. You are liberated from believing the mindstuff to be the totality of who you are. It is not that the contents change. In fact, the same things may be moving through awareness, but the point of view has changed. You have restored your true perspective as the container itself.

Yoga Nidra, in effect, takes you to a mini-enlightenment state. Each time you go there, the longer you can stay there, and the more this temporary state becomes a permanent perspective. This brilliant Yogic strategy is the foundation from which our expansive and formless Source can be realized.

Although not everyone is necessarily interested in Self-Realization, most people *are* interested in more happiness, more contentment and more peace in their lives. Yoga Nidra provides these benefits of greater peace and inner calm in the midst of life, regardless of a person's interest in recognition of Self. Yoga Nidra quiets inner noise. This makes the practice ideally accessible for those simply seeking greater relaxation and inner tranquility.

CHAPTER THREE

The Descent into Identification

Think of an ocean and its waves. The depths of an ocean are undifferentiated and have no form. Out of the depths of the ocean, waves arise. These waves come into individuated forms, as the body and mind do, but the waves are not separate from the ocean. They are the manifest aspect of existence. The only difference between the manifest, the wave, and the unmanifest, the ocean, is that the wave will eventually dissolve back into the ocean. It is impermanent. The ocean itself, however, remains the same.

The body and mind are the visible, manifest and embodied aspects of Source arising from the unmanifest or formless aspect of Source. The manifest aspect of Source is finite. The body/mind will live and die. It is impermanent and exists in time between birth and death. The unmanifest aspect of existence is timeless, eternal and unchanging.

When we become solely identified with *one aspect* of our existence, we become exclusively attached to the mind and body and live in forgetfulness of the eternal aspect of our nature. We become solely identified with the wave as the totality of who we are and overlook the ocean from which we have come. This forgetfulness causes us to lose our connection to Source and the inner peace and stability that come from it.

The *kleshas* (afflictions or obstacles), as outlined in the *Yoga Sutras of Patanjali*, map the process by which we have forgotten the formless aspect of our true nature and have become exclusively identified with the body/mind as the totality of "me." This limited view leads us into bondage and ultimately suffering. The *kleshas* explain the descent into identification with contents and the resulting consequences. Through greater understanding of how the problem was created, we can understand how the Tools of Yoga Nidra are designed to undo it. If we can understand how a knot was tied, we can also understand how to untie it.

Avidya (Ignorance/Forgetfulness)

Have you heard the saying, "We are spiritual beings having a human experience?" Who we are is unconditional, eternal consciousness manifesting through the human experience.

We are the ocean manifesting as a wave. The body is an instrument of this consciousness. The eyes, ears, senses and thoughts of the body are the mediums through which consciousness interacts with the world of form.

We might compare it to stepping into a character of a play. Consciousness gets to "play" the range of human experience via the body. When the character is joyful, it gets to experience joy. When the character is heartbroken, it gets to experience heartbreak. All the dramas of the human experience from childbirth to marriage to divorce, achievement and loss are fully experienced, fully allowed and fully lived—yet consciousness knows those experiences are not its totality. Rather, these experiences are like waves moving through consciousness. As such, it is all allowed, all lived, all fully experienced. There is nothing to resist. It is all part of God's play. And, like the keys on a piano, you allow and even enjoy every note life has to offer.

What happens, though, if you forget you are consciousness expressing itself through a character? What if you forget your true nature and believe you *are* the character? I imagine it as literally playing a role on a stage. Above that stage, the roof is open and you are connected to consciousness experiencing the human experience. You know you are the sky of awareness even though you are playing this role on the stage. But what if you forgot the sky of consciousness? What if you were only left with the body and the senses? It is as if the roof above you were to close up. There would be no connection to anything outside the box of human experience. You might feel cut off, alone, and the victim of the human condition with no connection or knowledge of anything outside this finite "stage." The stage would become the totality and limitation of your existence.

Now imagine how it feels to forget you are playing a role. You *become* the role. *It appears to be the totality of who you are.* If the mind and body feel good, *you* feel good. If body and mind feel bad, *you* feel bad. Experience that could once be enjoyed as part of the play of embodied existence within a silent backdrop of the sky of awareness becomes a deluge of events, feelings, and reactions that threaten to overtake you at any moment if not managed with all your might.

You suffer through it all, thinking it is all you, that there is nothing more. The experiences of life no longer feel like something to be fully allowed. They may feel like something to be feared, because there is no greater context of peace within which to experience them. From this limited perspective, it no longer feels as if you are "a spiritual being having a human experience." It feels like you are not that which is there before, during and after the experience; you *are* the experience.

Once the stage becomes the limit of your universe, you may feel something is not quite right. Of course something isn't right. You've forgotten the totality of who you are, but you don't know that. You are left with a nagging sensation telling you that you need more of something or less of something else. It is like that feeling you have when you go on a trip. You know you have forgotten something, but you don't know what it is. It leaves a lingering sense of unease which needs to be taken care of somehow. It is a feeling of "not being okay." "Something's wrong." Sometimes we interpret something is wrong "out there," sometimes we interpret something is wrong "in here" with me. No matter the interpretation, the feeling comes from the same place: a primal disconnection from Source.

Forgetfulness of one's true nature is called *avidya*. *Vidya* means knowledge. *Avidya* means lack of knowledge or ignorance. It is the fundamental mistake from which all others follow. We mistake the mind and emotions to be the totality of who we are. We take ourselves to be something we are not. This is the original error and the one Yoga Nidra solves. In Christianity, it is called *sin*. The literal meaning of sin is "missing the mark." This is where we miss the mark and suffer as a result. It is the original sin or originating error. However, from the Yogic point of view, this is not a permanent state and it can be solved.

Yoga Nidra re-establishes a knowing of our true nature as that which is there before, during and after experiences come and go. Here, we can allow for the full range of human experience to be held in a container of wholeness and allowing—just as a sky effortlessly holds all that is within it. *Without* this container, we feel lost in the world of contents, but *with* an essential knowing of Self as the container of all, we can effortlessly rest in the place *through which* all contents pass. We can remain steady and centered—established beyond the flux. This is Yoga Nidra.

Asmita (Egoism)

The body/mind is born in this world. Like a character in a play, it has a back story. The body/mind was brought up in a partic-ular family, with certain cultural and social norms and beliefs. This character has certain experiences, both joyful and painful, that have formed how the body/mind thinks, acts and behaves today. We could call these various influences "programming." They are the past experiences, learning and socialization that cause people to behave the way they do. This programming is not wrong or bad. In fact, it is necessary for the life of the body/mind complex.

All the things we have learned since childhood have ideally been to help us survive and thrive in the environment in which we have been placed. Our programming teaches us to discriminate when to cross the street and when not to. It tells us how to hold a knife so we don't get cut and what is safe to eat and drink. Programming also teaches us subtler things like how to act within social norms—how to get and keep a job, and how be a law-abiding, productive member of society. It also largely determines what we think, how we think, what our opinions are and what our worldview is. The body/mind is essentially programmed in much the same way a computer is programmed. It acts in accordance with what has been fed into it—either in this lifetime or other lifetimes.

This "back story" of the character in the play is what we commonly call the ego. It is the constellation of accumulated thoughts, beliefs and experiences we have come to call "me." As you can see, there is nothing wrong with the ego or the programming it carries. It is wholly necessary for functioning on this plane. We do not want to get rid of it.

So where does the problem arise? *When you believe yourself to be this and only this.* You identify with the mind-made programmed sense of self as "me." When identified with the character and its back story as you, you become it; and it becomes the limit of your world. The eternal Self, though still present, is forgotten. In its place, you call all of your experiences, feelings, thoughts and opinions "me." This is called *asmita* or egoness.

Raga and Dvesha
(Attraction and Aversion)

Once we lose touch with our eternal Self, we feel barraged by the un-ending waves of external experiences and internal reactions ceaselessly assaulting us. There is no rest; there is no peace here because by nature, things will always be moving through the container. Lived from the wave perspective, there seems to be no end—no way to get away from the onslaught of life except for short periods of time. We have no backdrop of wholeness from which to experience it all.

Now it *appears* the only way to quench that sense of unease is to *do* something. Make things happen. *Find* wholeness through the people, places and things on the stage. We can no longer let life happen as we did before when we knew ourselves as the ocean manifesting as a wave, enjoying the play of human experience. Life becomes something to be managed, controlled and steered to quell that inner sense of unease—to give us a measure of peace and stability. The ease that came from knowing Source in the midst of changing experiences is lost. In its place, we come to rely on resources rather than Source to give us the sense of wholeness we are missing.

In my experience, everyone the world over has this feeling. We all have the feeling we are missing something—that things are not quite okay—we feel overwhelmed or isolated. We are all yearning for a sense of peace—a time when all that noise inside will be quiet and we can deeply rest. Every person and every culture has a different way of attending to it—through relationships, money, success or recognition.

While the eternal Self is simply the background that allows things to come and go, we, as the character, cannot allow things to come and go because *they are us*. The container is space for it all to be, but if we forget that container, our happiness *depends* on the contents. The contents are no longer something to be allowed, they are something we have to manage. It feels as if the only way we can be happy is to make sure there are happy contents in the container. Pain and loss are the last things we want in the container. As a result, we no longer fully embrace and allow certain parts of the human experience. In fact, we do our best to avoid them.

If our whole life is made up of notes, like that of a piano, we become afraid of certain notes. The only way to be whole or to at least be okay for a little while is by managing the types of notes that are moving through our lives. Rather than wanting to experience the whole of life and all the notes it has to offer, the only way it seems we can manage to feel okay is to keep away the painful "bad" notes and try to get some "good" ones. We end up playing traffic cop with life, trying to hold on to certain experiences and allow them through, while we try to hold others at bay. We become attached to what we like and want in the container and are afraid of what we don't like and don't want in the container. *All because we have come to believe that the contents determine our happiness.*

Experience becomes less about its inherent and intrinsic satisfaction. *Experience becomes a means to manage the original discomfort we feel in life.* Food is not just about food; sex is not just about sex; work is not just about work. They become a means to feel good and avoid feeling bad. Sex, relationships, money, cars, houses, jobs, promotions and recognition become instruments to keep the pain of separation at bay.

It is as if, in our separation from Self, we go to the ego and ask it, "How can I feel whole?" "How can I feel happy?" Unfortunately the mind can only tell us to be happy based on the knowledge or experience it has acquired in the past. The mind biologically operates on a binary survival system: pleasure and pain.

Therefore, it is only capable of telling you how to be whole in the same way it keeps the body whole: reproducing pleasure and avoiding pain.

There are four basic strategies for happiness that the mind can give you:

1. It can tell you what made you happy in the past and to reproduce it.
2. It can tell you what made you unhappy and to avoid it.
3. It can tell you what you felt you lacked in your past and to make up for it.
4. It can tell you what society tells you will make you happy and to go acquire those things.

If you look at whatever your mind tells you will make you happy, you will be able to trace it back to one or several of these things. The mind is a closed system. It cannot open us up to anything more than what has been put into it. That doesn't make the mind bad; it means the mind is limited in its capacity to give us the answer we are seeking. When we live from the mind, the happiness we seek cannot be more than a refashioned version of our past.

If we follow the mind's solution, our whole life will revolve around keeping painful situations at bay rather than living life. We will do whatever it takes not to experience the pain of rejection, heartbreak, abandonment and failure. And, we invest our time in the antidote to pain—pleasure.

You can never be whole by being in relationship with half of life. Life is, by its very nature, composed of natural opposites. Each opposite informs the other. It is only because we feel sad that we can feel happy, or because we are down that we can experience being up. To expect to be up and never down is to put ourselves into a conflicting relationship with nature itself. The depth of the wave automatically determines the height of its pinnacle. The bottom defines the top. They are part and parcel of one another, just as when you pick up one side of the coin, the other automatically comes with it.

Life exists in natural polarity, like a pendulum. When the pendulum is swinging to the left, it is only gaining momentum to swing to the right. True happiness and wholeness come from our ability to be rooted in the stillness beyond the polar movements of life. When we pit ourselves against nature and try to make it so we will always be happy and never sad, we will always lose.

The instincts to seek wholeness through the mind and its binary system are called *raga* and *dvesha*; attraction and aversion. When we no longer live in harmony with the polar experiences of life, we are in duality. The mind operates in duality. We believe we will be happy when we succeed in getting rid of the uncomfortable. We believe that someday we will be able to be comfortable forever and ever. We dedicate our lives to that cause, but that day never comes.

Let's consider an example of *raga* and *dvesha* to understand this more fully. Reflect on what you want people to think about you. Make an internal list. Perhaps you want people to think you are smart, competent, organized and confident. Maybe thoughtful, loving, sexy, and caring. Perhaps spiritual, loyal, trustworthy and generous. Maybe all of the above. Now reflect on what you *don't* want people to think about you. Maybe you don't want them to think you are stupid, lazy, immature and needy. Maybe you don't want them to think you are cheap, greedy, superficial, selfish, dishonest, mean, crazy, judgmental or scared. Whatever your list, can you see how much of your life is occupied by getting people to look at you in a certain way and not look at you in a certain way?

Can you see how much stress we cause ourselves when we worry about being perceived in a way we don't want to be perceived and how much energy we expend to make sure that doesn't happen? This is an example of *raga* and *dvesha*. We want to feel good by making sure people see us in a certain way and avoid feeling bad by making sure they don't see us in certain other ways. Just these two things consume a tremendous amount of our life energy.

Now add to that, everything we are trying to secure to feel good and everything we are frantically trying to manage so we can avoid feeling bad. Think of it as your long-term internal "to do" list. What do you really want in your life? A relationship? Enough money to pay off all the bills? Perhaps friends, success, happiness, comfort, security, time, enlightenment? Or perhaps a house, a car and that new big screen TV? Now add to that all the stuff you want to make sure doesn't happen: bankruptcy, homelessness, illness, loneliness, rejection, unhappiness, aging, losing love ones, and dying alone. Can you see how we are all frantically running around after certain things that will make us feel better, secure and okay? And just as frantically running away from the things that don't make us feel good?

We run and run and run trying to make it all happen, convinced that if we can just get it all into place, everything will be okay and that niggling feeling inside will go away. Can you see that most of us are busy doing this most of the time? We are using all our inborn talents, energy, and potential to accomplish all this. This is what is occupying most of our existence.

We use everything we have, all our time, energy, talents, gifts and resources for one thing and one thing alone—feeling better, feeling okay. Finding something, *anything*, that will make the uncomfortable feeling inside go away, something that will make us feel good, whole, complete and content. That is the only thing we want and it is what drives this massive unending internal to do list.

Unfortunately, no matter how hard we run, we never seem to arrive for longer than a short period of time. The question is, "Why doesn't anything we do ever solve the problem?" The answer? You cannot solve a problem that doesn't exist! Can you ever solve a problem that doesn't exist? No! Because there is no problem in the first place! That means no matter what you do, you won't be able to fix it. That is exactly the case here. We have been suffering from a mass illusion that we are innately broken when we have never been broken at all. Therefore nothing we do to fix ourselves will ever work because there is nothing to fix! The real problem is that we are suffering from an illusion. It is a mirage. Nothing will fix a mirage because it is not real. *The only solution is to see it as a mirage.*

Our life is spent trying to fix what isn't broken. This is the big cosmic irony. *Nothing you do ever solves the problem, because there isn't one!* YOU ARE ALREADY WHOLE. YOU WERE NEVER NOT WHOLE. You only forgot that you were whole and still are whole. *If you are already whole, adding more will not make you any more whole.*

If you are already whole, can anything be added to you? Can anything be taken away from you? You are already everything. You are eternity itself. The issue is not that you are not whole; the issue is that you have believed yourself to be a limited version of yourself. In forgetfulness, we spend lifetimes searching for the thing that will restore our essential peace, not recognizing we have been whole all along. We simply forgot. Yet our focus is not on forgetfulness; our focus is on the belief that there is something *out there* that will make me feel better *in here*. In short, we've been searching in the wrong place.

If you use all your technical know-how, genius, talents, and energy to defeat an enemy in the forest, but they are not in the forest, will you ever succeed? No, because that is not where the problem is. Yet that is what we are all busy doing. We are firing all our ammunition—our talents, gifts and energy—at a place where the problem is not. Because the enemy isn't there, none of our talents or energies will ever solve the problem.

In fact, the more we do to become whole, the further we move from our essential nature. Remember our essential nature is comparable to the silence behind sound—the backdrop. The more we run, the more we do, the more we fill that space with drama, struggle, fear, worry, and stress. The more we DO in the name of being whole, the more noise we create. The more noise we create, the less we notice the silence behind it, and the further we move away from noticing the background. Life is filled with all the "stuff" we think we have to do and manage. There is no room for us to see who we are. This is the irony—the more we *do* to be whole, the further we move away from ourselves.

Yoga Nidra is release of all doing, all effort to be anywhere but where you are. It is a subtraction of doing. In the absence of doing, you notice you are already whole.

It is as if Source were the sun at our backs. We have forgotten it is there and we are running full speed away from it, in search of what is and always has been behind us all the time. No matter how far or how fast we run, we will never arrive. Why? Because the answer is not out there. *It is within us.* If we are not looking in the right place, we will never find it. The beauty of Yoga Nidra is this: no matter how long or how far you run into the world of form in search of wholeness, all it takes is turning around and the sun is right there waiting. You don't have to retrace your steps. Source is always there—at your back. It never left you. You simply have to look in the right place.

Stop looking outside. Turn around and look within. Stop running to be whole and recognize you are and always were whole. You were never missing anything. It was all an illusion. Rest into the sun that had your back all the time and recognize who you are and always have been.

The more you rest there, the less you NEED to do all the other things to feel okay. You can do them because you want to, but less and less because you *need them* to fulfill an empty part of you. *Then there is space for you to do what you came here to do—be a natural expression of yourself, rather than an expression of that which you felt you were missing.*

We often do things to make up for a false sense of lack, but that same doing can be life-affirming. It can be an expression of our wholeness. This is what our actions, talents and energies are meant to serve.

Abhinevesha (Clinging to Life)

Abhinevesha is the last of the *kleshas* or afflictions. Once we have identified with the body/mind as the totality of what we are, we believe that when the body dies, we die. Therefore we have a fear of death. This is similar to Freud's assertion that all fears stem from the fear of death. It seems natural to me that the body has a natural survival instinct. In fact, in Patanjali's *Yoga Sutras*, Patanjali writes, "*Abhinevesha* exists even in the wise." That is to say, even an enlightened person will have a natural survival instinct and an instinctual fear of death that is hard-wired into the body.

What *abhinevesha* also means is that we falsely invest our life energy in our self-image—our manufactured, man-made sense of self. We defend the thoughts, opinions, image, beliefs, likes and dislikes of this character—this manufactured self—as if it were us. When any of these elements of the manufactured self are threatened, we feel as if *we* are threatened, and we are often willing to defend our opinions with the same ferocity as our body. Everything we protect and fortify as our image to the world *is* me.

For example, when our work receives criticism, we feel hurt or defend our work because it feels like an extension of ourselves. The same is true of our opinions. In fact, many wars are fought and people are willing to die for opinions. It is because we have adopted them to signify who we *are* and our survival instinct expands to defend the life of those thoughts in the same way it defends the body. The more attachment we have to the image we need to project to the world, the more life energy it takes to fortify and defend it.

For some, the self-image becomes so strong, it becomes more important than the life of the body. Anorexia can be the result of many self-image factors, but one critical factor is when one's allegiance to the mentally-created image of the body becomes more important than one's own life.

The Story of Adam and Eve

The descent into identification through the afflictions or *kleshas* is not so different from the story of Adam and Eve being thrown out of the Garden of Eden. Adam and Eve lived in oneness with God, the Source. In a slightly different order than the *kleshas*, the story says that Eve ate fruit from the tree of knowledge of good and evil. This "knowledge" became the false knowledge arising from the mind seeking artificial wholeness through securing pleasure and avoiding pain (*raga* and *dvesha*) rather than through Source. Instead of being at one with God, they experienced separation from the whole. They lost their connection to God and were thrown out of the Garden of Eden. The awareness of their separation from wholeness is marked by the sudden self-consciousness of their own nudity as symbolized by the fig leaves covering their genitals. As a result of this loss of connection to God, Adam and Eve—and all their descendants—have to toil and struggle with life. Life is no longer peaceful as in the Garden when they were connected to Source. Instead, it is an effortful labor of sweat and pain.

When Adam and Eve are thrown out of the beautiful Garden of Eden, their connection to God, to peace, wholeness and oneness is lost. According to Yoga, this is the cause of human struggle, but it is solvable. In fact, Yoga suggests this is the purpose of being human. Source encompasses everything. Even though it manifests itself in myriad forms, it is still the common substance of all things. If this Source is everything, the only way for Source to experience itself anew is to forget its own nature and to rediscover itself. This, it is said, is the purpose of human experience: for Source to know itself. We travel away from Source, believing ourselves separate and alone, only to know ourselves as part of Source again. Yoga Nidra is a tool to return to the knowing of Source. It is the fulfillment of the soul's journey back to the place from which it came.

How Does Yoga Nidra Solve the Descent Into Identification?

In the *Yoga Sutras of Patanjali*, 2:10, it says, "These, the subtle ones, can be reduced by resolving them backward into their origin." Or, in another translation, "In subtle form, these obstacles can be destroyed by resolving them back into their primal cause." Do you remember the original problem from which all other afflictions arise? Ignorance. Forgetfulness of our true nature. If we can re-establish an experiential knowing of our true nature, we can resolve the other afflictions that arise from it.

Yoga Nidra stills the modifications of mind. It removes the clouds of struggle, effort, thoughts, emotions, worries, fears and memories that fill the sky. Yoga Nidra slowly takes us down into progressively quieter brainwave states until the sky is empty. In this state, we cannot help but notice we are the sky. We are the infinite, eternal, timeless Self. We recognize our connection to Source, to oneness, to wholeness. We realize we are and always have been that wholeness. We are restored to the Garden of Eden. The more we go there, the more we begin to live there and the less we are driven to secure pleasure and fear pain. We allow life to come as it comes and go as it goes, while knowing we are connected to something greater than all of it.

In the next chapter, we will learn how slowing the brainwaves assists in the stilling of mind and the experiential remembrance of our true nature.

CHAPTER FOUR

Yoga Nidra and Brainwaves
Understanding the Sleep that Awakens
Your True Nature

Every night when we go to sleep, the mind quiets and all its drama disappears. This is why sleep is so essential and so needed. It gives us a break from our crazy mind! Yet biological sleep only has the power to refresh the body. It does not have the power to awaken us to our true nature. Meditation is entering a state of quiet mind *consciously*. Yoga Nidra is a meditation technique. It is structured to drop the mind down toward sleep to deliberately enter a state where the mind is naturally silent and still.

A Yoga or meditation practice designed to still the waves of the mind so we can perceive what lies beyond it, is the "Yoga" we are referring to in "Yoga Nidra." *Nidra* means sleep. Yoga Nidra is a unique meditation practice because it rides on the natural process of sleep which is already built into our system. Sleep is not something we have to learn. Our body already knows how to do it. Ancient Yogis realized they could follow the same route, descending down into sleep states to *consciously* release identification with thoughts.

Yoga Nidra stills the waves of mind by taking us into conscious sleep states, progressively moving us through the same brainwave states as sleep. These brainwaves indicate less and less activity of the mind, creating profound states of meditative awareness—if experienced intentionally. Ancient Yogis realized that it was easier to use a process the body already knows to release identification with thoughts rather than struggling to learn a new one.

In Yoga Nidra, thoughts may be present, but they are not disturbing us in any way. In the space between our thoughts, we can settle into the eternal consciousness beyond the mind—and take this awareness back to the waking state. Even while awake, we begin to ground in the silent backdrop behind all that comes and goes. We cannot sleep our way to this state. In biological sleep, we are not cultivating the ability to bring the same state back with us to the waking state. This is why Yoga Nidra is *conscious* and *intentional* sleep.

In the ancient scriptures, the movement of the mind is described as *vritti* or waves (also translated as fluctuations). Interestingly, modern science also monitors the activity of the mind through measuring its electrical brainwave activity. Yoga Nidra takes literally Patanjali's *Sutra* from the *Yoga Sutras*, "Yoga is the stilling of fluctuations of mind." It "stills the waves of the mind" by stilling the brainwaves.

There are five major brainwave states: Beta, Gamma, Alpha, Theta and Delta. The additional distinction of the Gamma brainwave state has been added as scientists learn more about the brain. Brainwaves measure the electrical activity of the brain and the rate at which the electrical currents of the brain are cycling per second (measured in Hertz—Hz). The brainwaves can be observed with an EEG (or an electroencephalograph). Each type of brainwave has a purpose and helps us achieve optimal mental functioning.

Waking State *(Jagrat)*

Beta is associated with the normal waking state (Figure 1). Using the metaphor of a movie screen where the screen is the Self and the movie is the mind, the movie is most active in the waking state. The more active the mind's movie, the more difficult it is to perceive the screen. The wide range of potential brainwave activity while awake (Beta/Gamma) makes the movie seem very real and engaging. In life, the daily dramas, personality clashes, power skirmishes, details of living, working and getting our "to do" lists done seem very real. They grip our attention to the degree that we have a very hard time noticing the screen of silence behind them.

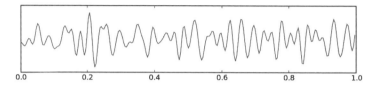

Figure 1: Beta Brainwaves 13-100 cycles per second.
Beta is associated with the normal waking state.

Beta Brainwaves are Associated with the Waking State: *Jagrat*
(*Vaishvanara* in the *Mandukya Upanishad*)

- Most identified with the character
- Least still
- Most driven by ego programming

In the waking state, we are most identified with the character and its unique programming. We view and interact with the world as the "real" world—a world that is solid and relatively unchangeable. Similarly, we interact with the feelings, emotions, reactions and thoughts that come and go in the waking state as equally real and consistent with the one character with which we have identified.

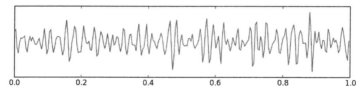

Figure 2: Gamma Brainwaves 40-70 cycles per second.
Gamma is associated with concentration and high IQ

In scientific journals, the definition and range of Beta and Gamma vary. Beta is said to range from 13-100 cycles per second, with Gamma as a subset of Beta (at 40-70 cycles per second). Regardless of range, simply note that Beta and Gamma cover the largest range of brainwave activity while awake.

The Gamma brainwave state (Figure 2), associated with high IQ, is found between 40 and 70 cycles per second (or Hz). It has been found that mentally-challenged and learning-disabled individuals tend to have lower Gamma activity than average. Gamma waves are important for learning, memory and information processing. It is theorized that the Gamma wave at 40 cycles per second (or Hz) is important for the binding of our senses to new input so we can learn and remember it. Meditation increases Gamma brainwave activity.[1] Additionally, greater Gamma activity in meditators is associated with greater empathy and compassion. The Gamma brainwave state is usually experienced while awake but interestingly can also be experienced in REM sleep.

Dreaming (Svapna)

The dream state is the second state of consciousness described in the *Mandukya Upanishad*. The Alpha brainwave state is associated with relaxed wakefulness all the way into dreaming or REM sleep. High states of Alpha correspond to a state of relaxed wakefulness. Brain activity begins to slow down and our thoughts come fewer and further apart. It is as if the movie on the screen is moving from "Die Hard" to "Driving Miss Daisy." Everything is calming down, quieting down. The volume of the movie decreases. In this state, it is fractionally easier to be less engaged by the movie and notice the screen itself.

As Dr. Hammond reports in the *Journal of Neuropathy*, "Alpha brainwaves (8-12 cycles per second) are slower and larger. They are associated with a state of relaxation and correspond with the brain shifting into an idling gear, relaxed and a bit disengaged, waiting to respond when needed. If someone merely closes their eyes and begins picturing something peaceful, in less than half a minute there begins to be an increase in Alpha brainwaves. These brainwaves are especially large in the back third of the head."[2] This is why most meditation techniques involve closing the eyes. Notice that the range of Alpha brainwaves is smaller than that in the Beta brainwave state (Figure 3). The Alpha brainwave state is a narrow bridge from wakefulness into sleeping and deeper states of consciousness. If one has difficulty dropping from Beta to Alpha brainwave states, it will be difficult to fall asleep.

Studies have shown that those with insomnia, excess stress and anxiety have less Alpha brainwave activity when awake. In these cases, Yoga Nidra can actually be good "exercise" for teaching the body how to let go of thoughts and fall asleep. Similar to gear-shifting, the body and brain need to be able to down-shift smoothly from accelerated brainwave states to slower ones. Developing this capacity through Yoga Nidra can be helpful for those stuck in high gear. It will also help create more Alpha brainwave activity while awake, allowing such a person to be more relaxed and better able to cope with life. Entering Alpha and Theta brainwave states accelerates memory retention and enhances learning. Compared to adults, children have much greater Alpha and Theta brainwave activity which allows them to digest and assimilate information from their surroundings at an astonishing rate. In the 1970s, this same phenomenon was introduced through the super learning technique in which people entered the Alpha brainwave state while simply listening to baroque classical music.

As we enter the Alpha brainwave state, we experience *relaxation* and ease. The body is often overcome with an overwhelming feeling of well-being associated with the release of serotonin into the system. In this state, the immune system is boosted enabling us to better fight off and recover from infections and disease. Here, we also begin to gain access to the subconscious mind. In Yoga, the subconscious is associated with the *Prana* or Energy body, which we will discuss in later chapters.

Dreaming occurs in the deep Alpha and high Theta brainwave states. We cross these same states in Yoga Nidra, but consciously so. In the dream state, identification with one concrete reality (or movie) becomes much more changeable and malleable. In a dream, there is no one constant reality. In one moment a dream reality might be a snow-capped mountain, in the next moment it could be a classroom. Even the character we identify as "me" in a dream is fluid. In any given moment we may be a woman, a man, a child or a bird. Our identification with one body and its set of thoughts, feelings and experiences becomes less rigid and more pliable. The "me" we call "me" becomes more transparent. Our attachment to it becomes looser. We are beginning to release identification with one character as "me." This is the bridge to total release from identification with the character.

When crossing the Alpha brainwave state in Yoga Nidra, you may feel as if you are hearing the guidance of a facilitator while simultaneously participating in a semi-dream state. Images, thoughts, and events may come and go, but in a disengaged way—as if observing these thoughts and images on a screen. Even though thoughts may be moving through in this state, they are more like background static as opposed to a foreground disturbance.

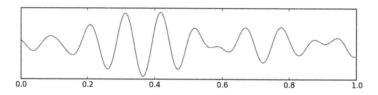

0.0   0.2   0.4   0.6   0.8   1.0

Figure 3: Alpha Brainwaves 8-12 cycles per second.
Ranges between relaxed waking and early stages of dream sleep. Relaxation, super learning, relaxed focus, light trance, increased serotonin production (intense feeling of well-being), beginning of access to subconscious (*Prana* body). Greater Alpha activity boosts the immune system. It has to do with ability to slow down and fall asleep.

Alpha and Theta are Associated with the Dream State: *Svapna*
(*Taijasa* in the *Mandukya Upanishad*)

- More malleable identification with character.
- Identification changes and shifts from dream to dream
- More distance and greater disengagement than waking consciousness.

Deep Sleep *(Shushupti)*

As we enter deeper states of meditation, we pass into Theta brainwave states. The brainwaves and movement of the mind slow down to the equivalent of a deep sleep state. Deep Theta and Delta brainwave states are associated with deep sleep, *shushupti*. The brain, cycling from 8-12 cycles per second (cps) in the dream state moves to a deeper state of silence at just 4-7 cps. Literally, Yoga Nidra is "stilling the fluctuations of mind" down to almost nil. This is a big shift from up to 100 cps in the waking state!

Theta brainwave states are associated with increased creativity, feeling relaxed and carefree. Artists, inventors and children often have more Theta brainwave activity, even in the waking state. This is also the state out of which creative solutions, inspirations and answers will often arise. If you have ever fallen asleep and awoken with an answer or solution to a problem, this is a result of entry into the Theta state. Along with the Alpha brainwave state, the Theta brainwave state is associated with increased retention of learned material and long term memory.[3] From early childhood to puberty, Alpha frequency increases but then starts to decrease with age. This can be prevented with mental training and is not age-related per se. People who can sustain a Theta brainwave state absorb information and learn very quickly. This is why children learn and retain information so easily. In the Theta brainwave state, memories are consolidated and "filed" in logical order so that information can be retrieved when needed.

Poor sleep appears to affect the brain's ability to consolidate memories about things that have been learned. Research suggests that the most critical time for the brain to consolidate information is the sleep period immediately following something learned.[4] Studies also demonstrate that memory accuracy in addition to memory strength is altered during slow-wave brain activity. Dr. Wilson, a senior researcher says, "What we think is happening is that during slow-wave sleep, neurons in the brain communicate with each other, and in doing so, strengthen their connections, permitting storage of specific information."[5] This could be an important use of Yoga Nidra to help the brain consolidate and accurately retain information.

While further study is needed, there is evidence that entry into the Delta brainwave state preserves cognitive abilities after trauma. It seems that slow-wave sleep induced immediately after a brain injury helps prevent axon damage and helps the brain retain normal brain function.[6] Even though the diagnosis of brain injury is increasing, very few effective, non-invasive and accessible treatments exist to prevent or even reverse compromised cognitive function. Yoga Nidra could be an important tool to enhance recovery from traumatic brain injury because of the slow-wave Delta brainwave state it induces.

In Theta brainwave states, we gain access to unconscious patterns and behaviors that, unbeknownst to us, guide our conscious actions, thoughts and behaviors (Figure 4). Thus, in this brainwave state, we can make potential changes in these behaviors. It is also the place where incomplete experiences can be integrated and completed at the deepest level, without even necessarily knowing what those experiences were or what changes happened. It has been determined that integration of emotional memories is, "Significantly correlated with the amount of REM sleep and also with right-dominant prefrontal Theta power during REM."[7] This same effect can happen consciously as we cross it during Yoga Nidra.

Studies suggest that meditation techniques alter Theta and Alpha EEG patterns significantly more than relaxation.[8] Entering the Theta state on a consistent basis is associated with positive brain changes such as the thickening of the prefrontal cortex, which has been identified to be denser in meditators.[9] Thickening of the prefrontal cortex is associated with greater ability to make conscious choices rather than habitual, preprogrammed ones and to manage reactions governed by the primal brain. It is also associated with greater ability to maintain calm and centeredness in the midst of increasingly stressful circumstances. In effect, this practice puts the brain and body in a more resilient state in which it is more resistant to becoming overstressed or being dragged into the drama of the movie.

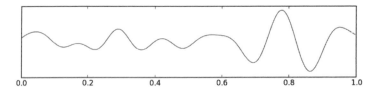

Figure 4: Theta Brainwaves 4-7 cycles per second

High Theta is associated with dream (REM) sleep. Deep Theta with deep sleep. Here we can see the waves of mind slowing down even more. Associated with increased creativity, feeling relaxed, and carefree. Artists and inventors have more Theta activity. So do children. Associated with increased retention of learned material (as children do) and long term memory consolidation. This is where emotional integration and completion of incomplete experiences can happen. This is where potential changes in behavior can happen through access to the unconscious mind. Thickening of the prefrontal cortex happens here.

Theta and Delta are associated with Deep Sleep: *Shushupti*

(*Prajna* in *Mandukya Upanishad*)

- May experience hypnagogic imagery, trance-like state.

- May hear the facilitator, but be unable to make sense of what is being said.

- May enter into a "gap" of nothingness.

- In the deepest states, the subset of objects in the awareness (body, mind, thoughts, past) which I have come to identify with as "me" is gone.

- The container is virtually empty.

Yoga Nidra and Brainwave States

The initial stages of Yoga Nidra happen between Alpha and Theta brainwave states. Here, dream-like thoughts and images are experienced at a distance. You may have thoughts in Yoga Nidra, but you are not interacting with them in the same way. They are distant from you, like a radio in another room. Though the voice of the mind is still there, it is not disturbing in any way; nor are you participating in what it says in the way you would in the waking state. It is just there, talking away—just as the radio does, *but you are not talking back*.

Often, at this level of Yoga Nidra, you may have dream-like images, thoughts, or feelings moving through. These often blend with the voice and guidance of the Yoga Nidra facilitator, creating a kind of wakeful dream. This is because the first level of Yoga Nidra crosses the dream state and can be experienced in a dream-like way.

Deeper states of Yoga Nidra happen in the Theta brainwave state. Experiences here can include drifting in and out of hearing the guidance of the Yoga Nidra. You may experience hypnagogic imagery such as colors, shapes, and lights or enter trance-like states. You may hear words, but you may not make sense of them in the usual way. The words are no longer being processed through the mind. However, the body is still responding directly and non-mentally to the directions given.

As Yoga Nidra takes you even deeper into Theta and Delta states, you may enter a gap of nothingness. It may feel like biological sleep, but when you are asked to come back at the end, you do. This is how you know you were, in fact, not sleeping in the same way you do at night. Your body is still receiving outside information while in the deepest and most profound of Yoga Nidra states. This is the distinction between biological and Yogic sleep. While the mind is silent as in sleep, awareness still abides.

In that gap, the fluctuations of the mind have slowed so much that identification with the character has disappeared altogether. In the waking state, identification with the body and its thoughts is strongest. In the dream state, it shifts to a more malleable and changeable state. In this, the deepest state, the subset of objects in awareness we have come to identify with as "me" is gone.

In this state, there is no separate "I." In Yoga Nidra, do you know what your name is? Do you know where your wallet is? What your political affiliation is? How much money you have in the bank? Is there even a "you" to be found?" The state of *Disidentification* with the character is so profound, we don't even know if the body is sick or healthy, if it is dying or not, if we are in jail or if we are in a mansion. It all disappears. The container is completely empty. In this place, you cannot help but notice you are more than all these things. You are that which contains it all. You recognize that you are one with the whole.

This profound release of identification with the body/mind is highly unusual in seated meditation and is typically experienced by only the most advanced meditators. These meditators may be able to create distance between thoughts and the body, but may rarely enter into prolonged gaps of awareness where all contents disappear and the sense of having a body at all dissolves. In Yoga Nidra, most people arrive at this deeper level of letting go within the first few times of practicing. Both meditation and meditation-based Yoga Nidra will take you there, but many find Yoga Nidra to be a very powerful and more accessible means to enter this space. Thereafter, the ability to enter this zone grows and people find their seated meditations are also imbued with these same qualities.

The deepest sleep states and Yoga Nidra states happen in the Delta brainwave frequency. Here, amazingly, brainwave activity can slow all the way down to 0.5 cycles per second. The range is between 0.5 and 3.9 cps (Figure 5). The fluctuations of mind are down to only the most basic survival functions. Since all other activity is shut off, this is the most restorative state for the body. When under anesthesia, when knocked unconscious or in a coma, the body is in a Delta brainwave state. The body, if injured severely enough, goes into a coma because this is the best state from which to heal. Medical professionals, as a last resort, now induce a coma with certain traumatic injuries in hopes of allowing the body to heal itself. Every time we go to Delta brainwave states in Yoga Nidra we are profoundly healing and restoring the body.

Every night, we cycle through the brainwaves several times. When we get a good amount of Delta brainwave sleep, we awake feeling particularly refreshed, alert and rejuvenated. It has been repeatedly proven that Theta and Delta activity tend to decrease as we age, and the tendency to stay in upper Alpha increases.[10] Yoga Nidra can help reverse this tendency and the sleep problems that can result. In Delta states of Yoga Nidra, human growth hormone is released. As we get older, growth hormone levels decline. Human growth hormone is essential to maintain proper metabolism and regulate the proportion of body fat to muscle. It influences the storage ratios of good to bad cholesterol and it is vital for proper heart muscle functioning. Growth hormone also maintains and corrects bone density and enables the growth and regeneration of all the organs of the body, including the brain.

In adults, low or absent growth hormone can cause emotional symptoms, such as tiredness and lack of motivation. All of this can be counteracted in the Delta brainwave state where growth hormone is released.[11] Delta brainwave states also reduce the amount of cortisol, a stress hormone, in the system. Cortisol accelerates the aging process and can be highly detrimental to the system, as we will learn in later chapters. Cortisol reduction reduces the rate at which we age.

Research shows that monks and meditators display more Delta brainwave activity in the waking state than usual and this is associated with empathy, compassion, intuition and spirituality. This is scientifically congruent with what Yoga Nidra seeks to achieve. We are training ourselves to go into deep brainwave states consciously, so that we may bring these states back to waking consciousness. The fact that we see greater Delta brainwave activity among meditators in the waking state suggests that the more we go into these deep meditative brainwave states, the more we are actually able to bring these back to conscious awareness and function in the world from this place. The resulting actions we take are initiated from greater empathy, compassion and inner balance.

Imagine that each time you practice Yoga Nidra, you move from the wave (the body/mind) to the ocean of formless consciousness. From that experience you see that all waves are part of one ocean. We are all one, and from there, compassion naturally arises for one another, for our planet, for all living creatures.

Yoga Nidra is not an escape from the world. The purpose is to teach you to live differently in the world. A Yoga Nidra practice of 45 minutes, even twice a day, does not necessarily balance out the other 22 or 23 hours of the day. Yoga Nidra is most effective when it empowers you to be effective and productive, yet internally steady in the midst of *life*—the other 23 hours.

Changes in meditators' brainwaves show that, in fact, this can happen in a measurable way.

Scientists used to believe it was scientifically impossible for a person to be in a Delta-predominant brainwave state and be able to walk, talk and interact with others in the conscious waking state. Swami Rama of the Himalayan Institute in Pennsylvania was one of the first Yogis in the West to use scientific instrumentation to verify the ability to be deep in Delta brainwave states while simultaneously being awake and functional.[12] Essentially, in Yoga Nidra we are training ourselves to do the same so that we can operate from a more relaxed baseline while awake. This is why one of the instructions in Yoga Nidra is to stay awake. This should not be a stressful task, but simply an intent put forth to your subconscious mind. Then let go and allow whatever happens to happen. In the beginning, some people have difficulty staying awake because the body is accustomed to being asleep in deeper brainwave states. Eventually, however, we can train ourselves to be awake but as deeply relaxed and distant from the mind as in sleep.

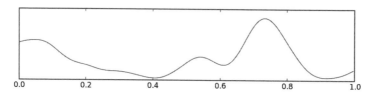

Figure 5: Delta Brainwaves 0.5-3.9 cycles per second
Associated with the deepest, most restorative sleep.
Experience: Dreamless sleep, complete loss of body awareness, Trance-like, non-physical state, may feel unable to move, associated with out of body experiences. Access to unconscious and collective unconscious.
Health: The most recuperative state for the body to heal itself. Reduces cortisol in the system – which is associated with accelerated aging. Human growth hormone (HGH) released in Delta. Anti-aging. Delta is the most refreshing sleep.

HGH is associated with:

- ○ Bone mineralization
- ○ Muscle mass
- ○ Fat breakdown and protein synthesis
- ○ Growth and regeneration of all internal organs
- ○ Homeostasis
- ○ Immune system

In the Delta state, we not only have access to the unconscious, but also to the *collective unconscious*. The collective unconscious, defined by Jung, refers to primal patterning built into the DNA of all human beings the world over. These are issues that are common to being human rather than more specific issues that are unique to each individual person—such as power, the search for wholeness, and being a woman or being a man.

Yoga Nidra experiences in the Delta state are usually associated with one's complete loss of body awareness. This is why, in the deep Delta brain experience, you may feel you cannot move, or it takes longer to come back to waking consciousness and the ability to move. Some may even have out-of-body experiences in Yoga Nidra, which are associated with the Delta state.

An out-of-body experience is when the Energy body remains connected to the Physical body, but *floats* out of the Physical body. This is a very healing state. The Energy body can see many things, travel, or journey, but remains connected to the Physical body. This is what some people call "soul journeying" and it is a practice in and of itself for some people. In Yoga Nidra, that is not the focus, but it can happen. There is nothing to be afraid of when it happens. In fact, children experience it spontaneously. One of the main benefits is that it allows us to see that the body is not the sum total of who we are. *We are more than the body.*

This expands our awareness to a greater sense of Self and begins to help us release our identification with the body as the limit of who we are.

Yoga Nidra Solves the Problem

The body and mind enter a state of *complete non-doing* in the Theta and Delta brainwave states of Yoga Nidra. The contents of the container are naturally and effortlessly stilled. In that space of nothingness, it is effortless to notice and rest as the container—the Source—that we are. There is nothing left *to do*. Only *to be*.

Remember that the problem Yoga Nidra seeks to solve is forgetfulness of our true nature and identification with who we are not. As we progressively descend through the three states of consciousness, identification drops away until there is nothing left but the space itself. The subset of objects in awareness that we habitually believe to be "me" is gone. The only thing left is the space of awareness itself. Here it is impossible not to notice one's true nature. That is all there is. The problem of mis-identification outlined in the *kleshas* is experientially solved. You do not just cognitively understand your formless nature, you *know* it, *feel* it, and *become it* experientially. This is a vital difference. We can all learn and study the scriptures. This is important. But until understanding becomes an experiential knowing through personal experience, it is only half of the picture. Yoga Nidra provides the living half. The scriptures are the map. Yoga Nidra is the journey.

The Fourth State of *Turiya*

Moving through the previous three states of waking, dreaming and deep sleep via the corresponding brainwaves allows easy access to *turiya*—the fourth state of consciousness. *Turiya* is resting as and kinesthetically experiencing the space of awareness beyond the other three states. It is the experience of the container, the background behind everything that is seen, heard, felt or experienced while awake, dreaming or in deep sleep. This is the ultimate purpose of Yoga Nidra: conscious entry into that deep-sleep space, the doorway to what is beyond the mind.

Once seen and recognized as our true nature, *turiya* eventually becomes noticed as the backdrop within which all other states are arising and dissolving (the container). In other words, the shift is made from the perspective of the contents to the perspective of the sky. *Turiya* is resting as the sky itself.

In the waking state, there can be a great many objects in the sky, and the sky has the capacity for all of it. In the dream state, there may also be many objects, but usually less substantial and at a greater distance; yet it makes no difference to the sky. In deep sleep, there is little or nothing occupying the sky; but once again, it makes no difference to the sky itself. For this reason, one could say *turiya* is essentially akin to enlightenment. It is resting as and noticing one's sky-like nature.

We have reinstated our nature as form *and* formless. Container *and* contents. Here we need no longer be overwhelmed by the flood of thoughts and emotions that move through the body and mind each day. All of it is held and seen in the container of awareness. Though nothing outside has changed, our *perspective* has, and from this place, we are better able to allow the changing ebb and flow of life to move through as we remain steadily connected to the unchanging Self that we are.

The more we recognize *turiya*, the less we are identified with, and bound by, the character and its acquired beliefs, concepts and limitations. We know we are Spirit playing the role of the character, but we are not held captive by the role. Our limitless nature simply expresses itself *through* the character rather than being identified and limited *by* it.

Yoga Nidra solves the ultimate problem that is the cause of all suffering: ignorance of our true nature and identification with who we are not. This is the first Tool of Yoga Nidra: *Realization*. It is the ultimate purpose for which Yoga Nidra was created. The process of *Realization* happens by degrees. As you practice Yoga Nidra, situations that used to bother you simply don't irritate you as much. You will find yourself less reactive to things that used to trigger you. Habits that seemed to run your life simply disappear. You will find yourself calmer and steadier in the midst of things that would have shaken your foundation. This effect grows over time and is a direct result of continuous entry into the state of *turiya*.

In Ayurveda, the sister science to Yoga, *turiya* is also known as the place where spontaneous and miraculous healing occurs. When we are identified with the mind, the body is affected by what the mind thinks and feels. Repeated thoughts and emotions to which we attach and believe, create chemical effects in the body and can contribute to disease. *Turiya* is evidenced by a complete release of identification with mind—including the subtle patterns that cause *dis*-ease in the body. The body's healing energy (*prana*), which is usually consumed by our thoughts and emotions, is now free to operate at its most accelerated and restorative level.

This is why, in Ayurveda, the definition of health is *swasthya*—to be seated in the Self. *Turiya* is where this happens. Even in medical science, a doctor intuitively knows the body will heal itself best when the mind and body are less active. This is why a doctor will always tell you to get plenty of rest when you are sick. Yoga Nidra is the most profound rest there is—not only for the body but also for the mind, which is usually holding the body's energy hostage. When released from the captivity of the mind, the body's natural energy can focus on healing.

This natural healing is like rebooting your computer when it malfunctions. Everything running on the computer is shut down. When we turn the computer back on, the entire system will often begin to work the way it should.

CHAPTER FIVE

Koshas: Mapping Embodiment from Formless to Form

Out of the ocean of formless potential rises a multitude of forms, as waves on an ocean. Each wave surges into form in a unique way, varying in depth, shape, amplitude and breadth. Each wave, though rising out of the same field of limitless potential, is differentiated but not separate. Each is part and parcel of the ocean itself.

Forms, like waves, live and die. They live in the world of time. The formless depths of the ocean do not live or die. The ocean is always there whether waves are present or not. It is timeless and eternal. Form and formless interact and interchange with one another in a ceaseless tide of waves moving from *formless to form* and from *form back to formless* with the ocean serving as the Source background potential from which waves can move into form.

In many spiritual traditions it is said, "We are all one." At the level of the ocean, we are all one. Even though the Divinity from which we all arise is the same, each one of us uniquely manifests as an embodied vehicle of the Divine. The Divine within us is Spirit. When formless Divinity moves into form, it does so through the building block of all matter—energy.

Energy is Manifest Divinity

Everything in existence, whether subtle or gross, is composed of varying densities of energy. A thought is composed of less dense energy, a chair of more dense energy. Physics verifies this. Einstein said, "Matter is energy reduced to the point of visibility."

In Yoga, the energy that serves as the building block of all things in material existence is called *Universal Prana*—life energy.

The same energy that animates all things also animates the human body. We call this *biological prana*. Biological *prana* is the Source of the body's life. When biological *prana* leaves the body, we die. This energy is innately intelligent and knows how to carry out millions of complex homeostatic processes which scientists have yet to fully fathom. Healing, digestion, respiration and circulation all function without us ever having to think about it. When given the opportunity, this energy is capable of miraculous healing and entry into subtler realms of consciousness.

Prana is formless Divinity made visible. It is the visible, manifest aspect of the invisible. The energy that animates your body is Divine energy manifesting through the body. This is what we call Spirit. *The same energy that vitalizes, maintains and heals your body is Spirit itself working in your body.*

In Chapter 15, Verse 14 of the *Bhagavad Gita*, Krishna, as the ocean of consciousness says, "I am the fire of digestion in the bodies of all living entities, and I join with the air of life, out-going and incoming, to digest the four kinds of foodstuff." This means the energy in you *is* consciousness. Energy is consciousness made visible. That consciousness is the force that is healing your body, breathing your breath, and digesting your food. That *is* the Spirit in you—and in all living entities. The Spirit in you doesn't just sit around. It is the energy force that keeps you alive and it primarily comes in through the breath. When we "inspire" the breath, we are drawing the Spirit force into the body.

The Spirit that is healing and maintaining our body has so much more potential than we give it credit. Healing and maintenance are just the very tip of its capacity. In fact, the Spirit, when freed, can become magnified. It can grow and accelerate. It can move from a biological force that maintains the body to a Spiritual force which will take us back to unification with Source.

The Integrative Amrit Method of Yoga Nidra is *Prana*-Based

The Amrit Method of Yoga Nidra is designed to work with the Spirit force of *prana*. It centers on freeing *prana* in the body so that *prana* can move from a biological healing force to an evolutionary Spiritual force. It stands to reason that if consciousness and energy are the same force appearing differently, then one will bring us to the other. In Yogic philosophy, these two aspects of Divinity are often referred to as *Shiva* (consciousness—the ocean) and *Shakti* (energy, consciousness made visible—the wave). Both *Shiva* and *Shakti* are inextricably connected to one another.

Just as a wave naturally returns to the ocean, energy (*Shakti*) wants to return to consciousness (*Shiva*). Rather than struggling to return to the formless, all we have to do is ride *prana* back to the Source from which it came.

In Yogic mythology, energy (*Shakti*) and consciousness (*Shiva*) are portrayed as a lover and her beloved. Both love one another with unspeakable intensity and want to return to an experience of oneness, the same as all beloveds do. Mind stands between the two. Instead of allowing *Shakti* to be reunited with her beloved, the mind steals her energy away. This is to say metaphorically, that the same fuel which feeds the Source, also feeds the mind. When the mind is agitated, upset and angry, it is burning the fuel of the Spirit. That energy is not available for the Spirit to return to Source. In the Amrit Method of Yoga Nidra, we want to quiet the mind so the energy of the Spirit builds enough acceleration and momentum to escape the gravitational pull of mind and return to *Shiva—Source consciousness.*

As you practice the Amrit Method of Yoga Nidra, you will find that each technique serves to quiet the mind and enhance the flow and awareness of *prana*. Time is given after each component to absorb the energetic effect. As *prana* grows and magnifies with attention, the mind is naturally and profoundly stilled. The energy released absorbs the mind and progressively drops you deeper toward oneness with your ocean-like nature. The beauty of an energetic practice is that it requires no effort other than *letting go of all doing.* In the absence of doing, energy is freed to do its evolutionary work.

Various styles of Yoga Nidra have different points of focus. Some focus more on concentration, others focus on working with emotions and thoughts. The Amrit Method focuses on *prana*/energy resulting in a powerful method to suspend the mind and merge into oneness. This is the hallmark of the Amrit Method.

The Amrit Method of Yoga Nidra is designed to move in a structured way through the subtle sheaths of embodiment, *koshas*, back to recognition of our formless nature. In order to understand how a Yoga Nidra is structured, we first need to understand the *koshas*. By understanding the process by which the ocean manifests as a wave, we can also understand how to track the process back to our ocean-like expanded nature.

The *Koshas*

The five *koshas* or sheaths (*Pancha kosha*) were first outlined in the *Taittiriya Upanishad*. The *koshas*, literally translated as "house" or "sheath", map the process of embodiment from unmanifest, undifferentiated potential (the ocean) into the physical form of the body (the wave). Each *kosha* is named as follows: *Ananda* (Bliss), *Vijnana* (Wisdom), *Mana* (Mental), *Prana* (Energy) and *Ana* (Physical) bodies respectively. Each body name is followed by the same suffixes: *maya* and *kosha*. We know *kosha* means sheath, and *maya* means illusory. These suffixes indicate that these are illusory sheaths of embodiment which may appear to separate us from Source, but in fact do not. Thus the *Ananda-maya-kosha* would mean, "The illusory sheath of bliss that appears to separate us from the whole." All of the *koshas* can be translated the same way. This is a subtle way of reinforcing that even though we are embodied, we are not and never have been separate from Source.

The *koshas* delineate the subtle process by which energy progressively condenses out of the soup of unmanifest potential and eventually densifies into what we know and see as the concrete and visible physical body. A metaphor to understand the *koshas* or bodies as increasingly visible and materialized sheaths would be to compare the Bliss body to ether, the Wisdom body to air, the Mental body to steam, the Energy body to water and the Physical body to ice. It is harder to affect or shape ice than it is to affect water. At the water level (Energy body), water will assume the form of whatever direction it is given, whereas at the ice level (Physical body), we would need to use a hammer and chisel to effect the same changes. As you will see, one of the primary Tools of Yoga Nidra—*Intention (Sankalpa),* makes use of this principle.

The process of embodiment first moves from formless into the most subtle condensation of energy at the Bliss body or *Anandamayakosha*. Think of the Bliss body as the first undulation of an ocean as it begins to swell toward a fully formed wave (Figure 6). This sheath is said to arise from the initial mutation from oneness to the sense of "me" as a separate and distinct entity from the whole of the ocean.

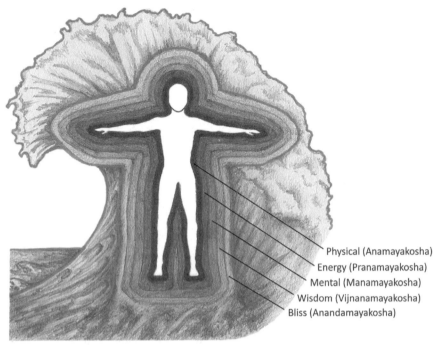

Physical (Anamayakosha)
Energy (Pranamayakosha)
Mental (Manamayakosha)
Wisdom (Vijnanamayakosha)
Bliss (Anandamayakosha)

Koshas emerging from the Ocean

Figure 6: *Koshas* **emerging from potentiality into embodiment just as a wave emerges from the undifferentiated potential of the ocean.**

Artwork by JoElizabeth James

The Bliss body or *Anandamayakosha* is the most powerful of all the sheaths, being the first involution into form. It is the finest veil standing between ordinary awareness and Source. In the *Taittiriya Upanishad*, the Bliss body is equated with the transcendental Self or Source itself, although subsequent Vedanta schools consider it to be the final veil surrounding the ultimate Reality, or Self. We will go with the latter here—the Bliss body as the final veil to ultimate Reality or Self. If Source is pure light and love, the Bliss body, as the thinnest veil receives the greatest luminosity from the Source. As each sheath gets denser and further from Source, the light of Source is less able to penetrate through these apparent veils of separation.

Anandamayakosha, the Bliss Body

The Bliss body is the junction between formless Source and form. It is the place where *Shiva* and *Shakti* or consciousness and energy meet and intermingle. It is experienced as a sense of purest silent joy. It is a space of abiding stillness and perfect contentment without cause or reason. There is no fear, desire or sense of inadequacy. The experience of love at the Bliss body is not emotional ecstasy, which has an opposite, rather it is a spontaneous opening of the heart that is so overwhelming, tears may come to your eyes. It leaves you with a feeling of great gratitude and oneness with everything. It is reflecting the Divine bliss of the Self.

The vast majority of humans will rarely experience the Bliss body while awake. One of those moments can be when we fall in love. The heart opens spontaneously and we feel at one, not just with the object of our love, but with existence itself. Besides during profound heart-opening experiences, *andamayakosha* most fully manifests during sleep, or sleep-like states. This is why Yoga Nidra is a powerful path to the Bliss body.

The Bliss body is the reflected light of Source. Its only difference from Source is that it contains a sense of individuality or "I am-ness"—a pure sense of being-ness. Contained within the Bliss body is the unconscious mind, or our individualized consciousness, called *chitta*. Like a computer's hard drive, it registers the impressions left by every life experience. These impressions are called *samskaras*. This is where all life's memories, experiences and images are stored. Core emotions, habits, attachments and impressions reside here. Deeper than thoughts, they are more like residual imprints left on mental pathways that continue to drive our motivations and tendencies from within. They include actions that have eventually become second nature to us through repetition.[13]

Chitta comprises the Causal body—another name for the Bliss body. The Causal body is the vehicle through which the individual soul reincarnates and is said to remain through rebirth. It contains *karmic* imprints carried over from past lives, but only a few are revealed in a particular lifetime depending on the environment. *Chitta*, or individualized consciousness, is not bad. It determines our distinct character, personality and mind.[14] However, some things held in our individualized consciousness are not helpful. Yoga Nidra can reach directly into this "hard drive" (*chitta*) and is a means to rewrite what is contained on it.

In its illuminated state, the *Anandamayakosha* reflects the bliss of the Source. When asleep to its Source nature, the *Anandamayakosha* operates through association with *chitta*—the storehouse of unconscious memories, impressions and tendencies. When we identify with these impressions (*samskaras*) rather than the Self, we experience our own mindstuff—beliefs, concepts and past—more than the transcendent light and love at the Bliss body. When identified with *samskaras*, these impressions and resulting tendencies can channel and direct the formless into form in both helpful and unhelpful ways. Yoga Nidra can be used as a tool to rewrite this programming directly at this critical changing station between formless and form.

Vijnanamayakosha, the Wisdom body

The next condensation of energy toward visible form, rising out of the ocean and toward a wave, is the Wisdom body or *Vijnanamayakosha*. *Vijnana* means "the power of judgment or discernment." It includes conscience and will and encompasses all the functions of the higher mind. The higher mind operates as discriminating intellect. It is also called *buddhi*. Its job is to discern between what is real and what is unreal.

The Wisdom body digests and analyses incoming sensory impressions received from the outer mind (*Manamayakosha*, the Mental body) and then extracts meaning from it. From this, our choices are made and subsequent actions are passed on to the body and organs of action to carry them out.

The Wisdom body holds a repository of information some of which is held outside of our conscious awareness. When working properly, this conscious and unconscious information is used to bring understanding, clarity of mind, good judgment, and discerning choices. The Wisdom body can function from pre-programmed conditioning or from beyond it. As a function of programmed perception, the Wisdom body is our intelligence—our ability to contemplate and engage in higher levels of thought such as philosophy, science, logic, and reason. However, *the Wisdom body, when unclouded by past programming, can operate from beyond mere intellect and can access true wisdom that stems from knowing Source itself. The higher knowing of the Wisdom Body has the capacity to perceive that the eternal is what is real and that the temporal is in passing and therefore unreal.*[15] This is not a function of acquired knowledge learned through books, but is known through *experience*. A Wisdom body opened to its higher potential brings intuition, wisdom, witness consciousness and objectivity.

When unobstructed, the Wisdom body acts as an inner divining rod that moves you toward truth and knowing of Source itself. It acts as your inner guidance system. In layman's terms, one might call it the "higher Self" or inner knowing. Some would call it insight, clear-seeing or deeper perception.

Undistorted, the *Vijnanamayakosha* is able to perceive with pristine clarity. Balanced, objective insight into any situation is available. It can see what is, as it is. However, adopted fears, beliefs, conclusions and interpretations can cloud the Wisdom body's ability to distinguish between the real and the unreal.

Often, this means we are not seeing reality as it is; we are seeing reality filtered through our past memories and beliefs. We no longer have access to insight or knowing because we cannot see clearly. We don't simply see a man or woman walking toward us, we see a man or woman who reminds us of pain we experienced in the past; so we avoid them. Or we see a man or woman as a potential partner because they remind us of our father or mother whom we loved; so we move toward them. We are not seeing what is, as is. We are seeing our fears and desires superimposed over that person. These fears and attachments compel us to act in certain ways. These tendencies are called *vasanas*.

Whatever is held in the Bliss body can affect the Wisdom body. This is because the *koshas* act in a hierarchical fashion—each more refined than the next, but influencing those below it. Therefore whatever is held in the Bliss body will, when attached to, affect all other *koshas*. Attachments and fears reside as *samskaras* in the Bliss body. Fear and attachment are the agents that most cloud the clarity of the Wisdom body. When we have no fear or attachment, we can give a friend solid, impartial and objective advice. However, when we are involved in our own story or drama, we lose our clear-seeing, particularly when we are attached or afraid of losing something we really want. Our clarity and judgment is clouded and we cannot discern what action is right for us.

Ultimately, what we consciously believe and act on can become an unconscious impression or a tendency held in the Bliss body. After repeatedly judging someone a certain way, we may continue to do so without even being aware of it. A conscious decision has become an unconscious way of being; automatically steering our thinking and behavior outside of mindful discrimination. Yoga Nidra is designed to take us to the Bliss body where we can affect this core programming even when it has become an unconscious pattern *outside* our conscious awareness.

In Yoga Nidra, we also work with the Wisdom body through witness. The *Dis-identification* gained through witness, creates space from past memories, beliefs and conclusions so that we can clearly see the present for what it is, informed by the past, but not clouded by it.

More gross than the Bliss and Wisdom bodies and moving more toward the full shape of the wave, is the Mental body. Though we cannot see the Mental body, it is more easily definable than the Bliss or Wisdom bodies. After all, we are able to identify thoughts and their effects as they come and go. The Mental body is called the *Manamayakosha*, or *the body made of thought processes*, and it is exactly that. In general terms, it is the outer mind that allows us to receive and digest sensory impressions from the outside environment. The Mental body is most connected with the eyes. When we close the eyes, we immediately begin to quiet the Mental body. The Mental body takes in data, and together with the Wisdom body interprets the information, which results in actions taken—with the Energy and Physical bodies acting as pawns of the subtler and more powerful mind and intellect.

In the *Yoga Sutras*, Patanjali says in 1.2: "Yoga is the stilling of modifications of mind." In Sanskrit, the words are, "*Yogash chitta vritti nirodaha.*" In Yoga Nidra, we are stilling the way the incoming senses (via *manas*—Mental body) interact with the unconscious pre-programming contained in the *chitta* which together cause fluctuations of mind (*vrittis*). Yoga is the stilling of these fluctuations of mind (*vrittis*). As these mental fluctuations or *vrittis* are stilled, our true nature is revealed. We have enough clarity to perceive the Self beyond the fluctuations of mind with which we are habitually identified. For instance, if we have unresolved feelings or conclusions about being "left out" stored in our *chitta* (hard drive) and we are the only one left with no seat at a picnic, the incoming information through the Mental body (*manas*) interacts with our past conclusions and beliefs (held in the *chitta* at the Bliss body), resulting in fluctuations or *vrittis* in the mind. The resulting fluctuations, or internal reactions, are stilled in Yoga Nidra so that we may perceive what is beyond it.

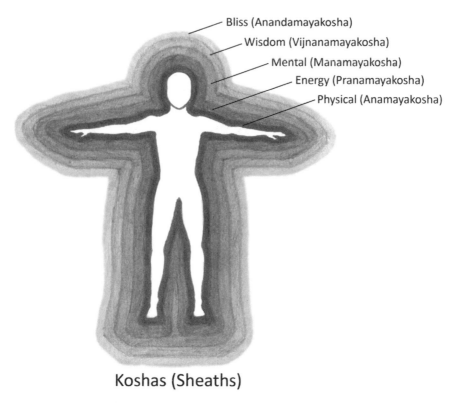

Bliss (Anandamayakosha)
Wisdom (Vijnanamayakosha)
Mental (Manamayakosha)
Energy (Pranamayakosha)
Physical (Anamayakosha)

Koshas (Sheaths)

Figure 7: *Koshas* (Sheaths)

Artwork by JoElizabeth James

Pranamayakosha, the Energy Body

The Energy body or *Pranamayakosha* is even more gross than the Mental body and more tangible (Figure 7). We can *feel* energy as sensation in the body very clearly. Even though we cannot see energy, the sensations in our body give us clear signals as intuition or instinctual signals. The difference between insight at the Wisdom body level and intuition at the Energy body level is physical sensation. The Energy body speaks through bodily sensation without language, such as gut feelings or impulses. At the Wisdom body level, insight can come in the form of knowledge and words. You might receive information from the higher Self, telling you what to do, what to say, how to act. It almost speaks through you. At the Energy body level, Source also speaks, but through the language of sensation. Keep in mind that even though we describe the *koshas* separately, they are an interconnected web. Everything is affecting everything else. So, our "inner divining rod" may speak to us through insight as well as sensation.

We feel the energy as sensation in the Physical body because the Energy body surrounds and infuses the Physical body. It is the energy or *Prana* body that serves as the mechanism by which *Universal Prana* enters the Physical body and enlivens it via the *chakra* system and the thousands of meridians or *nadis* that feed the organs and systems of the body. It is the *prana* of the Energy body that makes the heart beat, the lungs breathe. When the Energy body leaves the Physical body, the Physical body dies.

It is *prana* that maintains homeostasis and heals the body—and it is the same *prana* that is the visible aspect of the Divine that has the potential to take us back to the formless. *Prana* is the Spirit in you. In Christianity it would be called the Holy Spirit. It is that which connects the "Son" (you and I) to the "Father" (Source). When the *Prana* body or Spirit is very strong as a result of connection to Source, the *Prana* body can even become visible to the naked eye as a certain glow or aura emanating from around the body. This is depicted as a halo around saints and mystics in many traditions.

Anamayakosha, the Physical Body

Finally, the most condensed form of energy is the Physical body or *Anamayakosha.* It is the wave in full visible manifestation. *Ana* means "food" or "rice" because it is composed of the foodstuff we take in. It is tangible, visible, most dense, and least easy to change. The furthest from Source, it receives the least light and radiance. However, the more clarified all the bodies are, the more transparent and less dense all the *koshas* become, resulting in a visibly more radiant countenance and skin. You will see this effect when you begin to do Yoga Nidra consistently.

The Bliss body is also known as the Causal body. It is invisible and intangible—even to the subtle senses. The Wisdom, Mental and Energy bodies together are also called the "Subtle body." The Physical body is called the "Gross body."

The Amrit Method of Yoga Nidra focuses most heavily on the Energy body. The Energy body has the capacity to heal physically, mentally and emotionally at an accelerated level. The Energy body, unlike the Mental and Bliss bodies, is gross enough to feel and sense, yet—like water—is subtle enough to shape and change quickly and effectively. It is the place where we can affect the subtler Mental and Bliss bodies *and* the gross Physical body quickly and easily.

CHAPTER SIX

The Second Tool of Yoga Nidra: *Integration*

In the deepest states of Yoga Nidra, *resistances at all levels are released. Freed energy in the body is accelerated to its evolutionary level and begins to move back to Source, clearing and detoxifying unresolved blocks at the physical, mental and emotional levels.*

Not everyone is interested in Self-Realization. While *Realization* is more about recognition of the transcendent Self, *Integration* and the other Tools are designed to specifically benefit the body and mind. Maybe you or your loved ones just want to be a bit healthier, have a good night's sleep, manage high blood pressure or relieve stress. Maybe you want to have less worries and more peace. Yoga Nidra provides all this. The peace created in the body/mind is the first step. We learn to still the body/mind, we learn to manage it, and make it healthier and happier. Think about it. The healthier you are, the steadier your mind is. A steady mind is the basis for all further spiritual practices. The other Tools of Yoga Nidra (*Integration*, *Dis-identification*, *Intention*, *Relaxation* and *Restoration*) help still and steady the body/mind complex. This makes the final purpose of Yoga Nidra—*Realization*—much more accessible.

The body/mind complex is built of the *koshas*. Based on the beliefs, conclusions and incomplete experiences held at the Bliss body (*samskaras*), all *koshas* below it are affected. If we have a deeply imprinted experience that causes us to repeatedly conclude "Life is hard," or "Life is against me," that conclusion will filter our perceptions (Wisdom body), shape our thoughts (Mental body), direct our feelings (Energy body) and even drive the way we act (Physical body). These experiences, perceptions, thoughts and feelings will, in fact, affect everything.

Our next Tool, *Integration,* is designed to clear out the effects of such ideas and beliefs. If we have believed ourselves to be abandoned and unwanted, this thought and feeling will have imprinted itself not only into the psyche, but also into the meridians, muscles, cells, chemistry and biology of the body. It will have affected our perceptions, our thoughts and our feelings. Yoga Nidra helps clear the effects of the toxic conclusions we have adopted.

The Mind Usually Siphons Away Energy

The energy that enlivens our body is the Spirit in us. That energy has the potential to become a spiritual and evolutionary force returning us to Source. However, we often use up so much energy in the mind, we barely have enough energy left for healthy bodily function, much less exploring our spiritual potential.

Usually, the Energy body is at the mercy of the mind. Energy follows attention. Whatever the mind thinks, *prana* obeys. If the mind is agitated, energy (*prana*) is agitated. If mind is sad, *prana* is sad. If mind is distracted, *prana* is distracted. *Prana* is simply fuel. It takes the form and shape of whatever it is given—helpful or unhelpful—and gives it life.

When the mind is quiet and energy is strong enough, the usual subservient relationship between mind and *prana* begins to shift. *Prana* can accumulate enough momentum to escape the gravitational pull of the mind and can operate independently. When freed to do so, its intelligent, healing properties are accelerated and its biological properties are transmuted to evolutionary functions. Energy wants to return to Source. It knows the way home but is usually held hostage by the mind.

In Yoga Nidra, we want to accomplish two things: quiet the mind and magnify the power of the Energy body. The quieter the mind becomes, the more energy can gather and grow into a healing spiritual force. The converse is also true: the more we free energy in the body, the quieter the mind becomes.

You have probably noticed after a massage or yoga class that the enhanced flow of energy in your body creates a calm and steady mind. Similarly, in the Amrit Method of Yoga Nidra, we free energy in the body to help calm the mind. Rather than fighting with the mind directly, which only creates more conflict, we free *prana* as a gateway to create profound levels of stillness. This combination of heightened *prana* and quiet mind is what allows energy to merge back into the silent aware space from which it came. *Prana* is a force we can ride to consciousness. We don't have to *find* our way back to Source. *Prana* already knows the way. All we need to do is manage and cultivate this inner energy in such a way that it is freed to return home.

A wonderful story about a boy and his horse demonstrates this principle. In the story, the horse represents *prana—energy.* The rider represents the mind which usually directs that potentiality according to its wishes. One day a boy (the mind) decides to take his horse out into a vast expanse of nature. It is early in the morning and they ride and ride into the wild. As long as mind (the boy) is in charge, *prana* (the horse) follows its direction, using its ability to stride, gallop and jump in service of the boy. Together they cover miles of territory, jumping over streams, and galloping through the woods. After awhile, the boy becomes hot and wants to turn back. As he looks around to make his way back, he realizes he has no idea where he is, how he arrived, or how to return home. For awhile, he wanders around, trying to find a trail or some clue that will take him home. Finally, he realizes the futility of his quest. He (mind) simply doesn't know how to get back.

Then he realizes that while he may not know the way back, the horse (*prana*) does. Yet how to get the horse to take him home? He realizes if he can release the reins on the horse, it will take him home. At first, the boy only tentatively releases the reins.

The horse still feels the reins and waits to be told what to do. The boy realizes he has to let go of the reins *completely*. Only then will the horse (*prana*) realize he is free and follow his own inner guidance system home.

Now completely left to its own devices, the horse grazes here and there, waiting for further instructions. Then the horse realizes his rider is not giving him any direction. He walks a bit and then stops to see if he will be steered any further. No response. Then he walks a bit more and trots a little. After a number of starts and stops, the horse realizes that he is in charge and gallops all the way home, taking the boy with him! This is how the Amrit Method of Yoga Nidra is designed to work. *When the mind (the rider) is allowed to take a backseat to prana, the horse knows the way home to Source consciousness. All we have to do is trust it.*

Energy Experiences

As this energy begins to move toward Source, various energy experiences can indicate *prana* is carrying out accelerated restorative functions. Signs of increased energy flow at the body level include tingling, streaming, trembling, shaking, rocking, spontaneous jerking, or even a sense that you cannot feel the body or cannot move. Visual indications of the movement of energy include hypnagogic imagery, lights, or a visual cognition of nothingness. Psychic energetic experiences can include out of body experiences, and visitation from guides, family members or masters with whom you have a connection. It is also possible to hear sounds or receive wisdom and insight in these states.

It is very important to recognize that even though these experiences may occur, the power and benefits of Yoga Nidra do not depend upon any of these energetic or psychic experiences. Know that Yoga Nidra is working if you are experiencing deep states of stillness—even when thoughts are present. Unusual experiences can be an indication that energy is moving, but know that energy shifts are happening with or without these experiences.

Yoga Nidra is not about experiences. It is about recognizing you are the space in which all these experiences are moving. Otherwise, we are caught back in the contents, in the ego and what "I" *got* or what "I" *didn't get*, just as we were before. Be aware of this as it is a common trap on the spiritual journey. Sometimes people feel they need to have and compare experiences to prove how spiritual they are. Experiences easily become the new goal, and the true purpose of the practice, to recognize the backdrop behind all experience, is lost.

Through the release of *prana*, energy heals the body, clears the system and naturally steadies and stills the mind. Each time we go into Yoga Nidra, we experience this. We call this process *Integration*, the second Tool of Yoga Nidra.

When Free, *Prana* Heals the Body

When energy is freed from mind, it begins to operate at an accelerated level. It first begins to increase healing and restoration at the physical level. Now the healing force of the body is not limited to daily maintenance. It has enough fuel to heal long-term injuries, pain, misalignments and even chemical and mental imbalances. One could call this miraculous, but in truth, it is simply the healing power of the body finally freed to do that which it has always been capable of doing. I have seen people reduce and even stop the need for medication for pain, depression, anxiety, and insomnia through consistent practice of Yoga Nidra.

I had a student who had a car accident and whose involuntary nervous system would randomly change her body temperature, heart rate and blood pressure causing her to faint or potentially die. Doctors had no hope to offer her. I suggested that Yoga

Nidra might help. Now, a year later, she is able to function as a normal person in society. She says that Yoga Nidra saved her life.

Many diabetics note that their need for insulin is markedly reduced, and most people with high cholesterol and high blood pressure note significant drops in their numbers. Later in this book, we will look at scientific studies which explain how this happens during Yoga Nidra; but suffice it to say, the intelligence of the body knows exactly what to do. It just needs enough fuel to do it. This is what Yoga Nidra provides.

Another remarkable account is of a woman with severe scoliosis who was practicing Yoga Nidra. As she was lying on the floor, her body spontaneously adjusted itself and she heard a distinct "clunk." After the Yoga Nidra session, she reported her experience and explained that since her childhood she had scoliosis which caused her daily pain. She reported that in that moment during Yoga Nidra, she had no pain. Though the scoliosis never completely disappeared, the severity of her condition and the pain she experienced from it was reduced from that time on.

Another woman had suffered a stroke twenty years before, leaving her left hand curled into a fist. After just one session of Yoga Nidra, she showed the group her open hand, which had not opened for twenty years.

A 49-year-old woman in Yoga Nidra training had a traumatic brain injury when she was 15 years old, regressing her to the state of a 7-year-old. Eventually she relearned how to function, but she lost her memory of the time between the accident and her full recovery a few years later. After practicing Yoga Nidra during the training, her memory of that time began to come back.

Sometimes people will feel sudden stabbing pain, streaming, itching or some other sensation in an area that is or was injured, diseased or operated on. These are all indications that energy is moving in this area. Often people feel heat in an area needing healing. An area may even become visibly red for some hours after a Yoga Nidra. Once, a person who came out of Yoga Nidra had such stabbing pain in one of his knees, he thought he would not be able to get up. This was the same knee that caused him pain for years. Within an hour, he had no pain and his knee never bothered him again. Another student of mine had been in a car accident and experienced so much nerve pain in his foot he could not walk without shoes. After the Yoga Nidra, he came up to the front of the room, waiting patiently until I finished talking to another student. He said to me, "Look at my feet." He was not wearing any shoes! He reported this was the first time he had been able to stand without shoes since his car accident four years earlier.

Another student who had quit smoking many years earlier actually experienced the smell of smoke being exhaled through her lungs and released through the pores of her skin during a Yoga Nidra session. The smell was so intense she was concerned others around her in the Yoga Nidra experience would smell it. She felt this was her body releasing the toxic effects of years of smoking from her body.

This and many other stories, too many to tell, demonstrate the power of Yoga Nidra to free your body's innate healing capabilities. How many practices exist where you just lie down, breathe, and do nothing—allowing the intelligence of the body do it all? You don't have to do anything to make it happen and it all gets done. In fact, the reason it happens is *because* you are out of the way and are not struggling or efforting.

Prana Can Heal Subtler Mental and Emotional Imbalances

It stands to reason that if this intelligence can heal the Gross body, it can heal and integrate subtler aspects of the body/mind complex as well. I had a student heal herself from such severe trauma, she could barely stay in the room during the first weekend of the training. Three weeks later she was a different person—sharing with the group how she drove on the highway for the first time in 15 years. Anxiety, depression and other mood disorders can drop away with Yoga Nidra. The body knows how to bring these into balance when given the right environment to do so. Even a doctor does not heal a wound. He or she creates the right environment for *prana*, the healing energy of the body, to optimally do its work. That is why, no matter how great the surgeon, the rate of healing and success of the operation is largely up to the patient. Though I would never suggest to someone they use Yoga Nidra as a replacement for traditional therapies and medications, Yoga Nidra can be a powerful *adjunct* to treatment and healing. Working at the symptom level is often necessary, but Yoga Nidra will also help you simultaneously work at the root cause—whether physical, mental or emotional.

Emotional Integration

One of the most remarkable effects of Yoga Nidra is that it releases blocks at all levels—physical tensions as well as unresolved emotions. Emotions are simply constellations of energies that, like weather patterns, move through the body. Like clouds, emotions gather, form, magnify and dissipate. Imagine your body as a tube. We are comfortable with certain energy patterns moving through the tube of the body and mind. We can allow them to come and go, just as we can allow most weather patterns to gather without being disturbed by them. Allowed energies and experiences move in, through and out of the tube in a constant flow.

Have you ever noticed that when you feel sad and you *allow* yourself to feel sad, it passes and brings you back to equilibrium? This is because the energetic constellation of sadness, when *allowed*, moves in, through, and out. It knows how to integrate itself. It is like water that will seek its own level if allowed.

The energy patterns we allow vary from person to person. Someone born in an Italian or Spanish family may be very comfortable with the energy constellation of anger or confrontation as opposed to someone brought up in a very British or Asian family where anger and confrontation are not expressed.

When certain energies or acutely overwhelming experiences move through the tube, they can feel too overwhelming, uncomfortable, or unsafe for us to feel *at that time*. We might be afraid that if we feel them, we will be overcome by the feeling, drowned in it, and will never be able to find center again. Sometimes this can be appropriate. A child overwhelmed by a traumatic experience cannot fully feel it in that moment. It is not safe to do so. However, as long as the energy of that experience is *not allowed* to be felt, moved through the tube and then released, it will hang around.

We often think that events are what block the tube. Consider that it is not uncomfortable events or their corresponding energies that create blockages, but rather it is our *resistance to* them. Imagine water, as energy, flowing through a tube. If allowed, it flows in, through and out. When energy is intensely overwhelming, unsafe or uncomfortable, we don't want it to be there. We resist it, avoid it, and don't want to feel it. We shut down the flow. We try to talk ourselves out of it, distract ourselves with food, television, work or kids; or, we try to work it out in our minds. We do everything but allow that energy to be felt and flow through. The natural Gestalt—or return to wholeness—is never completed.

Energy does not block itself off. *We* subtly block it off because we don't want to feel the intensity of it. Imagine a particular energy flowing through a tube. If you block its flow, what will happen to it? That energy doesn't just disappear because we don't want to feel it. It circles back on itself. It goes into a holding pattern until the resistance is removed and energy can integrate by continuing through the tube.

A holding pattern of blocked energy can manifest at any level of density as it waits to move—from steam, to water, to ice. It may be visible in the body or invisibly held in the mind or emotions. We might not even know it is there until it gets retriggered by an event. We have all experienced how a present event can re-trigger old, unresolved pains of the past, adding fuel and often irrational over-reaction to a current situation.

In the deepest states of Yoga Nidra, all manner of resistance to the flow of energy can be released through the tube. As these blocks are spontaneously lifted, energy begins to flow once again toward *Integration*. This is a supremely efficient way to detoxify, clear and release past emotional baggage at all levels. The beauty of this method is that you never need to know its cause, why it happened or what it was about! It is simply energy that needs to move, and when it does, it is resolved.

Normally, we might think that in order to resolve an old block, we need to know what the uncomfortable energy was, its origin, when it happened, who caused it, and under what circumstances. Yet from an energetic perspective, we can see how events are simply constellations of energy moving through the tube and knowing its origin is not necessary for resolution. All we need to know is that it is here, and it hasn't had a chance to move through and be integrated.

However, sometimes the significance and meaning of what was released will appear of its own accord as insight, images, memories or as a kinesthetic sense. If this happens spontaneously, let it happen. Otherwise, it is not necessary to delve into the past. If you want to know about an image or symbol that appears to you during Yoga Nidra, ask your intuition for clarity. Then let go and see what comes up.

After-Effects of Clearing

As blocks are released and energy begins to flow through the tube, you may come out of a Yoga Nidra session feeling sad, angry, irritated or just a bit off. Rather than thinking that the Yoga Nidra is causing this, recognize it has been the catalyst to release blocks from your system before they build into something more significant. Think of it as taking out the trash. Everything you are seeing and feeling is on its way out. You don't need to know what the trash is. You wouldn't go picking through your trash to figure out the origin of each piece. What is coming up is simply arising to go away. All you need to do is relax, step back and allow it to move through.

Keep in mind that this release and *Integration* can also happen on a physical level. It is not uncommon to have a headache or feel nauseous when you first begin Yoga Nidra. I call this *Shakti flu*. *Shakti* is a word that indicates *prana* has accelerated from a biological to spiritual force. As this energy becomes strong, it will kick out anything from the system that is in the way of your spiritual awakening or optimal health. It can give you flu-like symptoms which generally pass within 24 hours or less. You can feel achy, sore, or feverish. These are impurities that have been held in your body. Your *prana* now has enough strength to kick it out of your system. You don't want or need this to be hanging around and serving as the basis for continued weakness in the body. Though temporarily uncomfortable, it is a much better alternative than leaving these toxins stagnating in the body. In other healing modalities, this would be known as a "healing crisis," which is actually an indication that the modality is working.

Visual and Bodily Experiences

As *Shakti* begins to move as an evolutionary spiritual force, experiences can include visions which can be ecstatic or disturbing as the system is cleared. Sometimes experiences will be very blissful and engaging. You might find yourself commenting on it, holding onto it, or trying to get there again. No Yoga Nidra experience ever occurs exactly the same way. It will be different every time. Rather than trying to hold on, simply allow it to happen. Be in it as it is happening rather than commenting on it. If geometric forms are drawing your attention in, let it happen. If you feel you are falling into the depths of stillness, let it happen.

Sometimes clearing happens in the form of a barrage of thoughts during or after Yoga Nidra practice. These are residual mental processes that finally have a chance to move through and unclutter your mind. If uncomfortable emotions come up, be the *witness* to what is happening. Do not be attached and try to hold on to the uncomfortable emotions, but don't react and be afraid either. Just let this be. Reacting makes the emotions stay. Watching what is happening allows the experience to simply come and go. Give yourself permission to come out of the Yoga Nidra at any time. You can squeeze your hands, bring your attention to the soles of your feet, or open your eyes with a soft gaze and go back inside when you are ready.

The same applies if these effects come up in dreams after Yoga Nidra practice. Dreams can be the body's way of clearing itself of mental and emotional debris. Yoga Nidra can enhance this effect. Know that whatever is being released in these states is freeing itself so that you no longer have to live with it inside you.

Yoga Nidra Is the Solution, Not the Problem

Most importantly, recognize Yoga Nidra is not the problem. It is the *solution*. Without proper understanding, it would be very easy for a beginning practitioner to think that Yoga Nidra is doing something bad to them. When we first get a massage, it hurts. We may feel a bit sore after or even feel the effects of toxic release. Over time, we come to understand that after those initial effects we feel more clear, relaxed and tension-free. We accept and know this about massage and are no longer deterred because of it. On the contrary, we know it is an indication that it is working! The same is true of Yoga Nidra. My friend and colleague, Eric Walrabenstein, once shared a wonderful metaphor with me that I will share with you.

Imagine you are taking a shower for the first time in your life. As you look at the dirty water pouring off your body, it appears as if the shower is making you very dirty. You see all that dirt going down the drain and may think, "If this shower is creating all this dirt, I'm never going to shower again. Showers are bad for me." Yet the shower did not cause the dirt! The shower is simply removing what was already there, but was never noticed. Now that the dirt is leaving, you are seeing it. It doesn't mean the shower is bad. The shower is simply revealing what is being released. It is the *solution* to the dirt, not the problem. Yoga Nidra is the shower that washes away accumulated toxicity.

CHAPTER SEVEN

The Structure of a Yoga Nidra

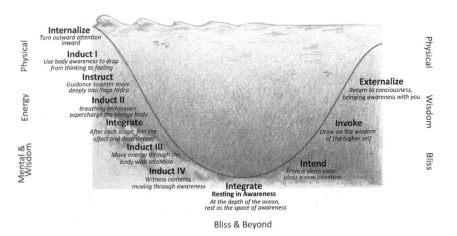

Internalize
Turn outward attention inward

Induct I
Use body awareness to drop from thinking to feeling

Instruct
Guidance to enter more deeply into Yoga Nidra

Induct II
Breathing techniques supercharge the energy body

Integrate
After each stage, feel the effect and drop deeper

Induct III
Move energy through the body with attention

Induct IV
Witness contents moving through awareness

Integrate
Resting in Awareness
At the depth of the ocean, rest as the space of awareness

Externalize
Return to conciousness, bringing awareness with you

Invoke
Draw on the wisdom of the higher self

Intend
From a clean slate, plant a new intention

Physical

Energy

Mental & Wisdom

Physical

Wisdom

Bliss

Bliss & Beyond

Figure 8: The structure of an Integrative Amrit Method Yoga Nidra experience.

Artwork by JoElizabeth James

The *koshas* (sheaths) map the process of condensation from undifferentiated potential into embodied existence. This map also lays out the route back to the Source from which we came. *A Yoga Nidra experience is structured to follow the map of the koshas back to Source.*

Imagine the ocean and the wave. A Yoga Nidra is designed to move us from the condensation of embodiment, the wave, backwards through the *koshas*, expanding our perception from a solitary wave to an experiential knowing of our ocean-like Source. A Yoga Nidra experience begins at the most gross body, the Physical body, and works backwards toward the subtlest body, the Bliss body, and beyond (Figure 8).

Physical Body: From Thinking to Feeling

We begin with the Physical body, employing such techniques as *asana* (yoga poses) or tension and relaxation. These techniques allow us to drop from the thinking mind to feeling in the body. Attention moves from the mind, which looks outward, to *prana* which allows attention to move inward. Then we heighten awareness of *prana* by connecting to more subtle sensations in the body. Practices such as Bumble Bee Breath or Palming the Face, help us begin to sense the body as cohesion of malleable vibrational energies. These techniques heighten the volume of energy in the body so it is more easily detectable. They help absorb the thinking mind into the feeling body.

Energy Body: Accelerating Flow

As we move into various breathing techniques, the flow of *prana* is accelerated. Breathing, also known as *pranayama*, is not just about the breath, but also about the control and management of *prana*. It is the most powerful methodology for pulling energy into the body and consciously channeling it to create specific effects. Various breathing techniques create different results— each therapeutic in their own way and each enhancing and amplifying the energy field while simultaneously pacifying the mind. The therapeutic benefits of each technique vary. *Sheetali* breath, for example, is excellent for balancing blood sugar. The complete three-part Yogic breath, a full diaphragmatic belly breath, is proven to be the most powerful for creating a para-sympathetic (*Relaxation*) response in the body and is excellent for a wide range of maladies including insomnia, stuttering, digestive issues, dementia and Alzheimer's. Knowing this, a skilled facilitator can begin to formulate therapeutic Yoga Nidra practices that optimize the health of the body and mind while taking us to the realms beyond.

The Second Half

After each component of an Amrit Method Yoga Nidra, we pay attention to its energetic impact. We call this the second half. The first half of the technique is willful and deliberate, but it is incomplete without letting go of doing and entering a non-doing state of being. In the second half we surrender to, and fully submerge the mind and body into the energetic impact of the technique. The more we pay attention to the residual magnetic effects of the technique, the more its effect multiplies, automatically absorbing and suspending the monologue of the mind. This allows the energy of the body to drop back into communion with consciousness itself. This experience of energy expanding beyond the boundaries of mind into a space of vast, empty stillness is profound for those who experience it for the first time. The cultivation, management and direction of energy for this purpose are key to reaching the depths of Yoga Nidra for which the Integrative Amrit Method is known.

The Power of Energy to Still the Mind

Kundalini Yoga is the branch of Yoga that focuses on the management and cultivation of energy as a tool to enter into communion with consciousness. Yogi Amrit Desai, my father, is a Kundalini Yoga Master who has gained energy mastery as a gateway to consciousness. I will share a small story with you to demonstrate the power of energy as a tool to enter meditative states. Once, my father and I, along with two assistants, were leading Yoga Nidra training at the Institute of Noetic Sciences in California. The Institute studies all manner of extra-sensory powers, and researchers were interested in studying the brain of a Kundalini Yoga Master. My father was asked if he would be willing to undergo a number of tests as such a Master. In one of the tests, they wanted to understand how the brain of a Kundalini Yogi in meditation differs from traditional meditators. What they found was that a traditional meditator takes about 20 minutes to get to the deepest meditative brainwave states. It took my father one minute or less to enter that state.

Each time they told him to open his eyes and come back, he did. Each time they told him to go back into the meditative zone, he would return within a minute or less. This is the power and depth that energy mastery can bring to your Yoga Nidra practice. It is a technique that can begin to serve *you* at will. Eventually, you will be able to close your eyes and in one breath, open the energetic channel to stillness. In one breath, you will find yourself in meditative depths—and will be able to emerge refreshed and ready to return to the world with a balanced perspective.

Energy Body: Directing Energy with Attention

Having used the breath to increase the overall available energy in the body, we now begin to consciously *move* that energy through the body. *Where attention goes, energy flows.* This magnified attention has the power to heal and remove energy blocks of any kind that may be held in the energy matrix of the body. Techniques such as "61 Points" move energy through the major *marma* points (sub-*chakras*) and meridians of the body. Other techniques, such as contrasting experiences of "heavy and light" or "cold and heat," allow us to begin to gain control over the involuntary nervous system which governs metabolism, body temperature, thirst, heartbeat, respiration and more. These are functions intelligently carried out by the body without our having to think about it. The involuntary nervous system is the designation that science gives to the functions of the Energy body. As we begin to pay attention to the Energy body, we can begin to direct it. This means we gain voluntary control over that which is normally considered to be outside of our conscious control.

Controlling the Involuntary Nervous System

Once, when I was a child, my father was on "The Mike Douglas Show." He was on the show with another guest who showed some incredible feats of extra-sensory perception. Then Mr. Douglas turned his attention to my father, asking him about the feats Yogis could perform. He said he'd heard that Yogis could consciously control their nervous system and involuntary functions of the body. Without any forewarning, he challenged my father, asking if a doctor could monitor him while he attempted to demonstrate such a feat on camera. My father did two things. First, he took his heart rate from normal to around 180; and then he brought it back down to normal in just a short period of time. More remarkable however, was that he changed his blood pressure in each arm so that when measured simultaneously, the doctor received a completely different reading in each arm even though they were being simultaneously measured! These are indications that we can consciously control the involuntary nervous system and gain mastery of the Energy body and its healing powers. Consistent practice of Yoga Nidra will help you develop this kind of mastery over the healing forces of your body.

Mental Body: Internalization, Concentration and Visualization

Much of the benefit of Yoga Nidra for the Mental body comes from the total internalization of attention and temporary withdrawal of the mind from the incoming senses. The Mental body is rejuvenated and strengthened through this total withdrawal. Additionally, the mental fire becomes steady and less pushed around by inner drives and outer senses through focus and concentration. Techniques such as "61 Points," breathing, and scanning the body, in addition to moving energy, train the mind to rest attention where it is placed, rather than where it is habituated to go. This is the first step to being able to direct the mind where we choose, rather than it running amok without direction or purpose. We can also harness the power of the Mental body through visualization. With relaxed concentration we can move attention and thereby consciously direct energy. Visualization is using the power of this relaxed focus to send healing energy to various parts of the body, and to subtler planes of mental and emotional healing.

Wisdom Body: Fostering Witness

When we work with the Wisdom body, the purpose is to foster an objective witness perspective free from identification with unconscious filters (*samskaras*) that normally affect the Wisdom body and all the bodies grosser than itself. This happens naturally as we progressively enter more expanded states. Magnified energy in the body automatically assists in bringing us to a neutral meditative space where we can be the witnessing observer to thoughts. Our perception begins to move from a constricted view to a wider-angle lens that can see and take in the whole picture without judgment. *The capacity of seeing clearly through the witness develops the strength of the Wisdom body and its ability to perceive truth, rather than the truth perceived through acquired filters, attachments and fears.*

In Yoga Nidra we can consciously foster the witnessing perspective through various techniques. One such technique is the use of opposites, where we learn to receive opposite words, such as pleasure and pain, from a sky-like perspective in which both are held and received equally. This empowers us to move out of our usual attachments and fears to the polar experiences of life. In actuality, the two poles of life are complementary opposites that together make up a total and wholly fulfilling experience of life. Although we tend to be afraid of pain, it is only in contrast to pain that we can fully experience pleasure. Without pain we would not know its opposite. Unending pleasure would become boring—and painful in its own way.

Allowing these complementary opposites to arise within the field of *witness* allows us to be relaxed with the ups and downs of life by staying connected to the unchanging field within which these opposites move.

Another technique we use is rapid images. Images have associations. Every image is linked to memories, recollections and experiences. From the meditative witness state of Yoga Nidra, we bring up various images. The purpose is to allow these images, and any related associations, to simply move through the field of awareness rather than engaging with them. When viewed from the non-participative witness perspective, the weight of identification is progressively released. We feel lighter and freer because we have let go of that with which we have identified. Dreams work in a similar way, but on the biological level. They provide a means for us to release and assimilate what we have accumulated during the day and throughout life. In Yoga Nidra, we do the same thing, but consciously.

Yoga Nidra teaches us to *witness* rather than react. We learn to *see* versus *dive into* the thoughts, emotions, and reactions moving through awareness. This capacity strengthens the Wisdom body and our ability to discriminate between who we are and the thoughts moving through awareness. This is a key skill we bring back to daily life.

Bliss Body and Beyond: Resting in Awareness

Remember that the *koshas* can be likened to condensations of energy rising out of the ocean of undifferentiated, unmanifest potential. As Yoga Nidra moves us back through the *koshas* toward Source consciousness from which we arise, we move deeper toward that ocean-like state. At each stage of Yoga Nidra, we drop down into progressively deeper brainwave states on our journey to the ocean of oneness. Each technique is designed to gradually expand awareness beyond the Physical body, Energy body, Mental body and Wisdom body. From here, we slip into the Bliss body—the storehouse of *karmic* conditioning (*samskaras*). The Bliss body corresponds with the deepest Theta and Delta brainwave states. It is a profoundly silent, deeply nourishing space of silence and feels like a place you would never want to leave. However, there is a space even beyond that. If you remember, each of the *koshas* end with the words *maya kosha*. *Kosha* means house or sheath and *maya* means illusory. All of the *koshas* are said to be illusory sheaths that appear to perpetuate the illusion of separation from Source. The Bliss body, as wonderful as it feels, is the thinnest veil perpetuating the illusion of separation from the whole. It still carries the subtlest sense of "me" with it. To glimpse our true nature as oneness, we must expand beyond even that.

The gradual process of Yoga Nidra naturally takes us to the most expanded sense of Self where we are no longer just the body, mind, perceptions or experiences, but that which precedes it all. *Now we come to the deepest point of Yoga Nidra; the point that all the techniques have been moving us toward—resting as pure potentiality—the very depths of the ocean.* In the deepest states of Yoga Nidra, the sense of "you"—that which you would normally call you—disappears. All that is left is the container. Temporarily, the contents, the body/mind complex we call "me" is gone, and we rest as that which abides beyond the temporal existence of the body.

Turiya is the space of pure consciousness. It is resting as the depth of the ocean which allows all waves to move through it. At the depth of the ocean, you see, know, and experience that every wave is part of one ocean. You are one. What appears to be matter is really not matter; it is all one energy, and one field. The ocean and the wave are one.

Turiya is not the same as Yoga Nidra. Instead, *Yoga Nidra is the doorway into the experience of turiya. Turiya* is something that is eventually experienced whether we are awake, dreaming or in deep sleep. Any state of consciousness is always accompanied by the backdrop of awareness, the underlying silence. *Turiya* exists as that backdrop of awareness regardless of the state of the mind. Eventually, even while awake or dreaming, you will have moments where you are resting *as* the silence while all permutations of mind simply move through like clouds on clear blue sky. Initially quieting the contents in order to *notice* the container is the first step.

This is the opportunity Yoga Nidra offers. A visceral, primordial knowing of one's true nature. It is not something that is read about in a book or speculated about; it is something you come to know and to rest in as the essence of *you*.

Enlightenment

In the Buddhist tradition, the word *Nirvana* literally means extinction—the temporary extinction of that which we identify as "me." It is the opportunity to experience that, when the mind and sense of "me" as a separate individual are gone, *oneness* appears. What remains is *you*. This experience realigns and re-unites you with your Source nature. It doesn't happen at the mental level, but far beyond it. You recognize you are so much more than this ephemeral body/mind. You are consciousness that appears to have consolidated into matter. From the Source perspective, you can see yourself, your life and everything that passes through you from the widest viewpoint. The more you rest as the biggest, most expanded Self, the less you will be at the effect of the one small part of you called mind. The mind is still there, but it is seen as one tiny pebble in the totality of eternity. From this vantage point, it is not that we no longer have a body/mind, it is just seen and interacted with from a totally different perspective. We are not IT, we *see* it. It is all allowed. Everything moves through like waves passing through the ocean. It all has its place and it is all okay.

Though nothing in the body/mind may have changed and although its circumstances may be the same, we experience peace. Peace with ourselves as we are and our life as it is. This is why the core *Intention* of the Amrit Method of Yoga Nidra is "*I am at peace with myself as I am and the world as it is.*" The more we live as the embodied Self from this perspective, the more "enlightened" we are. We are enlightened because we see the truth. We see the whole picture whereas previously we only saw part of it.

Dying to Be Reborn into Eternal Truth

When some people experience Yoga Nidra for the first time, they come out feeling that they went to a place they have never known before. Many have never experienced consciously losing the sense of "me." It can feel scary or confusing. They may feel that they "died." What temporarily disappeared was the ego, the sense of "I." If we have never felt anything beyond the man-made sense of self, it can be unsettling to know even that can come and go. There *is* something beyond it. Though potentially disconcerting, this speaks to the power of Yoga Nidra. It is as if you lived believing the world was flat for your whole life and then went off the "edge of the world" only to find it was not an edge after all. *There is an infinite existence beyond the edge of the mind.* In Yoga Nidra, we are able to experience it.

Eventually, we all have to let go of the body. It is a fact of life that what lives will die. What never dies is the eternal Self. In a certain way, Yoga Nidra is a mini "death." It is a mini-nirvana or extinction that prepares us for the ultimate one. We will all let go of this body and mind. It is just a matter of time. Yet if we know there is something beyond it, it will be much easier to let go when the time comes. For this reason, Yoga Nidra can be very powerful for those who are terminally ill or in hospice.

Though the body might have disease or not function the way it once did, the essential Self remains unchanged and eternal. This can make it easier to allow the body to run its course once we have done all we can. And of course, it is in these places that the most miraculous healing can occur if it is meant to do so.

Bliss Body: Planting *Intention*

As we move from the depths of the ocean, the deepest part of Yoga Nidra, we begin our journey back into awareness of the physical form starting at the Bliss body. Here, we have a unique opportunity to reach into the "hard drive" and reshape the way the past conditioning stored there is molding our potential. At this juncture, where potentiality moves into actuality, we can rewire any limitations we have been inadvertently reinforcing and recreating.

The Bliss body is also known as the Causal body because it causes and influences the shape of the bodies below it. It acts as a changing station for all things to move from the immaterial to the material. The Bliss body holds *samskaras*—past conditioning or impressions. These impressions are like channels that, despite all the potential outcomes we have the ability to create, keep us reincarnating the same results into reality in repetitive and predictable ways.

One could liken it to a vast body of water channeled through rivers, tributaries and lakes. Though water has the potential to flow anywhere, in any direction and in any fashion, it tends to follow that which came before. It will tend to follow the channels that have already been created. Water is pure potentiality. It will take any form and create anything. Yet, unconsciously, we insist on recreating the same reality over and over again. Here, at the Bliss body, we can deliberately rechannel that pure potentiality in any direction we choose.

Normally, when we use *Intentions* and affirmations, we use them in the waking state. This means we are employing them at the level of the Mental body. However, we know that what the conscious mind wishes, the unconscious mind has the power to wipe away. The unconscious mind is akin to the conditioning at the Bliss body. It lies outside our awareness, but influences everything we think and feel. Even if we consciously tell ourselves we will eat moderately or work out, the tendencies of the unconscious mind have the power to undermine the will of the conscious mind. Whatever changes we effect at the mental level happen because of will, not transformation. An internal fight will arise between the part of us that wants to overeat and the part that does not. Sometimes one part will win, sometimes the other part will win, but the body and mind are ultimately left in conflict.

When we use *Intention* in Yoga Nidra, we initiate *transformation* at the level of the unconscious or Bliss body. We go to the Bliss body, the seed level, where the core impressions are held and change them there. When back in the waking state, old thoughts may arise out of habit, but the desire to eat more simply falls away as a result of *Intention*. In fact, it falls away so effortlessly, we might not even notice the habit has disappeared. This is what we call *transformation*.

The effect of *Intention* is strongest when we use the waking state of consciousness to reinforce what was planted in the Yoga Nidra state. The more we reinforce the new channels created at the Bliss body through conscious behavior, thought and action, the deeper they will become until they become the way we naturally think and behave in the world.

The more you practice Yoga and Yoga Nidra the more you will observe its transformational effects. Things you might not even intend to change fall away. Things that used to bother you simply won't. If you found yourself getting irritated with a spouse or kids, you may find yourself remaining calm and clear. If you bite your nails, you might find yourself with long nails never having noticed when you stopped biting them. This is a radically different paradigm than the fight between will and the unconscious mind. In the old paradigm, part of you has to fight to win, but at some point the part of you that is winning will lose. You will find yourself swinging from one extreme to the other and experiencing inner conflict, frustration, self-judgment and guilt as a result. The shift needs to occur from other than the level of mental conflict. In Yoga Nidra, the shift is made at the core where there is no other voice to fight it.

Yoga Nidra is transformational whether you use *Intention* or not. What you no longer need simply falls away through the natural disengagement process that takes place in the meditative state. However, *Intention* is a powerful Tool. It allows you to work with specific issues you would like to directly and pointedly affect in your life using the power of transformation instead of inner conflict. It is a unique aspect of Yoga Nidra that differentiates it from traditional meditation. In later chapters, we will discuss *Intention* in more detail and learn how to use it in Yoga Nidra.

Wisdom Body: Invoking Presence

As we continue to move from the depths of the ocean back toward full embodiment, we move into the Wisdom body. Here we may call upon any masters, teachers, or guides to whom we feel connected. This may be felt as a Universal Presence. Guides, masters, even family members or mentors help us connect to our higher Selves. They help us connect to what we know to be true but often forget in the midst of our daily lives. Seeing and feeling a connection to something greater than ourselves helps us find our own inner knowing and inner guidance that is always available. As we move back into conscious awareness, this is something we want to bring with us.

It is quite common for those in Yoga Nidra to feel the presence of family members who have passed. In these subtle states of being, we can sense the presence of those who are near us, embodied or not. These moments of connection can be very precious and reinforce the knowledge that things are happening all the time outside of our conscious awareness.

Mental, Energy and Physical Bodies: Externalizing Awareness

At this point in the journey back to full embodiment you begin to come back to the wave: the mind and body. Slowly returning back to the body, there is a deep stillness. The mind is often very quiet at this time, your senses expand, your capacity to feel heightens and you are connected to an abiding sense of being. Though you are established in the body, you have brought a knowing of consciousness with you. The more you go there, the more you begin to live from there. You begin to establish a new relationship with reality.

Returning to the Waking State

After a Yoga Nidra, it often takes time for the mind and body to be fully functional; so it is a good idea not to rush into doing anything. Within 15 minutes or so, the body feels refreshed and the mind will operate with clarity and focus. Yogis say that 45 minutes of Yoga Nidra is as restorative as three hours of sleep. This is because we consciously accelerate access to the same slow brainwave states we experience in sleep. These states are deeply restorative to the body. Yoga Nidra can be used as an antidote to sleep deprivation, insomnia, and exhaustion. These restorative effects of Yoga Nidra are exponentially increased through the profound release of identification with the mind that is constantly and continuously hemorrhaging our life energy. The more we rest as the expanded, unfettered Self, we don't just experience the effects of Yoga Nidra for an hour or two. The body/mind becomes modified and entrained to notice this underlying sense of peace *all the time.*

CHAPTER EIGHT

Karma

To fully understand the solution Yoga Nidra offers to the body/ mind complex, we need to understand the root cause of most problems affecting us. That root is *karma*. Most of us think of the word *karma* as "good *karma*" or "bad *karma*." *Karma* is neither good nor bad; it is simply a natural law. In the Bible it is said, "As you sow, so shall you reap." Very often when we hear this, we think of it as punishment. That is not so. Rather, it is a natural law, just as gravity is a natural law. It has natural consequences. Gravity is not out to get you. It simply acts the way it acts within its realm of influence. *Karma's* realm of influence is our body and mind as well as other objects that live and die. Just as gravity predictably tells us how objects will behave on Earth, *karma* tells us how objects moving through awareness will interact with one another. How they will interact is very simple.

In the world of form, objects act according to the Universal Law of Cause and Effect. Every action will have a consequent reaction. Think of billiard balls on a table. If one billiard ball hits another one, the action of one will create a reaction in another and so on. The relationship of actions and reactions, even on a billiard ball table, become very complicated very quickly. This holds true in human lives. We may try to figure out the cause of effects we are experiencing, but because of the interdependency and interrelationship of so many objects interacting with each other, we can rarely discern the cause. Whether we can see the cause or not, *karma* tells us there is always a cause to every effect. It can be virtually impossible to figure out why external events are happening to us. It is more helpful to observe and understand the internal aspect of *karma*, to observe *ourselves* and the cause and effects *we* create through the way we choose to respond to events and the effects our responses create.

Karma, while neither good nor bad, can be helpful or unhelpful. The ways we choose to act can lead to a more still, quiet and balanced mind and life, or our actions can lead to more noise, clutter and agitation in the mind. We don't need to be afraid of *karma*, but we do want to understand how it works so we can make the best of it. Gravity is not against us, but if we don't understand how it works and act in accordance with its laws, it will not be helpful.

Understanding that one can step off of a stair, but not a sky-scraper, is important to know when acting in accordance with gravity. If we were to step off a skyscraper and plunge headlong into space because we didn't understand gravity, it would not be the fault of gravity. It would be our own self-caused suffering because we did not understand how to live in accordance with that law. In the same way, we need to understand the law of *karma* so we can understand how we are creating our own self-caused suffering through misalignment with its laws. In other words, we want to fully understand how our actions create effects that are either helpful, moving us toward the recognition of our true nature, or unhelpful, creating more drama and obstructing our ability to notice our true Self.

Karma comes down to this: "Who you are is the result of who you have been. And who you will become is the result of who you are now." See how simple it is? Simple consequences, no punishment involved. The problem is that we are not aware of who we are being now and how it affects who we will become. We don't realize the more we criticize our loved ones, or gossip behind others' backs, the more we are becoming that person. When we receive the effects of how we behaved, we suffer—not realizing that we ourselves are the cause of the effects. This is the law of *karma* as it relates to our self-caused suffering, and this is what we want to bring to light.

What Does *Karma* Mean?

The word *karma* literally means action. It delineates how action and reaction happen in the world of form. There are always two components to any action, one external and one internal. First, an external event, situation or circumstance occurs outside of us when external factors collide with one another. Then there are internal factors—*how we react* to those external events. These two components determine how the body/mind takes action in the world.

The mathematical formula is: external events plus internal reactions equal the action taken.

EXTERNAL

+

INTERNAL

OUTCOME (action)

Unfortunately, we are not always aware of how the internal aspect of *karma* affects the actions, behaviors and choices we make. For example, imagine you are laid off work. That is the external event. How you react to the event will determine the outcome. One person might be internally worried, anxious and fearful due to losing their job. The outcome may be sleepless nights, desperately searching the Internet for any and all jobs, and telling all their friends they are on the verge of being homeless! Another person with the same external circumstances could bring a completely different internal reaction to the event. They may be thrilled to finally have some time off to work on creative projects. The event is the same, but the outcome is completely different based on what each person internally brings to the event.

Though this seems obvious, most people don't notice that their *internal response* to any event is what determines the outcome they experience. If we are laid off and cannot sleep, we will usually say it is *because* we were laid off. We look at the *external event* as the cause of the outcome that we experience. However, this is not so. Ultimately, *how we handle* the event, how we choose to see it and react to it determines the final outcome—*karma*.

Karma Is Not What Happens to You. *Karma* Is How You Are with What Happens to You.

This simple formula has powerful implications. It means that ultimately, our internal response to external events is what determines the outcomes we experience, NOT the event itself. In essence, it means *we choose our karma*. No matter what comes to us from the outside, we have the final say on how it affects us. Often, I will hear students say that they cannot do anything to change their relationship because their husband or wife is not willing to change. That is the external circumstance. Using this *karma* formula is very empowering. It means that regardless of the person we are with, we have the power to change *our experience* of the relationship. We can still ask for the external to change when it is possible, but even when we don't get what we desire on the outside, it doesn't mean we are stuck. We have another option. We have the power to change our internal response.

There is a story about an alcoholic father with twin sons. When the sons grew up, one became a raging alcoholic. When asked why, he said, "Look at my father." The other son never touched a drop of alcohol. When asked why, what do you think he said? "Look at my father." Both had the same external circumstances. But each had a completely different *karmic* path based on how they chose to be with the external circumstance. That choice, though perhaps unconscious, changed the course of their lives completely.

Ask yourself; what is unconsciously driving your choices? Are these choices changing the course of your life in the direction you want? Right now, the internal aspect of *karma* is largely unconscious and automatic for most of us. We don't even realize we react in certain ways to events that determine who we will become. A pessimistic person always brings the same internal viewpoint to any external situation thereby unwittingly recreating the same experience over and over. The power of Yoga Nidra is in becoming aware of this internal aspect of *karma* and making conscious use of it rather than being the victim of these unconscious attitudes and the outcomes they automatically create.

Samskaras

The internal aspect of *karma* is unconsciously directed by our *samskaras*. *Samskaras*, literally meaning "grooves" or "impressions," are the internal aspect of *karma*. *Samskaras* are past pre-programming "magnetically" registered in *chitta*—the "hard drive" carried in the Bliss body. These impressions from our past—the collected snowball of experiences, events, interpretations, beliefs, cultural, religious, social and familial inputs—affect the way we perceive events and how we react to life.

Samskaras can even come from past lives or be acquired from family members. These past impressions shape how we are inclined to behave in the present moment. They will tend to shape our action—or *karma*. These unconscious, internal impressions can unwittingly recreate the same reflexive outcomes, actions, or repetitive behaviors over and over again.

Much of our past pre-programming is helpful. Actually, 99.9% of our *samskaras* are necessary and useful. They drive our behaviors mechanically so we don't have to think about them. Based on the cultural environment in which we were raised, we have learned not only how to survive but also how to thrive in our environment. An Eskimo in Alaska will have programming that allows survival in the wilderness in sub-zero temperatures. A person who was born in New York City will have programming that allows survival on dark streets at night. Each has learned and assimilated ways of behaving that are instinctive and automatic to help them do well in life. This extends to things like keeping a job, social norms, following the law and so much more. These are helpful *samskaras* and we don't want to get rid of them. There is only a small percentage of *samskaras* that work against us—but they tend to do so unconsciously and consistently. We need to become aware of these.

Here are some external *karmic* inputs. Notice how you would respond to each one. How would you think, feel or behave?

You are walking down the street and someone of the opposite sex looks you up and down.

Your father gives you a compliment.

Your mother gives you a compliment.

You hear footsteps behind you in an empty parking lot.

A teacher you trust gives you a compliment.

You have a sudden pain in your chest.

Depending on your internal programming (your *samskaras*), you will tend to behave in a very specific and predictable manner based on certain variables. For instance, if you are walking down the street and someone looks you up and down, your response depends on how the other person looked at you, if you find them attractive, or if you are single or not. Your reflexive response to these variables will cause you to behave in a certain way without even necessarily being aware of it. It all happens in a split second and you move on.

This is not a bad thing; it is simply a neutral observation of how things work. Often, it works in your favor. If you hear footsteps behind you in an empty parking lot, your programming will tell you how to behave depending on the time of day, the area you are in and if there are other people within shouting distance. Your programming might have you be extra cautious, put your hand on a car alarm, or otherwise prepare to defend yourself should it become necessary. This is a good thing. It is part of the learned experiences and education that help you take care of yourself in the world.

Notice also that your response is based on experiences you have had or things you have learned or heard about. If you have pain in your chest and your mother died of a heart attack, it could mean something different to you than someone who has no association with that feeling. If you have been mugged in the past, you are likely to be much more cautious overall than someone who has never had that experience. See how that past is affecting how you act now? While helpful to a point, these past experiences can become unhelpful. A person whose mother died of a heart attack or cancer may live in fear that the same thing will happen to him or her. A person who was mugged might never go out at night because of the fear of being mugged again. Now, it has become a limitation to living a full life. *Samskaras* generally become unhelpful when we move from past experiences *informing* our present actions to *restricting* our present actions. A mother dying in a particular way could affect how we take care of ourselves, or it could become the source of our own fear of dying the same way. Being mugged could give us a healthy sense of caution or keep us from being able to enjoy a night on the town.

Unhelpful *Samskaras*

Most *samskaras* are neutral or helpful. Those we want to work with are those that have moved from *informing* our potential experience to *restricting* it. Notice the variation in your response to your mother, father or a teacher giving you a compliment. Each is based on your past with them. Can you see how the past colors how you are with them now? If you had a great relationship with your dad, you might take the compliment as a given and receive it as a sign of the love you have always felt from him. Maybe with your mom, the relationship was always strained. If she gives you a compliment, can you see how this current circumstance is colored by your past and would therefore cause you to behave differently with her than with your dad? The externals are more or less the same. What's different is the internal conditioning that is unconsciously shaping your perception and driving your reactions.

I once had a student who believed that if her mother gave her a compliment it would mean her mother wanted something from her. This caused her to react defensively to her mother. Instead of receiving the compliment as a sign of love, her response to her mother was more like, "What do you want from me?"

Remembering our formula—external plus internal creates the outcome—can you see how the internal *samskaras* of the past may be driving her to behave in certain ways that limit her expression and relationship with her mother? By acting defensively with her mother, she is recreating the same relationship over and over without even realizing it. How powerful would it be if she were able to bring that inner aspect of her *karma* to light and deliberately redirect it? At least the potential would be there for a different kind of relationship. By deliberately and genuinely choosing a different response to her mother, she is sowing the seeds of another outcome. If we can bring this internal aspect of *karma* to light and make conscious and deliberate use of it, we can more powerfully direct our *karma,* our life, in the direction we want it to go—rather than leaving it to the unconscious programming of the past. When we alter our ways of automatically behaving, we give others the space to do the same. Though there is no guarantee the other will change, amazing things can happen when we energetically shift the light in which we see another. When we let go of our defensive position, it can change how the other relates to us too. Somehow, they sense it and are no longer thrown into their same old behavior patterns. The door opens for something different to emerge. The future is no longer a recreation of the past.

All the Tools of Yoga Nidra, including *Realization*, help us work with the internal *karma* that is unconsciously and automatically causing us to behave in certain unhelpful ways. At the level of the body/mind complex, *karma* is really the only problem we face. It is affecting us at all levels.

Koshas: Unhelpful *Samskaras* Affect the *Koshas*

Wisdom Body

An unhelpful *samskara* can limit our perception. The Wisdom body is what allows us to discriminate between the real and the unreal, but if our past is coloring our present, we live as if the past is happening now. Not only do we perceive through the filter of the past, but we may also try to resolve the past through the present.

Imagine that, as a teenage girl, your best girlfriend had sex with your boyfriend behind your back and that your girlfriend was blonde. This *samskara* is invisibly held in the Bliss body. Let's say years later you are dating someone. You mutually agree to break up. A month or so later, he begins to date another girl—a blonde. The truth of the situation is that you are no longer together, but what might you see or experience? Instead of seeing "what is, as is," you might see what you experienced in the past. It may feel as though you are being betrayed again in the same way you were in the past. Though you can tell yourself it is not the same and try to rationalize around it, that is not your *experience*. You experience the *past being replayed in the present*. These impressions are so deep and subtle, every time a similar situation arises, you are thrown back into the past. When we live with a lot of activated *samskaras*, we are rarely experiencing the present moment as it is. We are reliving the past through the present. Even though it is not real, we relive it as if it was. Once we adopt the past as the present, we are at the mercy of it again.

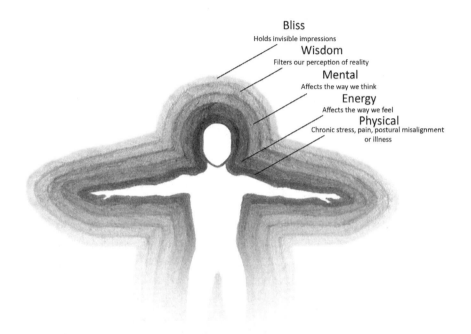

Figure 9: How unhelpful *samskaras* affect the *koshas* at all levels.

Artwork by JoElizabeth James

Once the Wisdom body is no longer able to distinguish between the real and the unreal, it affects all the *koshas* below it (Figure 9). We *think* we are being cheated on (Mental body), and *feel* as if we are being cheated on (Energy body), so our energy flows in accordance with those feelings and our body experiences the pain of the past again (Physical body). It is not a real pain. It is a phantom pain. The event passed long ago. What remains is an impression, that when attached to, causes us to relive the experience time and time again. This is the *karma* we recreate for ourselves. It is the internal component we bring to an external event. It affects us at every level of our being and causes us to repeat the past over and over.

Mental Body

Once perception is skewed, thoughts will follow. Thoughts will tend to circle around the false perception. If we are a bit more aware, we may try to think our way out of it, telling ourselves this isn't real and not to feel that way. No matter how much we might try to use the mind to talk ourselves out of that unpleasant feeling, it will be difficult because it is being generated from the unconscious Bliss body, which is subtler than the conscious mind.

Energy and Physical Body

Simultaneously arising with the triggered *samskara* and false perception are the feelings around that unresolved event. We know we have these feelings because they appear as the movement of energy or sensation. These sensations will give rise to even more thoughts, bolstering the feeling of re-experiencing the event. Eventually, if repeated and reinforced enough, or suppressed and not integrated, these energies can even materialize in the Physical body as a headache, nausea, knot in the stomach, pain in the heart, or tension in the throat. Now imagine this perception is held and persistently repeated for years and years. Eventually it becomes a habituated circuit which densifies into chronic stress, de-sensitized areas, deep-seated tensions, postural misalignment and even pain or illness. Though this is not the only cause of health issues, it can certainly be a significant contributing factor as we will explore later in this book.

We Are Constantly Interacting with Each Other's *Samskaras*

It is interesting that, without even realizing it, we are often not relating to one another in the present moment at all. We are relating to one another's past incomplete experiences. Continuing with the "blond *samskara*", let's say you decide to be a better person and befriend this new girlfriend of your former boyfriend. Even though on one level you want to move beyond the past and let go, your unconscious Bliss body might prompt you to make a few choice remarks about "blondes." Your new friend hears about it. Now *her samskaras* are triggered! Maybe in her past, she has been betrayed by envious girlfriends talking behind her back. When she learns about what you said, her old *samskara* of being betrayed by her girlfriends comes to the forefront and she is no longer interacting with this situation as it is now. She is experiencing you as if you were the people in her past. Her reaction is not just about now; it is about every time she felt the same way in the past. It helps to understand this when interacting with others. In a certain way, *we are all just interchangeable characters in each other's plays.* The reactions we bring up in others are not always about us, but are often about what we represent from that person's past. Understanding this can make it easier not to take things so personally.

So what do we do? If not by will, how can we get to these things that are unconsciously causing us to relive our past *karma* over and over? We can use all the Tools of Yoga Nidra. To fully make true shifts in life, the change needs to come from our entire being—all the *koshas* from the Bliss body to the Physical body. We cannot feel one way and pretend to feel another way. Though the intent is good, it doesn't serve anyone. We need to be willing to identify, face and shift these core patterns at every level of being and as a whole person. This is exactly what Yoga Nidra can help you do. It will help you access the Bliss body where these core *samskaras* are held, and start to rewire them. Shifts that happen here transform your whole being from the Bliss body to the Physical body. So the next time a similar situation comes up, you will be more able to genuinely observe and allow old impulses to pass through without engaging them. Like the Japanese Martial Art of Aikido, you will be able to stand back and let these impulses pass through. The use of *Intention* during Yoga Nidra allows you plant new impressions and tendencies, which, like seeds, will grow and develop over time. These will help you become the person you want to become, rather than the person your past has unconsciously shaped you to be.

Although the process may appear linear, keep in mind that effects can occur in any of the bodies, all of them simultaneously, or in a different order. For example, if a *samskara* is triggered, it may immediately be felt as a direct hit to the Energy and Physical bodies as sensation and only later do thoughts come in. You might see your ex-boyfriend with the new blonde girl, and you might feel it as punch in the gut. Only after, will your thoughts and feelings kick in. Or without even knowing what the trigger is, you may suddenly experience a physical symptom that seems to arise out of nowhere. You might find yourself suddenly feeling nauseous, or with a headache and not make the connection until later. Nevertheless, the principle is the same: subtle and unseen *samskaras* have the power to affect all levels of your body, mind and being. Though this seems overwhelming, it is actually good news. All you need to do is work with the single cause that is manifesting in various forms at all these levels.

Work at the Root of the Plant, Not the Leaves

A wonderful analogy is that of a plant. A plant has many stems and leaves; many "effects" arising out of a single root. Thus we seek a healthy root. You could spend a lifetime working with all the effects of *karma* individually. You could work with all the tensions in your body and all the health problems you come across. You could work with your emotions and thoughts and the myriad directions they take you one by one. You could work with keeping your body energy flowing. And you could work with each of your perceptions and interpretations about the world one at a time. Taken singly, you could be busy for a lifetime. However, seen as the result of one root issue, the solution is much simpler. Each of these issues is like a leaf on a plant. You could try to work on each leaf individually, polishing it, watering it, feeding it, or, you could work at the single root that is the foundation of it all. Change the root and the entire plant simultaneously changes. This is how the Tools of Yoga Nidra are designed to work—at the root.

The Answer is in the Problem

Before we can fully understand how to neutralize or manage the effects of unhelpful *karma*, we need to understand more fully how it works. By understanding the process by which a problem is created, we can also find the solution to undoing it. The answer is in the problem.

The basic principle of a *samskara* is that it becomes stronger and deeper through the process of repetition (and weaker through withdrawal). Science says the same thing: "Nerves that fire together, wire together."

Samskara means "groove" or "impression." Every time we do something, we create a corresponding groove or tendency. A groove begins very lightly, like a finger traced in the sand. With each repetition, that groove becomes deeper and deeper. The deeper the groove becomes, the more likely we are to follow the track or groove that has already been created. If you imagine water as pure potential, you would see that as water moves over the earth, it will tend to follow the grooves that have already been created. And the deeper the groove, the more likely water will flow that way. The more water flows that way, the deeper the groove becomes, until it seems that the water has no choice but to flow the way it is flowing. The groove of the Colorado River flowing through the Grand Canyon doesn't appear to have much choice but to flow the way it is flowing.

Our first actions begin as conscious and deliberate acts, but if repeated enough can move toward unconscious and automatic as the *samskara* gains momentum. The more we repeat a way of behaving, the deeper and more automatic that behavior becomes until, of all possible behaviors, we will tend to choose the same one repeatedly. Eventually it gains its own life and we feel we cannot be any other way.

The water flowing through the Grand Canyon no longer "thinks" about it. It simply flows automatically along the path that has already been set. This can work to our benefit or detriment. Whether the groove or way of behaving is helpful or unhelpful it will become deeper with each repetition. Just as the water flowing through the Grand Canyon, at some point it may feel like we have no other choice but to behave in accordance with the way our *karmic* grooves are channeling our behavior.

Let's say you are someone who takes control of things. You see things that need to be done and you just take charge and do them. You think, "No one can do it the way I want it done, so I might as well do it myself." The more you take charge and do things yourself, the more you will tend to be the person who does everything. At some point, that *behavior* may *own* you. You may no longer be choosing it consciously, it is just what you do—and it has become what other people expect from you. Of all possible options and ways of being, you have chosen one way of being. Over time, this groove will become deeper and deeper until no other option seems to be available other than to be the one to "take charge." In truth, there are many options in any given moment. You can say "no," you can delegate, you can pick and choose what you want to take charge of or not take charge of. Unfortunately when you get stuck in a *karmic* groove, these options are not apparent and you become limited without even realizing it has happened. Perhaps you feel resentful and exhausted and wonder why you are the one doing everything again. Yet when asked why you don't delegate, what might you say? "I can't do that!" Trusting someone else to do something doesn't even compute as an option. It is not that you are truly incapable of delegating to others; it is just that while there were once many options, there is now only one repeated way of being. The momentum of that groove has become so deep that it feels as if the river has no choice but to flow the way that is predetermined for it. Options give you freedom. Feeling as if you have no options is restricting. It is not that you should never take charge, but wouldn't it be nice to be able to consciously choose to take charge when you want and to make other choices when you don't?

What if you are a People Pleaser? Each time you say "yes," that tendency will become deeper until it can become a constraint to your potential. Why are you saying "yes?" You have learned it gets approval and appreciation while avoiding conflict and disapproval. At some point, when you tell your friends about all the things you are doing that you really don't want to do, your friends might ask you, "Why don't you just tell them you can't do it?" To which you will probably reply, "I can't!" Not because you are incapable of getting those words out of your mouth, but because no groove has been made to take you down that path. It is unknown and unfamiliar territory compared to what you know and have always done.

Can you see how this is limiting? Nothing is right or wrong. But you are denied the choice in any given moment to act in accordance with how you want to be. Your habits have already been decided for you. This is what we seek to restore to you with the Tools of Yoga Nidra. This Yogic teaching on *samskaras* is validated with science. Neural pathways of the brain shape themselves to our behaviors. The more we do something, the stronger that neural pathway becomes while alternative pathways tend to wither from disuse. This means that of all possible actions to undertake, we will lean toward the one we have taken before, rather than the "road less traveled." Our *karma*, or action, will tend to follow the same route over and over while other potential options will tend to fall away from our conscious awareness and perhaps not even appear as options at all.

This is how past *karma* with which we are identified, shapes who we become. Possibilities are potentials. If you feel your only option is to say "yes," your potential to be empowered is limited. If you feel your only option is take everything upon yourself, your life expression is stunted. For those who are paying attention, this effect will eventually be felt energetically and physically. Like a river, our life has already been channeled and directed unless we consciously choose to direct it elsewhere. Our two best options for directly working with the way *karma* shapes our lives are through the Yoga Nidra Tools of *Dis-identification* and *Intention*.

Initially, Yoga Nidra helps us *dis-identify* with our ingrained circuitry and disengage from our usual tendencies long enough to widen our lens and gain access to other possible solutions and actions. When we are stuck in the depths of the Grand Canyon, we cannot see anything but the habituated route laid out before us. However, if we go to an elevated perspective above the canyon, we see the river has many options and ways to flow.

Intention is essentially creating a new, more helpful groove that, when repeated, will become the new pathway the brain and body will follow. It is a Tool to rewrite our *karma* and consciously direct the field of possibility in the direction we want it to go.

CHAPTER NINE

Creating the Space to See
The Third Tool of Yoga Nidra: *Dis-Identification*

Yoga Nidra creates distance between you and the thoughts and habit patterns that usually direct behaviors and affect perception. This space allows room to choose to engage or disengage from unconscious and automatic mental habits that cause us to see and act in pre-programmed ways. By watching versus engaging in behaviors, we can weaken their effect on us and move them back from the unconscious and automatic to the conscious and deliberate.

Dis-identification is an earlier stage of *Realization*. The first movement toward *Realization* is the *Dis-identification* between you and your thoughts, impulses and behaviors. Here, you may not have completely transcended identification with thoughts, impulses and tendencies, but you have at least unhooked from them. You can witness and observe them. There is enough space between you and them that you can choose to engage them, not engage them or do something different altogether.

Instead of automatically and unconsciously saying "yes" out of sheer momentum and regretting it later, you can opt for what is most appropriate for the moment. Rather than mechanically taking responsibility for everything, you have the option to delegate to someone else. This may seem inconsequential, but once you have learned to master *karma* in these small ways, it will change the entire look and feel of your life.

Yoga Nidra supports the process of *Dis-identification* through its meditative nature. Like the lens on a camera, it helps us zoom out, broadening our perspective and creating a gap between us and our thoughts. We call this the *witness* or observer. From this perspective, we begin to see our thoughts, rather than believe and automatically act on them.

Being able to witness thoughts dis-engages us from the typical inverted power relationship with the mind which tells us what to do and what it wants while we jump to it. The mind is not bad, but it was meant to serve us. We are not meant to serve it. Imagine that the mind is like a dog. Right now that dog may not be your pet. It may be your boss! Have you ever seen a dog pulling its master where it wants to go? That is the relationship a lot of us have with our minds. We unquestioningly do as it bids us. Our habitual relationship with the mind is to go wherever it leads. When it wants to stay awake and worry, that is what we do. When it wants to obsess, that is how we are steered. When the mind wants to eat chocolate, we obediently obey. The mind sends us on coffee delivery and we dutifully trot down to Starbucks to fulfill its wishes! Most of us don't even realize we have a choice in the matter. We don't even realize the voice of the mind *is a voice*. *It is not who we are, and we are under no obligation to act upon it.*

Meditation and *Dis-identification* with thoughts help us solve this inverted power relationship. They recreate a healthy relationship with the mind, so we have a mind rather than it having us. They train the mind to "sit" and "stay" wherever and whenever we tell it. We have a mind that is trained well enough to *serve us*. We can use it when we need to, but put it aside whenever we choose. *Dis-identification* helps us *witness* and watch rather than engage with the impulses and thoughts of the mind. This weakens its hold. Once we break the old pattern, we can train the mind to do as it is bidden and place its attention where and how it is asked.

Burning *Karma*: Healing the Groove

To interrupt the momentum of programming as it acts on the mind, we need to decrease the depth of the groove (*samskara*). Let's look at how this works. Assume one night you are watching TV. The thought comes up, "I want ice cream." Notice first that a thought is a subtle thing. It has no power other than the power we give it. That thought may become stronger and stronger until, at some point, it has enough intensity to cause us to do its bidding. That invisible thought has the power to propel us off the couch, to the refrigerator, and maybe even down the street to the local food mart to get the kind of ice cream we want. *But only because we have given the thought the power to do so.*

On the first day we eat the ice cream, we create a groove, a tendency. On the next night, are we more likely or less likely to have ice cream? More likely—right? Of all possible courses of action, we will be slightly more likely to follow that one. Up to this point, our action is still conscious and deliberate. On the first night, we deliberated over the choice of having ice cream. Maybe we went back and forth. Maybe we even got up and sat down before finally putting on a coat to go get ice cream. We had to consciously get up and make a choice. The second, third and fourth nights, we are likely to slip more easily and with less hesitation toward ice cream as the groove becomes more entrenched. If we were to fast-forward two weeks down the road, we wouldn't even be thinking about whether or not to have ice cream. We might walk in the door, flip on the TV, pull out a spoon, grab the ice cream from the fridge and start eating without even thinking about it. The conscious and deliberate action would have moved to the unconscious and automatic.

At this stage, the *samskara* has the most momentum and has become a programmed reflex action. So how do we undo the habit? How do we lessen the groove and move what has become

115

a mindless action outside of our awareness back under conscious management?

One of the basic principles of Yoga is, "*Where attention goes, energy flows.*" The converse is also true. What we withdraw attention from grows weaker. Any attention, even negative attention, feeds a habit. You might feed the habit of eating ice cream, which clearly ingrains the habit. Yet fighting it also gives it energy and attention. In a subtle way, the issue is still about ice cream or no ice cream. You still act under its effect. In order to truly be free from and weaken a *samskara*, we need to withdraw attention and energy from it. This is why disengaging is so powerful. We are not fighting the *samskara*, nor are we feeding it. We are simply not giving it any energy. *If we withdraw the fuel it feeds on, it will die.*

Literally, we are starving the pattern. When we do this, we will feel a "burn." Initially it will feel uncomfortable, and we will want to go back into the familiar and comfortable pattern. If we do, we are back in the cycle. However, if we can get through the burn, let the mind scream for what it wants, and let the body be with the discomfort, then it will begin to weaken.

Think of a child having a temper tantrum. That temper tantrum is comparable to what the mind does inside of our head. It wants what it wants and will scream its head off until we act on it. We have treated the mind like a spoiled child. Since we don't know how to deal with it, we give it what it wants so it will be quiet and won't be disturbing. In the end, though, we are teaching the mind that if it screams loud enough, it will get what it wants.

You cannot fight a child screaming for what it wants. The more you fight, the more they fight you. It only fuels the fire and makes things worse. The only thing you can do to retrain a spoiled child is to withdraw energy. Do not feed the behavior one way or the other. Let the child scream, cry, and wail. Be willing to be with the discomfort of the child screaming its head off. Eventually, it will learn it is not going to get what it wants and will quiet down. That is exactly how the mind works. If you want to burn *karma* and retrain the mind, you need to be willing to let it scream and cry when it doesn't get what it wants. Withdraw from feeding it any energy. Don't fight it or judge it. The mind, which has been the instrument of your old programmed *samskaras*, will learn it is not going to get what it is habituated to getting and will eventually quiet down. Now you will be able to set the mind and your choices in the conscious direction you want them to go.

This is what we call "burning" *karma*. We could also say we are weakening its power through *withdrawal of attention and energy*. In Yoga, this is called *pratyahara*. If you want to "burn" an ice cream *samskara*, you need to practice *pratyahara*. On the first night you choose not to have the ice cream, the mind will want it all the more. The body will want to respond to what the mind desires because it has become habituated to a taste and feeling. This is a biologically ingrained *samskara*. As you begin to withdraw from the ice cream, the impulse to have it will increase. However, if you move through this burn and do not give in to the impulse, you will find the impulse weakening over time. The groove heals over and the habit begins to automatically move backwards from the unconscious and toward the conscious and deliberate. A few weeks later, you may not even think about ice cream when you come home. It is as if the *samskara* never existed. If the thought and impulse should arise again, it is typically from a more disengaged place where you can see the thought and impulse and have the space to re-engage with it or not.

We can use this principle of disengaging energy and attention with any *samskara*. However, depending on how firmly entrenched the *samskara* is, and how physicalized it has become, re-engaging the behavior even a little can potentially activate the groove to its fullest extent. This is different for everyone.

This is why total withdrawal from the triggering substance or situation can be appropriate. For example, an alcoholic can go through the process of healing the *samskara* or groove and if they abstain from alcohol completely, the impulse and thoughts around it will remain at a distance that enables them to maintain abstinence. However, one drink can potentially re-awaken the groove at the place where it left off and result in binge drinking or "falling off the wagon."

Even when withdrawing from patterns of behavior in relationships, it can be helpful to completely withdraw from the triggering person or circumstance for a time, and in some cases, for good. This allows us to regain our footing free from the effects of the *samskara* before we try re-entering from a different place. Perhaps you are unable to stand your ground with a particular person. It might be "over your edge" to practice your new way of being with them and the pressure may be so great, that it is not the best place for you to learn. You may need to withdraw for a time and build those skills elsewhere under less pressure. You always have the option to come back into the situation and exercise your new muscles at a later time.

How Does Yoga Nidra Help Us Gain Conscious Control over Our Tendencies?

Our tendencies are not the problem. Our relationship to them is. If we can see them, without the need to act on them, it is as if they do not exist. This is what the process of *Dis-identification* does in Yoga Nidra. We are not fighting the tendency, we are simply changing our relationship to it. We are witnessing and observing impulses without the need to do anything. We learn and understand that just because they exist, we are under no obligation whatsoever to act on them.

From this witnessing perspective, we can weaken our *samskaras* and "burn" *karma*. Normally, the momentum of our habits is so strong, it kicks in at a pre-mental level. Only after we have acted do we realize what we've done and said "What was I thinking?" For example, we might have an ingrained groove around overeating. Even though we may tell ourselves to eat moderately *before* we get to a meal, *at* the meal our conscious cognition disappears. Our pre-cognitive conditioning kicks in and we overeat. Only afterwards do we come back to consciousness and ask ourselves, "Why did I do that?" Trying to use the mind to catch something that is happening at a precognitive level is very difficult. We need to find a way to slow things down, establish more distance and to create a gap between us and how we usually act.

This is what Yoga Nidra does. It slows things down. It creates a wider *witnessing* perspective from which thoughts and impulses are seen. The greater the distance from the impulse, the less need there is to act on it. Though the impulse may still be felt, there is enough space to consciously withdraw attention and energy. This withdrawal starves the old *samskaras* and makes them weaker, distancing them even more. Yoga Nidra will not do all the work, but it gives us enough space to do something other than our *karmic* tendency. We can begin to choose our *karma*—our action—rather than having it chosen for us.

Removing the Sunglasses

My friend and colleague, Eric Walrabenstein, does a wonderful demonstration with sunglasses. I will share my version of it to demonstrate the power of *Dis-identification*. *Samskaras* are essentially thoughts that are meant to move through the sky of awareness but, for some reason, are held onto and believed. They do not pass through and instead are adopted as truth. Without realizing it, they become a filter through which we see the world. These "sunglasses" are firmly planted and become the lens through which we see life. If we have been hurt in the past, we will see life through the lens of, "Will this hurt me?"

The problem is that we don't realize we are wearing these glasses. We forget they are there so we believe what we perceive is reality. Usually, the glasses we adopt are the experiences we fear the most. Instead of letting go of our past, we unconsciously hold onto it. We might say, "I never ever want to experience that again, so I'm going to be on the lookout to make sure it never happens again." We keep it around to remind us of how bad it was so we don't have to feel it again. While this seems to make sense, the irony is that by holding onto it, looking through it, and living from it, our lives are shaped by it. We are recreating the experience over and over again rather than letting it move through.

The sunglasses we wear determine what we see reflected in the world. Imagine that a friend walks by as you are sitting at lunch having a meal. He or she looks at you, doesn't say anything and continues on. The reality is a friend walked by and no words were spoken. However, depending on the glasses being worn, we each perceive something different. If we have adopted a fear of anger, we will perceive that the person is angry with us. If we have adopted a fear of abandonment, we will perceive that they no longer like us. If we are afraid of rejection, we will feel rejected. What we are seeing is *who* is seeing. We are seeing what *our sunglasses* are. *We are not seeing reality as it is.* This is why it is said that life is a mirror. It is showing us who we are through what we are seeing.

We Try to Think Our Way out of Thoughts

Next, we go about trying to fix the problem we have created through our own altered perception. The way most of us try to solve this is by trying to think our way out. We put more thoughts on top of the original *samskara*, or conclusion. If our glasses cause us to believe someone is angry with us, we will place all kinds of thoughts on top of the original perception. "Are they angry at me...?" "What did I do...?" "Well, if they

aren't going to tell me what's wrong, I can't do anything...."
"Well, maybe they are having a bad day...." "I should be more
understanding...." Each of these thoughts is akin to piling on
sunglasses, one after another. Pretty soon we can't see anything
at all!

Of course the most interesting thought we put on is "You know
what? I forgive you." This is most humorous because in this
scenario, they haven't even done anything! It is all a story we
developed in our own minds from our own faulty perceptions.
We imagine a slight and then forgive the other for something
they never did in the first place!

You Cannot Solve a Problem with the Same Mind That Created It

Do any of the added thoughts ever touch the original *samskara*?
No. None of these ever remove the original *samskara*. They are
layered on top of it which only adds to our distorted perception.
Einstein said, "You cannot solve a problem with the same mind
that created it." No matter how much you try to think your way
out of a situation, you cannot resolve the original issue.

Yoga Nidra and *Dis-Identification*

Yoga Nidra has the power to dislodge the *original samskara*
and all subsequent thoughts that follow as a result. Through
Dis-identification we move back toward the sky-like space of
awareness itself. We begin to unhook from that which we have
attached to and adopted. Close up, these issues appear real and
monumental; at a distance, they appear less substantial, more
manageable, and less overwhelming. *Not only do all the thoughts
about the event move further away from us, so too does the original
adopted perception itself.* The sunglasses once tightly fused to our
vision of the world, begin to loosen and move away from us. We

witness what is passing through rather than looking at the world *through* thoughts and fears.

From a *dis-identified* perspective, we *can* gain access to and observe the original *samskara*—a fear of anger in this example. We can see all the thoughts that arise in response to that fear. They are all witnessed in the light of awareness. Although the fear and thoughts may still be there, they are seen as being at odds *with one another*, rather than at odds with *you*. You are the one who is witnessing the fear, *and* the subsequent thoughts about the fear, allowing *both* to simply move through awareness.

We have all experienced this whether we recognize it or not. We have all had issues that we have revisited over and over again. At some point, sheer repetition gives us the capacity to identify the recurring issue, the habitual thoughts and reactions that follow, and the discernment to recognize the path they will inevitably lead us down if we engage them. We develop the ability to allow it all to pass without engaging it. Things that used to "get" us—old expectations or voices in our head that used to upset us so deeply—are simply observed with an "is-that-so" perspective. Internally, the attitude is, "Here it is again. Interesting." We let it come and go. We've been around that *karmic* cycle enough to know there is no cheese down that tunnel, and we cease and desist. Yoga Nidra accelerates this process, allowing what might have taken years of circling around the same issues to be resolved in the light of expanded meditative perspective.

The beauty of Yoga Nidra is that we don't even need to know what the "glasses" are. We don't need to figure it out or analyze it. Whatever we are attached to, known or unknown, will naturally move away from us and will cease to affect us in the same way. This is different from traditional psychology where it is often assumed that we cannot work with the issue until we know what it is. It is also one reason why Yoga Nidra can be such a powerful adjunct to traditional therapy.

Dis-Identification Strengthens the Wisdom Body

The process of *Dis-identification* in Yoga Nidra strengthens the capacity of the Wisdom body. Most people don't realize they have the option to ignore the habits and impulses of the mind. They think the voice of the mind *is* who they are.

Recognizing that we are not that voice, that we are the ones who are *aware* of the voice is tremendously empowering. We have a choice to go with the mental voice and its impulses, or to go in a completely different direction altogether! The Wisdom body has the ability to take discriminating, conscious and deliberate action outside the forces of mind and the unconscious *karma* that drives it. This is the force of your own consciousness manifesting as a will greater than the mind.

Just as we can place attention on things outside us—a plant, a window, a pen, we have the same power to place this force of consciousness anywhere we choose inside us. We can place it on a thought, on a sensation or an image. We can withdraw attention from things that don't serve us and we can place our attention on things that do. This seems so simple and obvious, but most people do not realize they have this ability. Or they only rarely exercise it.

When we are really ill or when something tragic happens, notice how we are able to withdraw immediately from everything else that is unimportant. When the tragedy has passed, we step right back into the habit of being run by the everyday drama of the mind. Once we begin to see that our thoughts are simply things we can put our attention on, withdraw from, and redirect, we gain mastery over life. Our thoughts and impulses no longer own us. Yoga Nidra helps us gain this mastery by helping us *see* our thoughts rather than *being* our thoughts. From there, the choices are ours.

CHAPTER TEN

Rewriting *Samskaras*
The Fourth Tool of Yoga Nidra: *Intention*

Through the conscious use of Intention, we can steer our life in the direction we want to go, rather than where our habits tend to take us. Intention (Sankalpa) is unique to Yoga Nidra meditation, compared to other forms of meditation. We can use Sankalpa to consciously target and affect shifts from the subtlest states of being. We then reinforce these subtle shifts and deepen them through our choices and actions in the waking state.

Intention is the conscious placement of energy in the direction we want it to go. We know *samskaras* are internal impressions left on the body/mind complex causing it to tend to act in certain ways, both helpful and unhelpful. Unhelpful *samskaras* drive our tendencies toward limiting behaviors in a precognitive, reflexive manner. Unless redirected, they become the default setting from which we live, steering our life and creating outcomes, or *karma,* we do not intend.

As Yogi Desai teaches, "Without direction, your life will continue to be driven by these same pre-programmed beliefs, behaviors and habits. Whenever you perceive similar threats to your self-image, comfort or freedom, you reach into that storehouse of experiences and respond as though the current situation is the same as in the past. By believing it is the same, the outcome cannot be any other way. Driven by the distorted perception of memories, you are perpetually trapped in the same responses to life. You continue to be a victim of your own fears and attachments, glued to your self-image through your identification with your thoughts, emotions, opinions, beliefs, likes and dislikes."[16]

All experiences of existence, like clouds, were meant to pass through the sky of awareness. Sometimes, instead of an experience moving through the space of awareness, we hold onto it, believe it, perceive and live from that place. It acts as an unconscious intention at the Bliss body, creating visible effects in the other *koshas* through our thoughts, words and actions.

I once had a student who, as a child, overheard her parents fighting. During the fight one of them made the statement "Maybe we shouldn't have had children." This was a passing thought said in the midst of a difficult and stressful period in the relationship. While I am quite certain the thought came and went through the parents' minds, and was forgotten, it did not pass through their daughter's mind. Her conclusion, based on that sentence was, "I'm a mistake." That thought got stuck and she was caught in an impression lodged in the Bliss body. It began to influence the way she viewed her entire world. From that time on, she began misperceiving the world through the lens, "I'm a mistake. I wasn't really wanted."

This misperception became her reality. No longer was her Wisdom body perceiving the truth, it was perceiving through an adopted reality. The more she repeated it, the more real it became. The Mental body, following the lead of the Wisdom body, perpetuated the misperception through repetitive thoughts which only served to validate and reinforce the original conclusion. The mind would think thoughts like, "I have to make up for being a mistake." Her actions in relationships were often driven by proving herself to be lovable and worthy as if her essential being was somehow deficient.

This was all based on one experience, one impression which ended up determining the trajectory of her life. Everything that followed stemmed from a conclusion made long ago. Once believed, an impression will not only drive our energy to reflexively and repeatedly think and act in pre-programmed ways, it will eventually trickle down to influence the physiology of the body.

In this case, her whole demeanor radiated the conviction, "I don't have the right to exist. I don't deserve to take up space." With the continued practice of Yoga Nidra, she suddenly began to own her own body and the space she inhabited. She didn't make it happen, it just happened. It was remarkable to watch the effect on her whole demeanor as she was released from the *samskara* that had once molded and shaped her whole life. In fact, the next time I saw her in another training, she approached me smiling, happy and gregarious. She looked so different; I didn't even recognize her until she told me who she was!

Many unhelpful *samskaras* cause us to dedicate our lives to solving problems that have already passed. We may have heard and believed a remark made in passing and subsequently created our whole life around it. Perhaps someone once said we were "chubby" or a bit "slow on the uptake" in class. Our life might still be a reaction to that event. Perhaps we are busy verifying that the original conclusion is true—or proving that it isn't true. The question is whether this is what we want our life to be about. Do we want or need to prove something to someone who has already long forgotten what they said? Is that really what we came on the planet to do? Aren't we here to be an expression of ourselves rather than an expression of our unfinished past?

A student once shared that her father was a heroin addict. Her belief was that if she had just been a little more lovable, her father would have chosen her over drugs. Every relationship she entered, she found herself trying to resolve her *samskara* by trying to get her partner to choose her *first* in the way her father did not. When this didn't work, she felt rejected, which only reinforced her original conclusion of not being lovable enough. *Her life was steered by the continuous perception and attempted resolution of a past problem in the present moment.* Driven by the past, her future was already set.

It is like being on a boat that is on autopilot. The direction of our life is determined by the last setting on the boat, and it is still setting the course of our life. For some of us, the last setting might have been proving to our parents we are good enough. Twenty, thirty, even forty years later, our parents may have passed away; and we may *still* be trying to prove that we are good enough.

In the words of Yogi Desai, "Unless we know where we are going, our life will be driven by our unconscious tendencies. If we are not conscious, our life will be left to the devices of a haphazard, rudderless guidance system at the effect of whomever takes control; our highest potential one day, and our weakest *samskaras* on another. What is needed is clarity and stability of focus. Most of us have never considered what we truly want from life. We have a plan, direction and vision to actualize our business, but not one for the actualization of our life."[17] This is what *Intention*, also known as *Sankalpa*, or *determination*, does for us.

If we are living at the effect of unconscious tendencies (*samskaras*), our life has *already been predetermined* to a certain extent. *Sankalpa* means "determination", and is designed to help us *consciously determine the course of our life rather than the one our unconscious has chosen for us. Intention*, or *Sankalpa*, is a Tool to take the boat off autopilot. Rather than allowing the boat to be navigated by the last default setting, *Sankalpa* puts our hand on the tiller and deliberately sets our attention and actions in the direction we want to go. In short, *Intention* is a Tool to withdraw energy and attention from where we don't want it to go and place energy and attention where we *do* want it to go. It moves us from a pre-determined outcome to one that we consciously and deliberately create through the conscious use of our free will.

Yoga Nidra: The Art of Transformational Sleep

Goal vs. *Intention*

An *Intention* is different than a goal. An *Intention* is a direction, but without attachment to a particular end result. When we are heading in a direction, like north, we don't know exactly what it will look like, but we know the direction we are headed. Even if we end up going south, east, west or taking all manner of detours, we can still be heading north. In this sense, an *Intention* is "reality friendly." We can be heading toward a particular destination, say eating moderately, but even when we get off the road at times, we can still be moving in the direction of moderate eating. It is like taking a wrong turn. We know the direction we need to go, so even when we get off, an *Intention* allows us to just get back on the road and keep on going in our intended direction. If, on the other hand, we had a *goal* of eating moderately and failed to do it, we might put ourselves down, beat ourselves up and create such inner conflict that we might eat even more! *Intention* allows us to learn from our detours without judgment and conflict, and simply keeps us moving in the direction we want to go.

A goal comes *with attachment* to a particular result. As such, it can carry inherent stress and conflict when the desired result is not achieved to 100% satisfaction. If we *intend* to walk across the room, but do not quite get all the way across, it is not a failure. We can still be moving in that direction. However, if we have a *goal* of getting to a particular place and do not arrive there, it is deemed a failure.

Intention is a skillful way of taking action in the world. It moves us toward things we would like to achieve in life and allows us to enjoy the journey along the way. Often, when we have a goal in mind, everything becomes about getting *there* and we miss *here* in the process. If we need to get a project done, our children, colleagues and all our interactions can quickly feel like obstructions to our goal. Instead, we want to be able to enjoy the journey, the kids, our friends, the process of work and the interactions we have. The idea is to move toward our *Intention*, and even if we don't get the results exactly as planned, we still have the satisfaction of having lived a fulfilling life. Otherwise, we run the risk of postponing our happiness and missing our life altogether.

The distinction between a goal and an *Intention* is important when we begin creating Intentions. An *Intention* is a direction. *It doesn't mean you have to practice it perfectly. It simply means that is the direction you want to steer your ship.* If you are considering the *Intention*, "I accept my body as it is." You might say, "Well, I don't feel that way right now." That is okay. That is the *direction* you want your attention and energy to flow.

Where Is Your Attention? Put Your Attention Where You Want It to Go.

The power of *Intention* stems from conscious direction of attention. Remember, *"Where attention goes, energy flows."* Very often, people think they are putting their attention where they want it to go, but they are not. We say we want more money, but we tell our friends how little money we have. We say we want to relax more, yet we tell everyone how overwhelmed we are. We want to be more fit and healthy, but all our attention is on how much we hate our bodies. We think this self-flagellation will motivate us to action, but ultimately it only creates inner discord.

Your mind fighting with itself is registered as conflict, not change. Your Energy body will take whatever form it is given. If you are fighting with yourself or judging yourself, you are telling your Energy body to take that shape. That is exactly opposite of what you really want to create. Fighting turns energy in on itself and creates inner stress and conflict. In the end, it is you who loses, every time.

In order to avoid this, we need to *redirect* our habits rather than *fight* with them. We need to deliberately guide attention and energy to our greatest and best expression versus fighting the worst. Rather than hating what you dislike, grow what you love. Growth comes not by fighting what is wrong, but by loving (putting our attention on) what is right.

Rather than fighting with smoking, put your attention on seeing, feeling, knowing and wanting radiant health for yourself. Rather than putting yourself down for eating junk food, put your attention on loving your body by listening to it and caring for it. When you do this, an amazing thing happens. Your attention moves from the perceived obstacle to the vision. Instead of energy feeding the perceived block, energy feeds the vision you have created for your life.

In Yoga Nidra training, we do an exercise to demonstrate what happens when we put our attention and energy on a block versus a vision or *Intention*. Consistently people are amazed at the fact that when they put their attention on their arm, which represents the block, it actually becomes stronger. When they withdraw attention and energy *from* the block and focus on their *Intention*, the block becomes weaker. Though the block, for example self-rejection, is not removed—placing one's attention, energy and vision beyond it ceases to make an issue of it. When we focus on the obstruction, all our attention becomes about the struggle with the obstruction. When we focus on the vision, the obstruction is there; but its effect is diminished in light of what we are really moving toward.

The Power of *Intention* Placed In Yoga Nidra

We have already discussed the advantages of placing an *Intention* during Yoga Nidra. If we use an *Intention* or affirmation in the waking state, we are essentially layering thoughts on top of an existing *samskara*. While awake we can say to ourselves, "I accept myself as I am," but our unconscious programming may still be saying, "No you don't." Really nothing has changed—we are just adding more conflicting thoughts. In Yoga Nidra, we are not just layering on top of the *samskara*, we are actually *rewriting* it. We are creating a new groove at the subtlest state of being that, when reinforced, will become the new way pure potentiality is channeled. Water is akin to pure potentiality. It will take any form, direction or shape it is given. The Bliss body is the direct junction point where unmanifest potentiality is shaped into manifest actuality. Through the conscious placement of *Intention* at the Bliss body we give this formless potential a *new pathway* to manifest itself into actuality. We are creating a new channel for the infinite potential of water to follow. To access that infinite potential we must enter the place where formless potential meets form.

In Yoga Nidra, we have direct access to this interchange at the Bliss body. We place the *Intention* after we have rested as the sky-like space of awareness itself. We have fully disengaged from all other *samskaras* and are in neutral gear. Just like a standard automobile, we need to move into neutral gear before we can fully shift to any other. The same is true of Yoga Nidra. We are essentially a clean slate free from the influence of other programming. From this clean slate, we direct our energy fully into the gear we want. In the absence of any conflicting voices, attachment or fear, the new gear or direction engaged at the Bliss body is fully embodied and imprinted at every *kosha* without any other interfering influences or contradictory messages.

One could also compare *Intention* to writing a new program in a computer. If other programs are operational, they will interfere with the new programming. This is what happens when we try to use affirmations and *Intentions* in the waking state. Yoga Nidra allows us to rewrite our programming from a blank slate without the influence of any other factors. This is its power. This does not mean the old programming we had was bad. In fact, for a time it was probably needed and even useful to a certain extent. At some point, though, that old programming is outdated and needs to be upgraded to something that is more appropriate and useful to the world we are *in now* versus the world from the past.

The Difference Between Yoga Nidra and Hypnosis

Many people ask about the difference between Yoga Nidra and hypnosis because of their common power to rewrite from the subtler levels. Both hypnosis and Yoga Nidra are powerful tools that use the subtle to work with the gross. Generally, hypnosis is focused on optimizing the workings of the body/mind complex: thoughts, behaviors, habits and beliefs. Yoga Nidra works with these same things, but in a greater context. The context is one's own *Self-Realization beyond* the body/mind. We use Yoga Nidra to optimize the state of the body/mind to gain health, self-mastery and to calm mental and emotional drama. However, this is just the beginning of the potential of Yoga Nidra. Its ultimate purpose is to recognize the Self that *transcends* the limits of body and mind. We are calming the body/mind to eventually recognize what lies beyond it.

Hypnosis is more about *reforming and optimizing* the body/mind structure, while Yoga Nidra is about *transforming and transcending* it. Its benefits transform the body/mind, but are not limited to it.

While in hypnosis we may learn to stop smoking or be more confident at work, Yoga Nidra goes further. Why do we want these things? We want them so we can experience our own wholeness. *Yoga Nidra is designed for you to KNOW your own wholeness*—the wholeness that resides beyond the mind.

The most obvious difference between the two is on a physiological level. The brain state of Yoga Nidra corresponds to meditation. It is an extremely unusual state in which both halves of the brain are operating simultaneously as one whole. Usually the two halves of our brain are operating more independently, yet in coordination with one another. In Yoga Nidra, the *yin* and *yang* of the left and right brain become one unified whole. This virtually unified, sequential and synchronized movement of both halves of the brain is detectable in medical imaging tests such as PET scans of those who are experiencing Yoga Nidra.

In hypnosis, the brain activity is different than in Yoga Nidra or in meditation. In hypnosis, left anterior executive functions are suspended; and the right posterior part of the brain is activated.[18] Access to the brain is different than in Yoga Nidra. *The changes we see in* Yoga Nidra *come from unification with the whole.* In hypnosis, it seems the changes come from putting aside the left brain, which usually dominates, in order to gain access to the right brain. In Yoga Nidra, changes happen from a state of Oneness. In hypnosis, it appears the changes happen from submerging one aspect of mind so the other can function more optimally.

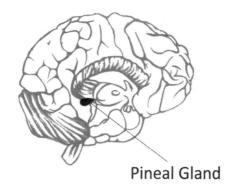

Pineal Gland

Figure 10: The Pineal Gland

Artwork by JoElizabeth James

Importance of the Third Eye

The *third eye* plays an important role in the Integrative Amrit Method of Yoga Nidra. The trigger point, located between the eyebrows, relates to the prefrontal cortex as well as an area located at the geometric center of the brain, about three inches in toward the center of the skull, and is most often associated with the hypothalamus, pineal and pituitary glands (Figure 10). The hypothalamus with the help of the pituitary runs most of the involuntary systems of the body. The pineal gland is noted for its solitary status within the brain. It is a photosensitive organ and an important timekeeper for the human body. The pineal gland produces melatonin, likely the same substance Yogis refer to as *amrita*, the nectar of immortality which takes you into the time-transcendent state of unification. Melatonin regulates sleep, biorhythms of the body and also the biological clock that determines how fast we age.

In the *Upanishads*, a human being is likened to a city with ten gates. Nine gates (eyes, nostrils, ears, mouth, urethra, and anus) lead outside to the sensory world. The *third eye* is the tenth gate and leads to inner realms of *consciousness*.

As Yogi Desai writes, *"The sense of sight comes from the two physical eyes, which look outward where they confirm duality, leaving the subtle worlds beyond your abilities. The vision of the physical eyes is confined to input of the five senses, time, space and duality. Only the Third Eye penetrates and transcends the illusion of duality. The single eye looks inward to union and sees all with the penetrating vision of unity behind apparent multiplicity. When you expose your entire body/mind to the aligning and integrative power of the Third Eye, all conflicting, fragmented parts of your being are brought into balance, functioning synergistically restoring harmony and health."*

"The purpose of Yoga Nidra is to open the Third Eye that sees life at its core, permitting Divine grace to pass through and integrate in the human form. It is the link between the human mind and Divine potential. Just as a radio transforms invisible electrical energies into

audible sound waves, the Third Eye is a pathway across which time-less immortal unity consciousness passes to the time-bound mortal manifestation of body, mind, heart and soul."

"In terms of actualization of Intention, the Third Eye is the gateway which links the immaterial to the material. Also known as the Ajna chakra, which means 'to command,' profound shifts can be initiated and all intentions and affirmations actualized through this channel. This channel is only open when you step out of the field of duality and conflict. This is accessible to you through Yoga Nidra when you are deeply relaxed and established in the Third Eye during the practice. Then, your whole being is free from changing, controlling or managing the experience. You move out of your own way and create an opening for potential to actuate intention into material reality. Here, there is no duality. There is no attachment to your desire coming to fruition or fear that it will not. There is a shift from seeking the rewards of doing, to receiving the grace of being. When the power of Yoga Nidra is combined with the command center at the Third Eye, you become whatever you think, feel, hear, speak or act in this state." [19]

Once, my father was asked to participate in a manifestation experiment. He was seated in front of a random particle generator that was shooting particles onto a screen. The experiment was to see if he could change the mathematically random way in which the particles were hitting the screen. The experiment was to determine if attention and focus could alter the random movement of particles as building blocks of matter. If so, it would imply attention does in fact influence the nature of matter itself. The instructions were to focus on the screen and concentrate on creating an organized pattern. My father said he would do the experiment, but he told the scientists that it wouldn't work the way they were asking him to do it. They asked him to do it anyway. Dutifully, he focused his visual gaze on the screen and concentrated on structuring the way particles hit the screen. Nothing happened.

Disappointed, the researchers said nothing as they began to shut down the equipment. Just then my father said, "But it can be done." Pausing, and looking a bit doubtful, the research assistant reset the machine and gave him permission to do the experiment his way. My father closed his eyes, bringing his attention to the *third eye* and allowing energy to move inward toward consciousness itself. Within a few moments, he was clearly empty of any aspect of his personality. He entered a non-doing space from which the power beyond his personality could take the lead. At the *third eye,* he simply set a non-verbal, effortless *Intention* for the particles hitting the screen to organize themselves. Sure enough, the scientists conducting the experiment could see a change indicating a shift from the purely random movement of particles to an organized pattern.

This is the principle we are discussing. To change the outside, access the command center within. Don't struggle to change the outside. *The external is simply the visible effect of the invisible cause. Go to the invisible cause and the effect will naturally and automatically shift.* We achieve this by going within to the *third eye*—the junction point between formless and form. This is what is happening in Yoga Nidra. This is exactly the opposite of what we would normally think.

The movie, *The Matrix*, touches on this point. At the *third eye,* we begin to see that everything appearing solid, dense and unchangeable is simply a physical manifestation of energy. When we can truly see, without a doubt, that everything is composed of energy, we have the power to shift and change it. Yogis have been known to demonstrate this power, though it is warned against in scriptures because it is so tempting for the ego to get involved.

In *The Matrix*, Neo gains superhuman powers over time as he begins to let go of his perception of reality as fixed and permanent. He begins to see that all things are simply composed of one infinitely malleable energy field that can be shaped at any time. Finally, at the end, he perceives his own body as a matrix of energy, and the bullets moving toward his body as an expression of that same energy—all part of one thing—and infinitely malleable. In the absence of fear, he recognizes he has the power to direct and shape it all. The only limit is what his mind tells him is and isn't possible. That is what we are touching on when we work with the *third eye* in combination with the Bliss body and *Intention*.

Once we develop the capacity to go to the *third eye*, we begin to develop a deeper perception of ourselves and others.

As Yogi Desai explains it: *"Established in the Third Eye, you receive penetrating insight, propelling you beyond your physical, emotional and mental self. It opens a new psychic world where you are able to feel, see and experience things that are not of the physical world. You may see auras, spirits, guardian angels and visions. You can sense energy fields around people. You can feel it when someone speaks an untruth because your insight penetrates at different levels. If you have penetrated your own levels, you have the facility to penetrate that of others. When you clearly see how your mind plays games, how you were blocked and became unblocked, you also receive insight to see into others. Because you saw it in yourself first, you can see it everywhere. Now there is compassion for all."*[20]

Do We Need to Have an *Intention*?

When we enter the timeless state, our time-bound habits and *samskaras* dissolve back into their timeless, formless origin and we are spontaneously freed from them. *In such a practice we are embodying* Spirit *rather than the time-bound mind.* This realignment with unmanifest Divinity gives rise to spiritual protection, profound healing and paradigm shifts passing through and integrating into the fabric of human form and structure.

The re-alignment between form and formless allows necessary healing to happen. We do not need to make this happen nor do we even need to know what shifts are happening.

Therefore, in truth, we do not *need* to have a conscious *Intention*. Spirit, knowing what is best, will do it for us. However, if we consistently find ourselves caught in conflict—perhaps with a family member, co-worker, or in a stressful situation, we can then create a specific *Intention* to help actualize a shift with that particular person or situation. We can only use *intentions* when we can observe and identify what is not serving us. However, aware or not, Yoga Nidra is always working outside of our conscious awareness to resolve and release invisible underground seeds which are automatically and involuntarily acting upon us.

Types of *Intention*

There are two basic types of *Intention*: primary and secondary. A primary *Intention* is a statement of who you are, whether as formless Source *or* as the manifested embodiment of that Source. A primary *Intention* speaks to the fullness of who you are as the immaterial or the material. An example that speaks to the immaterial consciousness that you are would be: "I am the silence behind all that moves through awareness." An example of an *Intention* that speaks to the essential quality you bring to the world as an embodiment of Spirit would be: "I am a healing Presence."

Secondary *Intention*

A secondary *Intention is a path clearer.* A secondary *Intention* is designed to remove whatever inhibits the realization of our primary *Intention*. These could be perceptions, ways of thinking, speaking or acting that keep us small. These behaviors obstruct our ability to perceive our true nature and subvert our fullest and most powerful expression in life. A secondary *Intention*

helps dislodge and redirect entrenched behaviors and perceptions to more helpful habits that support full self-expression and
a recognition of our true nature.

A secondary *Intention* generally manages three major areas: attitudes, habits and external stressors. We want to manage our
attitudes in a way that supports us. Attitudes include things we
repeatedly think or conclude about ourselves. For example, we
might consistently fall into an attitude of regret. As thoughts
are moving through awareness, when a regret thought moves
through, we tend to grab it, hold on to it, internalize it, and
repeat it over and over. In order to neutralize this *samskara*, we
need to withdraw attention and energy from it and redirect it.
We can do this by consciously redirecting our *attention* to an
Intention such as, "I trust the path that has brought me here."
When you direct attention toward your *Intention*, the energy
and attention you place on trust makes it grow stronger and
more powerful, while regret automatically withers through lack
of attention. This is such a simple, yet underutilized Tool. And
the power of Yoga Nidra only adds to the strength and success
of *Intention*. Below are several examples of the redirection of
energy through the Yoga Nidra Tool of *Intention*:

Thinking Pattern	*Intention*
Resentment:	*I release those who I hold responsible for my happiness.*
Helpless:	*I rest in the power that resides within me.*
Not Enough Money:	*I recognize the ways the universe is already supporting me.*
Self-Judgment:	*I am at peace with myself as I am.*
Self-Doubt:	*I trust my ability to see clearly and make choices that serve me.*

Yoga Nidra: The Art of Transformational Sleep

A secondary *Intention* can also address visible habits. These include things we do and ways we habitually act that don't necessarily serve us well. Here are some examples:

Habit Pattern	***Intention***
Burnout/Over-giving:	*As I take care of my own needs, I take care of others.*
Overeating:	*I love my body by feeding it nourishing foods.*
Procrastination:	*My time is a valuable expression of me.*
Controlling/ Perfectionism:	*As I let myself be as I am, I let others be as they are.*

A secondary *Intention* can also address situations causing stress. When confronted with a stressful situation, we often have a default "go to" behavior to deal with it. Sometimes this go-to behavior leaves us feeling disempowered and frustrated. If we can change our internal response to stressful situations to something empowering, then we will no longer be thrown off by the external situation itself.

Let's say you have a boss at work that makes you feel unsure and less confident. Every time you are around him or her, you feel insecure and uncertain even though you know you do your job well. That is the external circumstance. However, what you may not be seeing is how you are being in the situation. Do you tend to try to please this person to get their approval? Do you not speak up when you disagree? Do you become passive aggressive and simply go back to your desk and feel sorry for yourself? Then ask yourself, "How do I want to be in this situation instead?" Maybe it is speaking your point of view calmly and clearly, free of any expectations. Changing the internal, *how you are* in the situation, may not change the other person, but it will help you shift how *you feel about yourself* in that circumstance.

What if you have a son or daughter who is irresponsible? Notice how you tend to be with them. Are you judgmental? Do you keep your heart closed until they do what you want? Or are you too easy going because you want them to love you? How you are being could be contributing to the outcome. By asking yourself how you want to be in the situation, you can redirect your own response and help create a different outcome. One possible *Intention* could be, "I set family boundaries with calm, clarity and conviction." At the very least, you can feel more aligned with yourself even if the external situation doesn't change. You are opening the door to do what you *can* do and taking charge of what *is* within your sphere of influence. This stance of internal alignment can give you more empowerment, greater clarity and personal ease than before.

How to Create an Effective *Intention*:

Once you have an idea of what your *Intention* might be, it should be as effective as possible. There are five qualities of an effective *Intention*:

- It Resonates.
- It is in the Present.
- It is Positive.
- It is Concise.
- It is About You.

Resonates

Above all, an *Intention* should resonate with all aspects of your being. Once you get the right *Intention*, it should feel as if you have hit the nail on the head. There will be a corresponding "click" in the body that will tell you it is the right one. Sometimes, you come upon an *Intention* that brings tears to your eyes. Not tears of sadness, but tears of knowing. This is your strongest indication of having found the right *Intention*.

Initially, as you learn to work with *Intentions*, you may not feel this click. Start with the *Intention* you have, but be open to another version, or a different intention being revealed to you. You might go into a Yoga Nidra with a specific *Intention*, but another one may spontaneously arise. Go with the one that spontaneously arises as it is coming from the Wisdom body and is likely the one with which you will resonate the most. Even in the waking state, you may find that just the right word or phrase suddenly pops up out of nowhere. Choose the *Intention* that feels like the closest fit, and then let the rest reveal itself over time. If, over time, the *Intention* no longer resonates with you, you may need to formulate a new one or refine your current *Intention*.

Present

In order for an *Intention* to be most effective, it should be stated in the present tense as if it is happening now. An *Intention* is only effective when it resonates. In order for it to resonate, you have to feel the words being embodied into every cell of your being. Your whole body should say "yes." The only place you can feel that resonance *is now*. State the *Intention* in the present moment as if your whole body were experiencing that truth NOW. With *Intention*, you are directing the feeling, sensation, or energy to create a particular result. Your Energy body takes the form of whatever direction you give it through feeling and sensation.

This is not so different from *mantra* chanting. Each *mantra* is specifically chosen to create a particular frequency or energetic vibration which channels manifestation via energy in specific ways. *Mantras* are chosen according to the energetic frequency needed to create a corresponding shift. This is exactly what you are doing with *Intention*, only the language is not Sanskrit, it is your mother tongue. However, the vibration of the words themselves, when deeply felt in the present tense, will gain their own power and will begin to shape and direct your energy. The present tense has vibration and power that the future and past tense do not. This is how you phrase your *Intention* to maximize its potency.

Positive

From a Yogic perspective, an *Intention* does not always need to have positive words in it, but it should *feel* positive for you. Said differently, the *Intention* should be more integrative than positive. In Yoga, up and down are seen as two natural complementary opposites that together create one whole. Your *Intention* should feel as if it is helping you move into a better relationship with the *whole* of life, rather than using one aspect to escape the other.

Your *Intention* should either reinforce an aspect of yourself you want to grow or help you develop a more relaxed relationship with an aspect of life with which you struggle. It depends on what is appropriate for you and what is in sync with your needs in the moment. For instance, your *Intention* may be, "I allow myself to experience joy," or "I accept sadness as part of my humanity." Just do not use one to cover up the other. If you are unable to be with the discomfort of sadness, your *Intention* should be centered on *accepting* the sadness, rather than *covering up* that sadness with an intention that says, "I am happy."

In other traditions of working with *Intentions*, the facilitator will say the *Intention* needs to be positively stated because the body will register the negative wording. From the Yogic point of view, if the intention is *felt* as positive, it will energetically be received as positive even if it has a word like "sadness," "struggle" or "anger" in it.

This principle allows you to use wording in the *Intention* that specifically resonates with your needs. For example, it might be much more resonating for you to use "I release all struggling," than to use "I am relaxed." If releasing all struggle gives you the feeling of letting go and resonates in your being, that is the one to use.

Your *Intention* will be most powerful if you avoid words like "not." Instead, use words that create the feeling you *want* to feel. For instance, instead of "I am not angry" or "I do not get mad," choose "I remain calm and steady."

Concise

It is important to be able to recall the *Intention* when you need it in Yoga Nidra, and in life. This *Intention* will be your *mantra* to help you get back on track when you need it. If the *Intention* is too long and unwieldy, it will be hard to remember and will lose its power. Generally, the shorter the better. However, if you have a slightly longer *Intention* that fully lights up every cell of your body, go with that.

If your *Intention* is too long, look for the core word or phrase within it. You don't need to say everything in your *Intention* as long as you know what that core word or phrase means to you. Just saying the phrase will bring up the fullness of meaning in your body.

Often, I further shorten my *Intention* for use in daily life to just one word or one image. This is very useful when I need something simple to interrupt the momentum of thought or action. Rather than saying, "I am at peace and remain steady in the midst of stress." I shorten to "steady." Then, when I find myself just about to react to someone's behavior, all I have to do is pull up one word: "steady." Since I already planted this in my Yoga

Nidra, my body already knows how to go back to that state. With just that one word, I am able to drop back in and maintain internal steadiness instead of reacting as I might normally do.

Some people find that words don't work for them, but an image does. In that case, create your *Intention* by visualizing yourself the way you want to be, or by calling on the image of the ocean, a bird—or anything that creates the energetic sensation you want. Eventually, an *Intention* can be completely silent—felt as wordless, non-mental sensation received at all levels of body and being.

About You

While it is possible to manifest anything from the subtle to the gross, what you manifest may not be helpful to your Self-Actualization. With attention and focus you could manifest more money and more abundance. However, the question is, in service of whom, and to take care of what? Having more money is not good or bad, but if it is used to cover up a deeper fear of not having enough, it is not really doing you any good. *In the Amrit Method, the purpose is not just to manifest what you want, but to use the principle of manifestation to serve your highest expression and Self-Realization.*

Specifically, this means your *Intentions* are focused on shifting your relationship to your own unhelpful *samskaras*, rather than using circumstances or things to cover them up. You may have an *Intention* that your husband will treat you like a princess, but that *Intention* may be keeping you from doing your own work of seeing that you already are a "princess" and worthy of love. This is where your *Intention* needs to go. If you have an *Intention* that your boss will give you a raise, you may not be working with the underlying issue of feeling you don't deserve that acknowledgement. If you only focus on getting the promotion, but not on the fears around it, you haven't done the inner work.

In the Amrit Method, we always want to try to work with our internal beliefs and attitudes around circumstances and things. This is why we call it an *integrative Intention*. We are shaping *Intentions* to move us toward an internal state of *Integration*, harmony and peace regardless of external circumstance. We are working with the internal aspect of *karma* to affect our experience of life.

Yoga Nidra is a sacred practice. It is a practice about you—not them. We can certainly do what we can to effect external change, but we cannot always rely on things going our way. What we can always change is *how we are* with external situations. This practice is about *your* transformation and evolution whether external circumstances change or not. That is why your *Intention* needs to be *about you. Once you shift yourself, you will change your experience of all relationships and circumstances simultaneously. You are the one common denominator in all your experiences of life.*

Taking Your *Intention* into Yoga Nidra

Once you have your *Intention*, take it into your Yoga Nidra practice. Some guided Yoga Nidra experiences will tell you to bring your *Intention* into your awareness. If they do not, I suggest bringing your *Intention* into your awareness just after you get settled and have closed your eyes. Then, as you feel yourself in the deepest state of Yoga Nidra, bring it into awareness again. Finally, at the end of the Yoga Nidra, when you are lying on your side, bring your *Intention* into your awareness for the last time. Many people are so deep in Yoga Nidra they do not recall being asked to place their *Intention*. Do not worry. The work is being done outside of your conscious awareness. *When you get out of the way, there is room for grace to do the work for you.* Once your *Intention* has consciously or unconsciously been planted, you can strengthen it by reinforcing it when you are awake. In the next section, we will look at how to use *Intention* in daily life.

CHAPTER ELEVEN

Using Your *Intention* in Daily Life

It is important to understand that using *Intention* in the waking state alone potentially adds yet another competing thought to the mind. In Yoga Nidra, we plant *Intention* at the root, the Bliss body, when all other voices are silent. Then, when we are awake, we can *reinforce* that *Intention* at the level of mind.

While awake, old tendencies arise. You might observe the tendency to speak in an angry tone, for example. Yoga Nidra not only withdraws energy from where you don't want it to go, weakening your old *samskaras*, but also places attention where you want to grow and develop—nourishing the new direction you want to create for your life. You are not fighting anything—not even yourself. You are simply rechanneling the flow of energy in ways that serve you. So, for example, instead of allowing energy to be channeled toward being angry, you direct and channel energy toward, "I speak to people in a calm and steady manner."

Whenever you can catch yourself in any stage of an unhelpful behavior, interrupt it. Even if you do not catch yourself until *after* the old behavior has transpired, learn from it. Observe what triggered you as a scientist would—with curiosity, without judgment of yourself. Set the determination that next time, you will act in accordance with your *Intention. Each time you withdraw attention from where you don't want it to go and redirect it toward your Intention, you are creating your own life, rather than the life unconscious karma has created for you.* It may not seem like much, but suddenly you will find your life moving in a different direction altogether.

Don't worry about the times you fail, just keep moving in the direction of your *Intention*. Each time you do succeed, you are deepening the groove and giving it the momentum to become your new default behavior. Instead of your old behavior being the rule, it will become the exception. When you do fall back, you will immediately feel the effects and it will no longer feel good or natural to you.

Making Choices

You can also use *Intention* as a divining rod to make choices that support your direction in life. If you want to feed your body with nutritious foods and your friends ask you to go out for dessert, you can use *Intention* to help you make that choice. Will going out for dessert serve your *Intention*? Can you go out for dessert and still fulfill your *Intention* with your choice of dessert? Can you enjoy the company of your friends and have a cup of tea as your dessert? Rather than automatically going with preprogrammed habits, an *Intention* will allow you to align your action and choices with what you want to create.

Let's say your life's purpose is to express your creative energy and you are offered a job as an insurance adjuster. You can use your *Intention* to help you gain clarity. You might say no to the job, or you might see if there is a way *to bring* creative energy to this job. You could see if this job will give you the freedom to express your creativity in other areas of life. Neither of these is right or wrong, and both will lead you toward the spirit of the life you want.

Karmic Seeds

Changing your *karmic* trajectory in the waking state with the help of Yoga Nidra is extremely effective. Once fully understood, it has the potential to transform your whole life. *Samskaras* are like underground seeds. Even after a gardener has weeded, invisible seeds remain which have yet to be exposed. It takes just the right mixture of sun, rain, temperature and nourishment to coalesce into the right conditions for those seeds to grow into weeds. People, situations and circumstances are like coalescing weather patterns. They create the right environmental circumstances for our invisible, underground seeds to grow into weeds.

Let's imagine you are married and your spouse forgets your anniversary, which is important to you. That is a weather pattern. In the same way temperature, humidity, light, shade and rain come together to create conditions for a seed to grow, your spouse can create just the right environmental conditions to reveal an underground seed in *you*. Perhaps the forgotten anniversary is the perfect weather pattern to reveal underground seeds of disappointment, feeling not respected or unimportant. What we don't realize is that these circumstances are not *causing* us to feel the way we do, they are *revealing* an underlying feeling which was already there in seed form.

These underground seeds are our *samskaras*. We have old impressions, unresolved feelings, and experiences we don't even know are there until someone says just the right—or the wrong—thing. Before you know it, your seed has become a weed. You might think you don't have any problems with feeling forgotten, until the right circumstances come along. This is not a bad thing. It is a completely natural thing. When conditions are right, what was unconscious and outside your awareness will move into consciousness. You will have a feeling or reaction. That first reaction is simply a visible manifestation of a buried seed. The beauty is that now you can see it and do something with it. Before, you didn't even know it was there, and therefore you couldn't do anything about it.

We Reveal Each Other's Concealed Seeds

It is said we make a soul agreement with our loved ones to show us what we need to learn. In other words, our loved ones are here to help reveal our underground seeds. And they do it perfectly. And don't we do it for our family members as well? We can push their buttons like nobody's business. What is interesting is that we often choose relationships we think will trigger us the least. We choose someone who will not irritate us, will always remember our birthday, and will always be loving and never critical. We choose someone who is a good weather pattern for us, but they end up being expert at surfacing what we are hiding.

Some of us are able to observe our surfacing *samskaras* without blaming the "weatherperson." More commonly though, we will tend to blame the person or circumstance who *revealed* it. "If only they had remembered the anniversary, I wouldn't feel this way." So we train them to be a better weatherperson so we don't have to experience that feeling again. This tactic keeps our underground seeds intact and does not allow us to grow. While it is appropriate to ask for external change from others, it is also important to recognize and address *the inner seed*. Instead of immediately looking to *change the other, we also need to look at what the other is helping us see about ourselves.*

Yoga Nidra practice allows us to reshape and neutralize our original underground *samskaras* so they are no longer triggered in the presence of external circumstances. Through *Realization* and *Dis-identification*, things you didn't even know were affecting you will spontaneously drop away. Old stories and beliefs you have held onto are cleared through *Integration*. And *Intentions* planted in Yoga Nidra will help redirect your reactions in more helpful ways. However, we are all human beings; and we are all still going to have reactions that are coming from our unresolved *samskaras*. So we need to understand how to work with them in the waking state as well.

We Tip the Scales Through Repetition

We have already discussed the repetition principle as it relates to *samskaras*. The more you repeat a thought or behavior, the stronger it will become. The more you withdraw from it, the weaker it will become. When a feeling of being forgotten and unloved is triggered, we generally have a particular way of dealing with it. The more we repeat that behavior, the stronger it will become, until of all options available, we will tend to go down the same route every time.

We could use the metaphor of a seed. The more we act a certain way, the more we plant seeds that will tip the scales toward continuing to behave in the same way. According to the principle of *karma*, "Who you are, is the result of who you have been. And who you become is the result of who you are now." That means the seeds you plant now will tip the scales toward who you will become in the future.

Let's say you come in the door anticipating your romantic anniversary celebration. You find your husband watching TV and eating spaghetti. Eventually, after standing in the doorway and scanning the room for telltale signs, you realize there truly is no surprise behind his blank look. The *samskaric* tendency will be to go to the behavior you have always presented—maybe being passive aggressive or angry but not speaking up.

You might go into the kitchen and bang the pots and pans, your hurt and displeasure clearly emanating from the kitchen. When finally asked what is wrong, you might say something like, "Nothing," while making it absolutely clear something is *definitely* wrong. Or if pushed a bit more you might respond, "You should know what is wrong; I shouldn't have to tell you." Every time you repeat this behavior, you are planting another seed. You are increasing the likelihood that of all your choices, this is the behavior that will be unconsciously and automatically predetermined for you. It can even become who you are without you even being conscious of it. You might see this with people you know. Maybe someone you know has played the guilt card so many times, it has become who they are. They don't even know they are doing it anymore.

There is nothing wrong with feeling disappointed that your anniversary was forgotten. This is just the invisible becoming visible. You cannot stop it from happening, nor should you. This is an opportunity. The real question is, "What will you do next?" Will you do what you have always done? Recognize that what you do next is tipping the scales toward who you will become. So make conscious who you want to become and plant seeds *now* that nurture that person.

Yogi Amrit Desai uses a wonderful example. He says, "What you want in the end must be present in the beginning in seed form." If you want a mango tree in the end, you cannot plant a lemon seed and expect a mango at the end. If you want a mango tree, you have to plant a mango seed. That is exactly what we are talking about here.

If, instead of going down the old path of becoming angry but not speaking up, we redirect with our *Intention* to speak up first—we are planting more seeds of communicating and lessening the backlog of seeds that will cause us to lean toward old behaviors. Little by little, we can change the entire course our life and our *karma* this way. What appeared entrenched and predetermined is seen as manageable and changeable. You become the master of your life, and you begin to consciously determine your own outcomes—your own *karma*.

Breaking the *Karmic* Patterns that Bind You

Let's examine a real-life example to demonstrate how to use these principles to change our *karmic* trajectory in life. Years ago, my friend Sally's basic *karmic* pattern was to "be nice." While this quality had its positive points, it also caused her not to state her needs, to avoid confrontation, and to give in to others' desires and wishes so they would love her.

Sally had a friend by the name of Ralph. Though nothing romantic ever emerged between the two, she had always hoped that something would...but the timing was off. A few weeks later, Sally suggested she and Ralph take a trip to New York City to take in some shows, go out for dinner and see the sights. Ralph agreed, but said he wanted to go out with a lady friend of his on one night, leaving the other night free for Sally. Sally, being the "nice" girl, agreed.

Upon arriving in New York City, the two took in all the sights, and had a wonderful time. That night, Sally said she would take the night off and watch a movie in the hotel room they were sharing while he and his lady friend had dinner. Ralph insisted Sally should come along and said his lady friend was looking forward to seeing her as well. Knowing Ralph and his lady friend had a romantic history, Sally was reluctant. However, staying true to her *karmic* pattern, she didn't feel she could say no.

Sure enough, the dinner was uncomfortable for Sally who could not help but observe the obvious connection between Ralph and his love interest. Using all her skills, she rallied herself to enjoy the evening, gave nothing of her inner feelings away, and was pleasant and engaging. That night, Sally thought she'd done a great job. She had kept her poise in the midst of a painful situation. She was proud of herself. The next night, she looked forward to a pleasant evening with Ralph as her reward for having made it through the night before.

The next day, Sally and Ralph took in a show, visited museums and absorbed the city atmosphere. Tired, they went back to their hotel rooms and collapsed on their individual beds. Ralph asked where she would like to go to dinner. Sally replied she would take a little nap and would give it some thought. Ralph said he would go down to the lobby and do some work. Sally awoke from her nap refreshed. With no sign of Ralph, she turned on the TV and began watching a movie. Just then, the door opened. As expected, Ralph walked in...BUT behind him was his lady friend from the night before!

Now let me just say as the weatherman, *"Thunderstorm Alert!!!"* Sally could feel it, but told herself to stay calm and not to make any assumptions. The two settled on the other bed affectionately. A tempest was beginning to build and Sally could feel an intangible, internal reaction building without even knowing what it was.

Then the storm hit. "So where do we *all* want to go for dinner?" Ralph asked. NOW all the conditions were right for Sally's dormant seed to grow into a weed. Her weed was to see herself as less important than others and to feel forgotten. So what was her *karmic* tendency in the midst of it? To do what she had *always* done—seek love and acceptance by pleasing others. Now, in these conditions, this feeling and accompanying tendency rose to the surface.

Swadyaya – Self Observation

We will pause for a moment regarding Sally's situation as we carefully examine what is happening, then we will return to learn how Sally dealt with her feelings.

To shift our *karmic* trajectory in the waking state, we have to be truly sick of what we've been doing. This means we have to be completely done with experiencing the results of our choices. If we repeat something unhelpful enough times, life will begin to reveal that what we are doing is not working. Until this is absolutely clear, we generally won't stop. Sometimes we might even see ourselves going down the same road, but we are not ready to stop.

This is much easier to see with other people than ourselves. We might know a loved one who cannot seem to help but get themselves into the same situations over and over again. No matter how much we warn them, advise them or try to help them, they just won't get out. I believe this is because they are not ready. They have not suffered the consequences of the action enough to be truly done with it. No amount of logic or argument will dissuade them from their path until they are ready to change it.

The same is true of us. Perhaps we have pursued a type of person or relationship over and over even though we know deep down it is not right for us. There are things we can do to fast-track the process of change. One of them is self-observation or, as it is known in Yoga, *swadyaya*.

We often take action thinking it will get us one result, while it really gives us another, but we don't stop long enough to pay attention to the *actual result* we receive. We only pay attention to the result we *expect* to get and don't look back to see if that really happened. It is like a mouse going down a tunnel expecting to get cheese at the end. Even though there is no cheese, the mouse is convinced there is, so it keeps going there over and over. This is what we sometimes do. We keep going down the same path over and over convinced the solution we are looking for is there, but it is not.

Swadyaya is paying attention to the result every time we go down the tunnel. The sooner we recognize that taking that tunnel is not giving us the result we want, the more quickly we will move away from it. Over time, we figure most things out, but consciously observing the actions we take and the direct outcomes they produce will accelerate the process. If we can see "Hmmm... every time I go down this tunnel, it doesn't work and I don't get what I'm really looking for," and consciously make note of it, we will naturally begin to move away from that tunnel. Not because the tunnel is "bad" or because someone told us not to do it, but because it *doesn't work*. Once we see, through our own personal experience, that the habit of going down the same tunnel is not giving us what we want, it will simply fall away.

There is a famous poem called "Autobiography in Five Short Chapters" from Portia Nelson's book, *There's a Hole in My Sidewalk: The Romance of Self-Discovery* that encapsulates this concept perfectly:

> *I walk down the street.*
> *There is a deep hole in the sidewalk.*
> *I fall in.*
> *I am lost...I am helpless.*
> *It isn't my fault.*
> *It takes forever to find a way out.*
>
> *I walk down the same street.*
> *There is a deep hole in the sidewalk.*
> *I pretend I don't see it.*
> *I fall in again.*
> *I can't believe I am in the same place.*
> *But, it isn't my fault.*
> *It still takes me a long time to get out.*
>
> *I walk down the same street.*
> *There is a deep hole in the sidewalk.*
> *I see it is there.*
> *I still fall in. It's a habit.*

My eyes are open.
I know where I am.
It is my fault. I get out immediately.

I walk down the same street.
There is a deep hole in the sidewalk.
I walk around it.

I walk down another street.[21]

When you know you have a *karmic* pattern you are not quite ready to let go of, just begin to notice it. Iyanla Vanzant, spiritual teacher and author, has a famous line, "You're not ready 'til you're ready." Until you have suffered enough, you may not be ready. Whether you are ready to change the behavior or not, begin to make a connection between what you do and how it makes you feel. The more this becomes clear to you, the sooner you will recognize this is not the path and the sooner you will be ready to choose a new one.

It is like a hot stove. Once you realize that each time you touch the hot stove you get burned, you will no longer go there. You don't even need to think about it, it will simply fall away. In Sally's case, each time she allowed herself to take second place, she paid a price. Finally, that night in a hotel room in New York City, she hit the wall. She was done. She had suppressed her own voice for years and for whatever reason, that day was the day she could not compromise herself one more time. She was no longer willing to hurt herself, suppressing her own voice and needs in order to be loved and accepted. She was no longer willing to "burn herself on a hot stove" by repeating the behavior over and over. She was ready.

Dis-Identification

Just being done with an old pattern doesn't mean we know what to do next. "Nerves that fire together, wire together." The way we have behaved becomes so automatic, we don't really know how to be any other way. In addition, our old way of being has so much momentum behind it, the same time-worn words may come out of our mouths before we even know it, thus compromising ourselves once again.

The third Tool of Yoga Nidra to help change *karma* in the waking state is *Dis-identification*. In the past, you may not have recognized what you were doing to yourself. Sally certainly didn't. It was there, but just outside her conscious awareness. Through the practice of Yoga Nidra, Sally's automatic and unconscious way of being began to move further away from her. It began to move back toward the conscious. She could actually *see* the behavior and the outcomes she was creating.

When we first see these behaviors, it may seem as if we are getting "worse." We will see all kinds of things about ourselves that were previously outside our awareness. When we see them for the first time, it can seem as if we are really "messed up." This is not the case. In fact, it is more helpful to see our behaviors and actions for what they are, for only then can we do something about them. *Until we see what we are doing, we are powerless to change.* The practice of Yoga Nidra gives you the power to see and change.

Making Space

Once the pattern is revealed, it is very important to *dis-identify* with the old trajectory by making space. The old way of being has such weight and acceleration behind it, it is important to stop yourself from saying or doing anything *until you have clarity*. Otherwise, you are very likely to do what you have always done.

This statement can be helpful: "Let me think about this and get back to you." If we can train ourselves to say this, before our automatic response, we can buy ourselves some time. That creates the space to choose differently.

In reply to Ralph's question about where do we *all* want to go for dinner, Sally said, "Let me watch the end of this movie and I will let you know." This gave her time to sift through her options.

Intention

Once you have space to choose, ask yourself what seed you want to plant. Remember, *how you act now will be creating who you will become in the future. Every choice you make now is planting a seed.* How do you want to grow? Who do you want to become? That will determine what seed you want to plant.

When we follow our predetermined patterns, we know exactly what to do and say. When we go "off script," it is like learning a new language. Behaving in a way other than what we have known for years feels unfamiliar, and sometimes even terrifying.

Even though we may *know* we are capable of speaking, we cannot even imagine ourselves saying what we need to say. The old pathways are deeply grooved. The new ones are unknown, feel unfamiliar and even dangerous. This is because our old ways of being have been our strategies to secure love, approval and acceptance. When we break these habits, we risk losing these things. However there comes a point at which the internal misalignment we create in the name of getting external approval is no longer worth the price. That is when we are ready to shift. But if we have always done the same thing, we can be blind to any other options. *We may see what doesn't work, but that doesn't automatically mean we know what to do instead.*

To get close to a new option, there are two things that can help. *Pratipaksha Bhavana* is a practice mentioned in the *Yoga Sutras*. It literally means, "Moving to the other side of the mansion." In this context you could use this principle by asking yourself, "What is the opposite of what I would normally do?" If the habit is to not speak up, the opposite would be to speak up. If the habit is to suppress your own needs so others will like you, the opposite would be to listen to your own needs. This principle assumes of course that you are employing "skill in action." Therefore if anger was the opposite of your habit of being nice, you would look for a way to use the energy of anger skillfully to set a boundary, rather than to blame or dump on the other person.

The other useful tool to get us in the neighborhood of a new way of being is *satya—truth*. The question to ask yourself would be, "What truth do I need to speak?" Do you need to say you are disappointed rather than walking away? Do you need to say, "I thought just the two of us were going out to dinner"? Very often there is something uncomfortable underneath that we don't want to say or acknowledge, so we go to a known behavior to avoid it. If we can align and speak to what is really going on, we will automatically interrupt the avoiding behaviors.

Try Out Your Options with Your Intuitive Knowing

As Sally considered her options, the first and easiest option that came to mind was to say, "I'm not feeling well. You two go out and enjoy yourselves." But then, what seed would she be planting? She would be planting the seed of *avoidance*. She had to consider whether this was the seed she really wanted to plant. Was that who she wanted to become? Someone who avoids telling the truth in a vain attempt to find their power?

She also considered the "truth" option with something like, "Well, I was looking forward to dinner with just the two of us." This would have been a viable option, but it was too big of a leap for her to make just then. It is important to respect our own edge when we are making shifts like this. If we push ourselves too far, it will feel too scary and we are more likely to do something unskillful as a result. Better to make a shift that is risky, but doable. Then, you will build your capacity over time without treading over your own boundaries.

It can be very helpful to try out your options through your body's intuitive knowing. When something is "on" and right for you, your body will tell you. You will feel a click, an inner resonance that says, "Yes, this is the right way for you to go." On the other hand, if something is not right, the body will tend to feel heavy, the heart closed, or the belly tight. These are all intuitive signals that this is not right for you.

In the end, Sally had to ask herself, "What do I want to be?" Her answer was "Empowered." She wanted to stand up for herself regardless of what anyone else did or said. If she were to express her disappointment at not having an evening with Ralph, her experience would be dependent on what *Ralph* did or did not do. The issue was not really about Ralph, it was about her. Sally asked herself what she would most like to do that evening if she were just listening to herself. To her surprise, an unexpected answer arose from an inner voice Sally had long ago become used to ignoring.

Finally, Sally spoke for that voice. All this time, while the movie had been running, Sally had been trying out the various "seeds" and using her discrimination to choose her next step wisely. Finally, it was time for Sally to speak. With an unsteady, wobbly voice, shrill to her own ears, she said, "You two clearly have a connection, and I think you should enjoy the dinner. I would like to do what really speaks to me this evening and that is to visit my friend Jake." Her quaking voice and trembling body were signs she was facing her fear and breaking a deeply ingrained *karmic* pattern. She was moving down an unknown path.

After that sentence there was silence. Sally got up, took a shower, got dressed, said goodbye and walked out the door. In the hallway, she felt an enormous force move through her body—as if something deep within her was shaking itself free. She could feel her whole body shuddering. That *karmic* pattern had literally ingrained itself into the muscles and cells of her body. Once she changed the pattern, it began to unravel the corresponding blocks that had built themselves into her body.

Over years and years Sally had repeatedly compromised herself. She had locked away her own needs—and her inner power with it. Yet that suppressed energy didn't just disappear. It was held in her body waiting for the day when it would be released and freed to move. What started as shaking became a deep burn. It took two weeks for Sally's belly to stop burning. The burning was all the years of suppression finally surfacing to resolve itself. In the end, the event had nothing to do with Ralph. He was just the weather pattern that provided the opportunity for Sally to release something deep within herself. This time Sally got it. She changed the pattern within herself rather than waiting for Ralph to change his.

This event was a watershed moment in Sally's life. The instant she aligned with herself, she planted a new seed. She created a new way of being in the world and that could never be taken away from her. It is like riding a bike. Once you know you can do it, no one can take it away. Once you have a glimpse of who you can be in the world, that knowledge can never be lost. You might forget, cover it up, or pretend it is not there for a while, but it is never lost. *Once you plant a new seed, you know you have the power to act differently, and no one will ever be able to take that away from you.*

Every time you choose to align with yourself, you deepen the groove. It is like water that begins as a single drop, but when repeated becomes a trickle, then a stream, and eventually a raging river that contains its own self-propelling force. *You cannot help but be the new person you have created yourself to be. It has become who you are.* There is nothing else but being aligned as a person who speaks their needs. If you occasionally drop back into your old patterns, it will feel uncomfortable and unfamiliar. The old way of being will become the exception, rather than the rule. Your body will tell you something is "off" and it will be noticeable.

Every time you plant a new seed, you are changing the trajectory of your life. It is as if you are changing your navigational direction one degree at a time until one day you wake up and realize that your life is heading in a different direction altogether. *This is how you change your karmic destiny. One seed and one degree at a time* This story and these principles seem simple, but if you practice them in conjunction with Yoga Nidra, they will change your life in the same way they changed Sally's.

Establishing a New *Karmic* Trajectory

Keep in mind when you begin to practice this, you may not be very skillful. You know your pattern very well. When you learn others, you are likely to go to extremes, overdo—like a bull in a china shop. Keep this in mind, and be as conscious and skillful as you can. It never hurts to write down how you want to be and what you want to say. Rehearse it a bit.

In Yoga Nidra, see and feel yourself behaving in this new way. Practice Yoga Nidra with this *Intention* and allow it to resonate with your being. Then, when you are awake and you see yourself going down the same old path, use your *Intention* to withdraw from the momentum of the old behavior and choose the new direction instead. Repeat your *Intention* as a *mantra*. Use it to help you deepen the new direction versus the old one. The fact that your *Intention* was planted in Yoga Nidra already started the process of moving the body/mind in the direction you want to go. Now it is just a matter of reinforcing it in the waking state by aligning action behind that *Intention*. The more you do this, the more momentum your *Intention* will gain, and the stronger the power of your *Intention* will become.

Your *Intention* is creating a new *samskara* which will allow words to come out more smoothly and naturally when situations present themselves. It will also help you get comfortable saying things you are not used to saying. The more you do this, the more likely you'll be able to broach a subject in a calm and collected manner. Otherwise, so much pressure may build up that your ability to communicate with delicacy will be overridden in the heat of reaction.

It might also be a good idea to let friends and family know you are practicing to break your old habits, whatever those may be. Let them know ahead of time that you might not do a great job, and see if they are willing to help you as you learn. This will help those around you be more patient, understanding, and even encouraging as you step into new ways of being in the world.

When We Change, We Create Weather Patterns for Others

You might be wondering what happened between Ralph and Sally after Sally's declaration and dramatic exit. Our *karmic* patterns don't arise in isolation, but rather co-arise with others. When we change the way we are, we create weather patterns for others and water *their* seeds.

When Sally was behaving as her sweet, kind, people-pleaser self, her way of being kept Ralph's seeds of fear of rejection and abandonment safely hidden. However, the moment she changed her behavior, these old, dormant seeds were revealed. His face went cold. He shut off completely. He acted as if Sally was dead to him, as if he didn't care what she did. This was *his* patterned reaction when he felt hurt.

On some unconscious level we know this, and this is very often *why* we don't change our patterns. We intuitively know how we need to behave around others to keep their seeds hidden. We play the game because we don't want to risk their pain, their anger or their reactions. After all, the reason we developed many of our patterns in the first place was to be loved. Changing the pattern puts that love at risk. However, there may come a time when we are no longer willing to pay the personal price to keep another comfortable. There may come a time when the pain of keeping ourselves small is so great, we are willing to risk the pain of being big.

When that time comes, we need to be willing to face the first reaction of the other person and be prepared for it. Just as our invisible seeds become visible, so will theirs. They may have a reaction just as we did. The more prepared we are for this and make space for it, the better off we will be. They may be momentarily upset or unhappy. However if they know you still love them and you have been as skillful as you can, they will get over it. Most people (but not everyone) want to grow. Keeping our patterns in place so we won't upset them may be underestimating their capabilities. We may be keeping them from their own opportunity to grow.

Sometimes, we may consciously and deliberately choose not to trigger others' seeds for all kinds of valid reasons. Sometimes it is just the better way to go. However, I still believe conscious and deliberate choice is more empowering than letting your habits choose for you.

As you change, it is not necessary to be abrupt or unfeeling to others. The way you relate to another is like a teepee. You lean on each other, depending on each another. A bond is created through the specific ways you rely on each other. If you suddenly pull away, you can imagine what will happen. However, if you make small shifts within their edge and ability to adjust, they are more likely to be able to shift with you with minimal triggering. Little by little you can move toward being more aligned with yourself, while aligning with others' needs as well.

Let's say you have become interested in a Yogic lifestyle, but your partner is not. You want to eat healthier foods, meditate and practice Yoga rather than watch football games and eat chicken wings. This could be how you and your partner show each other love. If that behavior suddenly changes, the other might feel love is withdrawn. If you change the weather pattern slowly—still watch games and eat meat, but also add in what you need and want in your life, the transition will happen more easily.

This one event in Sally's life changed her whole outlook on the world. It became the ground from which she sowed the seeds of her personal power. Her relationship with Ralph slowly changed to a more equal one. Ralph respected Sally and her opinions more, and Sally saw herself as someone to be valued. Take a moment to reflect on the principles illustrated through this story. Think about a circumstance where you find yourself behaving in a way that isn't helpful. How do you want to be in that situation next time?

Formulating a proactive plan of action initiates the process of planting a new seed and increases the chances of choosing the new intentional path rather than the old one. Your body and mind will already be programmed with the new, more helpful *samskara*. For the most powerful effect, plant this *Intention* in Yoga Nidra. See and feel yourself embodying this new way of being. Feel yourself aligned and resonating with this *Intention*. Then, when you need it, call on this same *Intention* when you are awake and use it to interrupt and redirect the pattern.

Primary *Intention*

So far we've explored using *Intention* to redirect patterns which automatically and unconsciously drive self-limiting behaviors. An *Intention* can release us from past habits and open us to new ways of being in the world.

However, there are questions still to be answered: If we weren't living our habitual patterns, what *would* we be doing? Who would we be? What *would* occupy our mind and attention? If we weren't so busy trying to get recognition, or worrying about what people think about us, or trying to prove to our parents we are good enough, what *could* we do with the rest of our lives? And in fact, what *did* we come here to do? I'm sure we weren't put on the planet to occupy ourselves with trying to get others' approval for 80 or 90 years. We came into embodied existence for a greater purpose. A primary *Intention* is designed to help us discover just that.

Just as the ocean is composed of its formless depths as well as its formed waves, there are two elements present in a primary *Intention*. First, a primary *Intention* speaks to our nature as the eternal, unchanging and timeless Presence that is the backdrop of everything that is seen, felt, heard, thought, imagined or experienced. It reminds us that no matter what may be moving through the sky of awareness, we are awareness itself. We are there before, during and after these experiences come and go.

A primary *Intention* helps us to disengage from whatever might be moving through and remember that we are the *witness* of it all. It helps us rest as the sky through which, "This too shall pass." It allows us to remain steady and grounded in the only thing that doesn't change—eternal Presence. Everything else is guaranteed to change. Presence is the one thing that won't. When we rely on anything else other than Presence to steady us, we are resting on shifting sands. It may appear that people, situations or things are letting us down, but in fact they are not. They are simply doing what they were meant to do—change.

Presence is love—unchanging, eternal, unconditional. It is always there; it never leaves. The more we know and rest in this place, the more we can let life flow. We can let events and circumstances come when they come, enjoy them for the time they are here, and let them go when it is time to let go. Rooted in the unchanging depths of eternal Presence, we can dance with the shifting tides on the surface.

Such a primary *Intention* could be, "I am the seer, the witness of all that is seen, unaffected by all that is in perpetual change." Or, "My Source is silent stillness." It grows our awareness of the eternal Self and roots us in it. Each time you find yourself losing that perspective in the waking state, you can use your primary *Intention* to steady yourself back into Presence.

While the first aspect of a primary *Intention* speaks to the unchanging, eternal Presence, the second aspect of primary *Intention* speaks to the ocean expressing itself as multitudes of waves. Each of these waves is part and parcel of the ocean, and yet each is uniquely shaped and molded in a way no other form is. Each of us is one of those waves. We are the ocean embodied—a unique expression of the Divine.

Yet most of us spend our lives feeling like anything but the Divine. We feel not good enough, smart enough, rich enough, thin enough or good looking enough. We spend our lives fixing what we think is broken—our past, our body, our personality, other people. We spend our lives looking at other people and deciding how we should look or could look. We are round-bodied and wish we were lean-bodied; we have lean-bodies and wish we were bustier; we are bustier and wish we were less so. We worry about every wrinkle, every spot, and every scar. We spend our time managing the places with too much hair and fretting over the places with too little hair. We worry about our sexual performance and if we measure up. We fuss about the right things to wear in order to cover up our body and make it look its best. We spend our lives dressing it up, parading it around, loving it, hating it, comparing it and fixing it. Yet we never ask ourselves one simple question, *"What is this body here for…what purpose does it serve?"*

Your body is a vehicle through which the Divine manifests itself. You are here to be an expression of that Divinity.

It is said that your spiritual journey cannot begin until you accept yourself. I believe this is why. Until you accept the body, the form, and the personality that is your vehicle, your life will never be more than trying to fix it. An entire life could easily be consumed by that. We spend hours, days, months and years waiting for perfection to arrive. We fix, we tinker, we judge. We think we can't be a great expression in the world until we are faultless. We tell ourselves that someday, when things are just right, we will start living.

Your power is not in your perfection. Your power is in your willingness to fully allow your imperfection to be a part of the wholeness that you are.

We tie ourselves up in knots waiting for the day when we will somehow arrive. The harder we try to live up to a manufactured ideal, the further we move away from ourselves, the less alive we are and the more stuck we become. The harder we try to be something else, the less we are ourselves, and the less powerful we become. Our whole life can literally be wasted, waiting for the day when we will "get there." If that day of arrival at perfection never comes, we may realize we've let our whole life pass by without truly living. To me, that is the ultimate waste of a life, when it could be so much more.

How many of us tell ourselves we will really start living once we are smarter? Once we have enough money? Once we've lost weight? Do you really think that is why you are here? To have money? To be thin? To be sexy? Do you think that is why you came into existence?

The word "perfect" comes from the Latin "perfacere," which means *complete*. When you know yourself to be complete and whole as you are, you become an instrument through which the Divine can shine.

There is joy and freedom and peace that comes from letting go of the shackles of who you *think* you should be and just letting yourself *be as you are*—flaws and all. That doesn't mean you don't do your best, it means you are no longer fixing the vehicle for the sake of the vehicle. You are refining the instrument to be a clearer, wider and more aligned instrument of Presence. The more you come into your own expression, the more you will want to do the things that support it. You are not *becoming* something else because you wish you were different; you are transforming into *being* a more powerful version of yourself—a fuller version of you.

We keep ourselves trapped in *becoming* through comparison. We look at another and think we should be like them. Newsflash. Everyone already has themselves covered, but no one can do "you" like you can. In the words of Oscar Wilde, "Be yourself; everyone else is already taken." What if you were to stand up and stop apologizing for yourself? What if you were to stand as yourself and say, "This is it. This is me. Flaws and all." Then you wouldn't be *becoming*. You would be *being*.

A tree, whether it is big or small, doesn't wish to be different than it is. It is a perfect expression of itself. It doesn't need to be anything other than that. Yet we insist on turning our back on God's creation in favor of our self-created manufactured ideal. Some of us not only turn our backs on God's creation, we actually hate the creation. How much pain do we inflict upon ourselves believing there is some essential mistake in our core being? *There is no mistake in the way you were made. How could there be any mistake in it? You are an expression of Divine Presence manifesting through everything in existence.* Did the Divine make a mistake creating apples, pears and bananas? No they are all wonderful, beautiful expressions and shapes we all get to enjoy. How boring if we only had one fruit! The shift is not in changing your body and mind. You have tried it long enough. It is about embracing the body you are in, and letting it be a vehicle for something greater than you.

It is said the reason we are here in embodied existence is for Presence to know itself. Presence, being like air, can only experience itself through a vehicle. It has no quality of its own until it moves through a form, just as air has no sound until it moves through an instrument. Presence knows and experiences itself *through* you and you experience Presence when you let it move through you.

Think of a drum, a flute, a horn and a guitar. Each has a completely different shape, yet each is a vehicle for the same thing—air. Air, like eternal Presence, has no qualities of its own. However, when that air moves through a particular shape and form, it creates a beautiful, distinctive and unparalleled sound, impossible to perfectly reproduce ever again. You are the instrument. You bring a quality into the world that no one else can or will ever replicate. You don't need to be like anyone else. Only one person can be like you—embrace it.

We could spend our life comparing the instrument we are to others, asking, "Why am I not like them?" "Why can't I be like that?" That is like a drum saying, "Why can't I be like a flute?" Or a guitar saying, "Why do I have to have strings?" We get so busy wanting to be something else that we never realize we aren't actually playing our individual melody. We're just waiting.

When we finally accept the instrument we are, we open the door to our true purpose; and play it.

Sometimes we think we're not ready or that the experiences we've had exclude us from being an instrument of something greater. To this I say, it is *because* of the experiences you've had that you are a unique, embodied expression of the eternal Self. Every experience has shaped the instrument that you are. Every dent, every scratch, every so-called imperfection *makes* you who you are and makes you a unique and incomparable addition to the whole. Those unique experiences shape the flow of air as it moves through the instrument, forming the unique and distinctive sound you make when Spirit moves through you.

The beauty of an "embodied" primary *Intention* is that it speaks to you as the wholeness that you are. It reminds you that you are an instrument of the Divine. Every time you accept the vehicle and stand in it fully, you become an expression of the Divine. If you accept the fullness of the wave that you are, you are embodying the ocean in you. If you occupy only part of that wave, you are not an expression of the fullness of the ocean. So ask yourself: in your heart of hearts, are you willing to put down your self- judgment and be who you are?

What do other people feel in your presence? How do they say you make them feel? What quality or experience do you want to bring to others above all else? These questions will help you discover your primary *Intention*. The basic and most profound one being, "I am here to be the fullest expression of myself." In the beginning, this was my primary *Intention*. It was most powerful for me because it put my attention and energy in just being the fullest expression of me without judgment.

Previously, I tried to be powerful by trying to be perfect. Yet there is no such thing as perfect. It is a moving target manufactured in our own minds. Instead of making me feel good about myself, the search for perfection left me with inner conflict and self-judgment. When I discovered my primary *Intention* ("I am here to be the fullest expression of myself") I found a vast hidden reservoir of presence and power within.

Then after a year or two, my primary *Intention* changed. I was increasingly moved to share that Presence in the world. Now my primary *Intention* is, "I stand in the power of Divine Presence." There are many underlying additions to that *Intention*, but I don't need to write all that down. I know what it means and it resonates with me. As long as it gives me the feeling in my body, the inner "click," I know it is the right one for me. Usually primary *Intentions* will change less often than secondary *Intentions*. Secondary *Intentions* change depending on the issues you happen to be facing.

You can use your primary *Intention* as your life purpose. It can be your divining rod to help you make decisions, guide how you behave, what you say and how you say it. It becomes the North Star of your life. Even if you don't live it perfectly all the time, it is still the guiding force that progressively allows Presence to be lived through your life.

Here are some examples of an embodied primary *Intention*:

I am a healing Presence.

I am here to empower others.

I am here to accept and love myself and others.

I am an expression of creative Spirit.

I am here to express the power of the Divine as it moves through me.

I am here to be the full expression of myself.

I am here to empower others with love, authenticity and clarity.

The more your life becomes directed toward a primary *Intention* such as "I am here to stand in myself as I am and my life as it is," the more that becomes the rudder that steers the boat of your life. Rather than the old voices of insecurity and self-doubt guiding your life, your life is given in service of something greater. The more you get clear and align with your primary *Intention*, the more everything that doesn't serve that *Intention* naturally falls away—like self-rejection, criticism, regret, resentment, and second-guessing your life choices. If you are here to express the power of the Divine as it moves through you, you will leave behind the small self who is uncertain and insecure. Conversely, the things that *do* move you toward your *Intention* will naturally grow—like gratitude, self-acceptance, contentment, and peace. If your life comes to a point where you can no longer stand in yourself as you are or your life as it is, that is an indication you need to make changes in accordance with your *Intention*.

Traditional Eastern philosophy defines "enlightenment" as *knowing oneself as the eternal unchanging timeless Presence*—the depths of the ocean. Yet wouldn't it be just as true to say that embracing and aligning with the expression of the wave *is knowing* the ocean? Couldn't this be a kind of enlightenment too? Not everyone is interested in knowing the eternal Self. Some find their full, whole expression in the world, not by what they do, but through the unique flavor and essence they bring to the world. To me, either one, is a practice of enlightenment.

SECTION TWO

Applying The
Ancient Secrets
of Yoga Nidra

CHAPTER TWELVE

The Fifth Tool of Yoga Nidra: *Relaxation*

Relaxation happens when we are aligned and at peace with the present moment as it is unfolding. We are content with how things are and nothing needs to be different than it is.

Relaxation Happens in the NOW

The most fulfilling moments of our lives can only ever happen *now*. We only experience fulfillment in the present moment. We may *anticipate* happiness in the future, or *remember* a time of contentment in the past; but it can only be *experienced* NOW. Any sensation, any feeling, including *Relaxation*, can only ever be experienced here. Food, sex, a great shower or a massage, can only be fully enjoyed *while it is happening*.

If you are not there for it, it loses its ability to fulfill and replenish you. You could be eating your favorite food, but if you are thinking of something else, you might as well be eating dust. A shower can deeply rejuvenate and nurture the body, but its effects can be easily lost in worrying about what you need to do next.

The more powerfully we can drop into the present moment, the more powerfully we experience *Relaxation* and its rejuvenating effects. Whether going for a walk, washing the car or playing with our kids, we are filled full by the moment when we are fully present and engaged in it. If we are divided from the moment, we miss the inherent and intrinsic joy and restoration every experience has the capacity to give us.

Most of us are not seeking *Relaxation* through the present moment, we seek *Relaxation* in the future. We postpone our own fulfillment and enjoyment for a future time. "Just this one more thing," we say to ourselves, "and *then* I'll be able to relax." We make our relaxation contingent upon getting more done. Only when the "to do" list is done, do we tell ourselves we can relax.

Oddly, in the name of relaxation, our life becomes about doing more. We run and run and never arrive. The more we get done, the more that list spontaneously repopulates. When we *do* allow ourselves to *momentarily* relax, something else arrives on the internal "to do" list and we are off and running again. We run, struggle, strive and scramble for the time when we will be able to stop. We leap-frog from momentary relaxation to momentary relaxation, which is hardly any relaxation at all. The problem with this is we are training ourselves NOT to be in the one place where *Relaxation* happens. Rather than being here, where fulfillment is, we are training ourselves to constantly look to the future. Everything becomes a rush to get "there," and we end up missing "here." We end up missing the one place where ease, peace and *Relaxation* are present. We are *doing* in order to *be,* but we rarely get to the *being*. We seldom allow ourselves the fulfillment that comes in the moment now.

The solution Yoga Nidra offers is to learn to find fulfillment in *every* moment. Rather than delaying our own ease, peace and *Relaxation* until the end, we learn how to be fulfilled more and more in the moments of our existence. It isn't that you cannot do, just *be present* while you are doing it. The more you show up for every moment of your life, the more it will fill you up. If you ignore everything along the way to your goal, those things will just become a means to an end and you will miss the beauty of living.

How often are we on the way to work or an important meeting and friends, partner, family or kids just feel like obstacles? We might still do or say the right things, but inside we are thinking,

"Yes, yes, hurry up. I need to be somewhere else!" Of course, life happens in time, but in every moment, we have two choices. Show up for the moment as it is happening and be fulfilled, or dismiss the moment in favor of something else. One will give you the fulfillment you are looking for now; the other will only give you temporary fulfillment at the end.

Do this experiment. Next time you are busy, be present to what you are doing and choose to enjoy it as you are doing it. Breathe, relax. Then when you need to move on and do the next thing, do it. Feel yourself walking, breathing, talking, and interacting. Then do the next thing. You will find something remarkable. You are capable of doing everything that needs to be done, but you can do what needs to be done in a relaxed way, and in a way that fulfills you.

Yoga Nidra is a powerful tool to help you come back into a fulfilling relationship with the present. The practice itself is about dropping from mind, which is busy doing, and progressively entering states of being in the now. We first begin with reconnecting with the body, then with the breath, then subtler still by sending energy and attention through the body. As a result we are fully restored to the present and the peace to be found there. Yoga Nidra brings us back to the bodily experience of the present so we can remember what it is to live from that place. We can feel our body when it moves, the breath when it breathes. We notice our speech and our action with *mindful* Presence. We can feel the subtle effect of the simple pleasures of life and be filled up by them. *We remember that doing is not a prerequisite to being. We can enter the moment and be filled full by it any time we like, no matter what we are doing.*

Resistance

We know fulfillment arises in the present. It arises when we are so absorbed in what we are doing that we are not thinking of the next thing. We are completely aligned with what is in front of us. There is no part of us that needs anything to be different.

Consider that unhappiness or stress arises only when we cannot be aligned with the moment—when we are divided and misaligned with the experience as it is. Most of us think *the cause of our stress is external*: the kids, our boss, traffic, or our mother-in-law. However, if we were to look more closely, we would see that it is not these people and things that are causing our stress. Rather, it is our *inability to be present and aligned* as experiences are arising.

A red light could be exactly the same on two days. On one day, you might have no problem with the red light. You might be relaxed and maybe even pleased to get a red light, so you can check out the adorable puppy in the car next to you. On another day, you might be at exactly the same red light. The light is no different, but *you are*. You want to be at work. While your body might be at the red light, the mind has jumped forward to needing to be at work. You are in one moment, but you are resisting being there. You don't want it to be that way. You want the situation to be different. You are divided and out of alignment with the present. I suggest it is this division and misalignment with the present moment that is causing us stress.

The red light is the external circumstance. It isn't different. What is different is *you* and your ability to *be with that external circumstance*. The hypothesis is this: if you can bring yourself back into alignment with the present moment as it is arising, you will feel more relaxed. Imagine that instead of being divided into the future at the red light, you bring yourself back to the present moment—to the breath, to the car seat, to music, to what you see. In the present, you are sitting on a cushy seat, looking at a light that happens to be red. Nothing is happening except in your own mind.

The degree to which you can come back to where you are (because you can't be anywhere but where you are in any given moment), is the degree to which you will experience peace and harmony within. Yogi Amrit Desai has a wonderful quote, "Nothing is a problem, until you decide there's a problem." When we decide that something about the moment should be different than it is, it can become problematic.

Consider your boss or colleague. Until you decide they should or could be different than they are, do you have a problem with them? When we attach to an alternate version of reality, we are dividing ourselves from this one. We start to fantasize about how it *could be* over *how it is*. Suddenly *now* doesn't measure up to our picture of how it *should* be and now reality is experienced as a problem. This is how we manufacture problems. According to Yoga, all problems are self-created. In Yoga Nidra, we can interrupt the process by which we generate and perceive problems.

Yoga Nidra, by its nature, drops us into an allowing space. Learning to rest as the sky makes it much easier to let events arise as they do and be with them as they are. From this relaxed place, you learn to relax and align first. Your airplane may be delayed, or your car dented. Reality is reality. Resisting won't change it. Starting from a place of *Relaxation*, you will find yourself able to handle situations and do what is needed from a calmer, more balanced place. You will be more at peace and relaxed with more and more aspects of your life.

Stress

What exactly is stress? Stress is classically defined as any "non-specific demand for change." We think of stress as being "bad" and relaxation as being "good." Actually, in healthy doses, stress is a good thing. The stress that is tension in our muscles allows us to stand upright. The "demand for change" that is education creates a stronger and quicker mind. The "demand for change" that is infection in our environment forces our bodies to become stronger in their ability to fight disease.

Good or healthy demand on the body is called "eustress." At some point, that healthy demand on the body can flip over into being unhealthy and counterproductive. While we know the pressure of education can be good for us, we also know that when the pressure becomes too great, the demand that made us perform *better* actually begins to make us perform *worse*. Instead of thinking more clearly and sharply, we cannot think at all. We cannot access any information, any answers or anything we have learned. Test anxiety is a good example of this. The demand that was working for us begins to work against us. This is called "distress," or unhealthy amounts of tension. We want to be able to increase the amount of demand we can sustain before eustress (good stress) becomes distress. The amount of demand we can handle before eustress becomes distress is called our "allostatic load."

Tension and Relaxation in Balance

When tension and *Relaxation* are in balance, the body can function indefinitely. Imagine your own hand. If you were to make a fist and release the fist in an equal and opposite manner, can you see how you could repeat the action almost indefinitely? Think of a muscle contracting completely and releasing completely. If those two actions are in balance, the muscle will work for life. The heart muscle will work for 70 to 90 years for most of us and is said to be designed to last 120 years.

Yet if the heart muscle has too much tension or too little tension, it cannot function efficiently and a heart attack will occur. The whole body is designed to work through a balance of tension and *Relaxation*. Any imbalance in this equilibrium sets the stage for disease.

Yogis knew this thousands of years ago. If you look at Yogic illustrations of the body's energy system (Figure 11), you will see the two major energy currents depicted as snakes, wrapped around a central channel. Obviously, this could well be the root of the medical symbol known in the West as the *caduceus*. In Yogic teachings, each "snake" represents an energy current. One corresponds to tension (*pingala*), which is the sympathetic nervous system, and the other to *Relaxation* (*ida*), the parasympathetic nervous system. The *pingala* current is positive and the *ida* is negative. When out of balance, the energy system of the body is compromised and is believed to set the stage for disease. Perhaps balance as the core of health and imbalance as a cause of ill-health is the deeper meaning of the caduceus as well.

Yogis believe that when these two currents are operating in harmony, the resulting energy field will not only generate radiant health, but also opens the third and central *nadi* or channel called the *sushumna*. When *ida* and *pingala* find balance, both energy poles operate as one unit and become energetically unified. This energy is now strong enough to not only heal and maintain the body, but becomes a Spirit-force capable of returning us to Source. When the *sushumna* channel opens, energy, as a unified Spirit-force, begins to involute back toward Source, merging at the crown or *Sahasrara chakra* (Figure 11). Thus, *ida* and pingala balance is not just for optimal health, but also creates the ideal state to realize one's true nature.

The *chakras*, meaning wheel or disc, can be thought of as energy transformers, transmuting the universal energy of *prana*—contained in air, light, water, thought, environment and food—into biological energy to feed, sustain and nourish the organs and systems of the body. Like the *ida* and *pingala*, they also serve a spiritual function because the energy they manage is Spirit energy. Thus the *chakras* not only serve a physical, but spiritual function as well, mapping the journey of the Spirit-force through various levels of development back to Source.

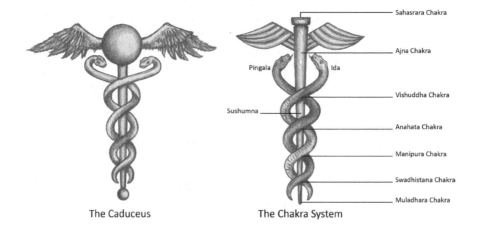

	Sahasrara Chakra
Pingala	Ida
	Ajna Chakra
Sushumna	Vishuddha Chakra
	Anahata Chakra
	Manipura Chakra
	Swadhistana Chakra
	Muladhara Chakra

The Caduceus   The Chakra System

Figure 11: A comparison of the caduceus, the symbol of medicine and the *chakra* system.

Artwork by JoElizabeth James

Returning *ida* and *pingala* energies to balance is the purpose of Hatha Yoga. "Ha" corresponds to the *pingala nadi,* "tha" to the *ida nadi.* Hatha Yoga is designed to balance these two elemental energies not only for health, but also for Divine *Realization.* Health and steadiness of mind is the basis of all spiritual practice. Yogis knew everything must begin here.

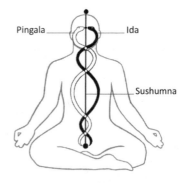

Figure 12: *Ida, pingala* and *sushumna* are the three primary energy channels (*nadis*) of the body.

Artwork by JoElizabeth James

Interestingly, the *ida* and *pingala nadis* are related to the nostrils and the halves of the brain. The right nostril relates to the sympathetic nervous system (*pingala nadi*) and crosses over to connect with the left brain. The left nostril relates to the parasympathetic nervous system (*ida nadi*) and crosses over to connect with the right brain.

Usually, we switch from right to left nostril dominance every 75 to 90 minutes, indicating a shift from left to right brain. However, after Yoga Nidra, you will often notice that you are breathing equally through both nostrils. This is an indication that "ha" and "tha" are in balance; both halves of the brain are operating in unity consciousness and energy is flowing through the sushumna (Figure 12). Yoga Nidra is a whole-brain experience generating the physiological and spiritual state of Oneness.

The tension of the *pingala nadi* ("ha") is perfectly healthy and normal. When the sympathetic nervous system is aroused, our heart rate, blood pressure and body temperature go up. The pupils dilate and blood moves to the arms and legs in order to fight and run. Think of a cat, which when feeling threatened by a dog, will go into full *fight or flight* mode. When the dog is gone, the cat will immediately lie down and go back to sunning itself. Now the cat is in parasympathetic mode. This total balance of tension and *Relaxation* is how our body was designed to function optimally.

After acute tension, the body should return to a complete recuperative state of *Relaxation*. As you can see with the cat, there are no aftereffects of the stress as the two states operate in perfect harmony. The *fight/flight* instinct of the sympathetic nervous system is completely restored to balance through the recuperative, restorative power of the parasympathetic nervous system.

However, excessive activity on the *pingala* (active side) combined with not enough recuperation on the *ida* (restorative side), sets the stage for disease. The reverse is also true. Excess inactivity or passivity on the *ida* side also builds a foundation for disease. In the West, this *ida* or *pingala* imbalance is known as *stress*. Whether the imbalance comes from too much doing or not enough, the net result is stress on the body and we know stress is one of the greatest epidemics in the West today, far outranking contagious diseases in first-world countries.

Chronic Tension and Disease

The problem is that most of us don't experience a complete balance between tension and *Relaxation*. We have become so adapted to carrying an accumulated backlog of tension, we don't even know we are living in a constant state of stress. Imagine an open flat hand representing you in a relaxed, neutral state. You wake up in the morning to a snow storm and find the car won't start. Imagine a bit of tension created in that hand, the fingers curling. You get the car started and cleared of snow but now you are freezing cold, wet and late to work. A little more tension in that hand, fingers moving toward a fist. You get to work and notice you have salt and slush stains from the snow all over your best suit—and you have to give a presentation to some very important prospective clients. More tension, moving toward a closed hand now. You manage to get the stains out and deliver your presentation. You rush home to make dinner and pick up the kids, who are irritable and intractable. Now your body is in a state of tremendous built-up tension—a fist in the grip of tension. Once the kids are in bed, perhaps you have a few moments to yourself. You may watch TV, or have a glass of wine. The fist loosens a bit, but the *Relaxation* you experience and the sleep you receive is not enough to relieve all the tensions accumulated during the day.

The following morning you wake up with an accumulated surplus of tension before your day even begins. The next day continues as the day before. Every day, day after day, there is an ever-mounting backlog of excess tension. We not only have the tensions from present day, but the leftover tension from the days, weeks, months and even years before. The fist never goes back to the flat hand. This is the state of *chronic stress*. It is estimated that a whopping 97% of people in Western countries are sympathetic dominant which means their bodies are operating under a state of constant and chronic stress.

Stress has exploded into an invisible, trillion dollar health epidemic, according to the *Huffington Post*. That's more than the cost of cancer, smoking, diabetes, and heart disease *combined*. Stress is a factor in five out of the *six leading causes of death*: heart disease, cancer, stroke, lower respiratory disease, and accidents. [22] This is critical information, yet somehow most of us are not fully aware of it. The body is like a car. Left in overdrive without regular maintenance or care, it only makes sense that some part of the body will give out. Anything driven hard enough will break down somewhere at some point. The body is no exception. The following symptoms are signs that the body has been doing too much and not balancing itself with the restorative, recuperative state.

Here is a short but by no means exhaustive list of symptoms that can be linked to stress:[23]

- Asthma
- Sleep disorders
- Depression/mood swings
- High blood pressure/cholesterol
- Diabetes/hypoglycemia
- Unexplained pain/weakness/fatigue
- GI disorders-irritable bowel, constipation, nausea etc.
- Epilepsy
- Back pain-especially low back
- PMS
- Hot flashes
- Erectile dysfunction
- Skin disorders (eczema, psoriasis)
- Fertility
- Sexual response
- Allergies
- Heart disease
- Chronic muscle tension
- Migraines/tension headaches
- Anxiety
- Heart disease/stroke
- Immune response
- Thought to be related to stress: certain types of cancer—stress can uncover cancer DNA

Understanding the Logic of Stress Symptoms

When we go into *fight or flight* response, digestion, appetite, satiety and metabolism are disrupted. Growth and reproduction, considered non-essential in a *fight or flight* situation, shut down. All available resources are shunted to the defensive systems of the body. It is logical that if the body is in a perpetual state of stress, digestion will be continually disrupted, as will growth, reproduction, fertility, hormone production, and the ability to enjoy sexual activity. Muscles that were meant to be tense for a short period of time begin to take a chronically defensive posture, leading to chronic pain, tension headaches, backaches and the like. Blood pressure doesn't just spike for a short period of time, you begin to live with high blood pressure all the time. You may become accustomed to breathing in a rapid and shallow manner, rather than the deep, full, diaphragmatic breaths associated with the *Relaxation* response. In short, the whole body adapts to living under constant levels of stress as if it was normal and the symptoms show it. As high blood pressure moves through the blood vessels, the elevated pressure creates rough spots. Fats and other debris in the blood accumulate in these areas setting the stage for heart disease and strokes. While acute stress can boost the immune system, chronic stress weakens the immune system and kills white blood cells. The ability to fight infection and produce antibodies is compromised. The immune system can become so hypersensitive and over-activated, it starts to fire indiscriminately—even at its own body. This we call allergies and auto-immune disease.

Severe or prolonged stress negatively affects learning, long-and short-term memory, math skills, language and problem-solving. In one study, adults with high stress performed 50% lower than adults with low stress.[24]

Stress is related to a child's ability to do well in the classroom. Unresolved conflict among parents, trauma, living in at-risk and dangerous neighborhoods all cause elevated levels of stress hormones in children *as young as two years old*. The stronger the degree of environmental conflict, the greater the effect on performance. Consistently, these kids show difficulty concentrating, problem-solving, retaining information and modulating emotion. All show significant disparities in standardized math and reading tests.[25] These effects are reversible. In four months, 106 at-risk adolescents from three high schools reduced stress, anxiety, hyperactivity, and emotional problems with meditation while increasing grade point averages.[26]

Cortisol

Long-term stress causes the release of cortisol in the body. It signals the body that it is under potential "famine" conditions, so the body begins to retain water and belly fat. Long-term release of cortisol affects hormones and blood sugar, setting the stage for type 2 diabetes. The chemical and hormonal conditions in the body caused by stress can lead to depression and anxiety. Related symptoms include deregulation of thought processes, memory, language, reasoning, and spatial perception.[27] Stress can cause hypersensitivity to even small demands leading to increased startle response and disproportionate mental and emotional reactions.

Yoga Nidra Rebalances Tension with *Relaxation*

One seemingly small thing, too much tension not balanced with *Relaxation*, can have many real and significant consequences. Eventually, if not addressed, it has the potential to define your whole life. Yogis knew this imbalance was the root of many diseases and Hatha Yoga is designed to address just that. Remember the list of stress symptoms. We could work with each symptom individually, or we could work with the single *root cause* of all these symptoms—the imbalance of tension and *Relaxation*. This is what Yoga and Yoga Nidra do. I believe this is why both Yoga and Yoga Nidra have been found to be so profoundly useful in dealing with the myriad symptoms of overstress ranging from infertility to headaches. Both practices address the invisible underpinnings manifesting as visible symptoms.

Yoga Nidra profoundly reduces the surplus excess tension accumulated in the body and breaks the feedback loop which is constantly throwing the body back into a hyper-reactive, *fight or flight* state. When the body has become habituated to living with a "closed fist," it is not enough to simply have a glass of wine or watch TV. The body needs to go to an Alpha brainwave state or deeper to begin to discharge the excess tension that has accumulated in the body and nervous system.

By initiating a parasympathetic, *Relaxation* response, we give the body an opportunity to return to tension/relaxation, ha/tha balance. In Yoga Nidra, we put the body in an optimal environment to prevent and even reverse stress-related illness *at the root cause*. Not only does Yoga Nidra work at the root of stress-related symptoms, but it does so at an accelerated rate. According to Yogic teachings, forty-five minutes of Yoga Nidra gives the body the same restorative effect as three hours of sleep. This means that Yoga Nidra can very quickly and effectively begin to reverse the attack of stress on the body.

While this restorative aspect of Yoga Nidra is in and of itself a powerful and compelling reason to practice, there is more. If we rebalance the excess tension in the body, but never ask ourselves *why* that excess tension has accumulated in the first place, we are likely to recreate it over and over. This is often why we get rid of one symptom of stress and another appears some time later. *We may have relaxed for a time, but we have not interrupted the process by which we are creating tensions on an ongoing basis. Relaxation* then becomes a Band-Aid to a deeper underlying habit that is causing stress—the habit of the mind.

Today our Stress is Mostly Psychological

The body is designed to be in true *fight or flight* for just 60-90 seconds at a time. While most of us do not live in the highest state of *fight or flight* arousal, we definitely subsist in some type of lower-level, hyper-tense state. We call it *chronic stress*. The question is, why don't we return to a full parasympathetic response—like a cat does—after a stressor has passed? The answer is the mind.

In ages past, we had 60-90 seconds to *fight* a life-threatening danger, or *flee* from it. If a tiger walked into the room, we would either run away and survive or we would be killed. Either way, the situation would be resolved in a short period of time. In modern times, most of us are rarely in true physical threat. The dangers are *perceived* and *imagined* dangers. These are dangers created through the perceptions and interpretations of the mind. The problem with this kind of psychological "danger" is that it comes, but it doesn't necessarily leave. Within a minute or two a tiger will either eat you or you will escape. Imaginary tigers—our worries, fears, and insecurities—may never leave until we consciously release them. They continue to hang around, recreating stressful effects over and over for as long as we choose to engage those thoughts. Since most of us don't know how to deal with our thoughts, their effects usually end up lingering for long periods of time and wreaking havoc on the body.

While the body has the capacity to recover from an event with a beginning and an ending, it cannot balance the fears manufactured by the mind which have a beginning, but often no end. The mind has the capacity to create more stress, more worry and more fear than the body can ever hope to balance. This is why, in modern times, the tiger we need to tame is the mind.

The mind is not bad. It is meant to serve us. It is a tool. However, when not well-trained, that same mind can work against us.

Therefore, any truly effective method to manage chronic stress needs to manage our relationship to stress-producing thoughts. Yoga Nidra is designed to do just this. It not only allows the body to discharge the surplus of tension, but also teaches us how to avoid building up excess tension in the first place. A massage, as wonderful as it is, is limited to releasing accumulated tension in the body. It cannot prevent us from recreating that tension over and over again. The power of Yoga Nidra is that is not only releases accumulated tension, but teaches us how to manage the mind—the primary agent of excess stress in the body.

Stress-Producing Mental Habits

In modern times, most of the stress we experience comes from the way we interact with our thoughts. Rather than defending ourselves from a true life-threatening situation, we use our life energy to defend against mentally interpreted threats. *Rather than defending our physical body, we defend the body of our concepts and beliefs.* Let's look at some of the common stress-producing habits of the mind and how we can begin to recognize and short-circuit them.

Resistance

Stress is resistance to what is. When we enter into conflict with how things are, we experience stress. When we are standing in a long line at the Department of Motor Vehicles, no one is assaulting us; *it is resistance in our own mind* that is assaulting us. This is the internal tiger. Nothing is happening out there; our mind is the culprit. It is our resistance to reality that is causing us stress, whether the reality is a red light, a delayed flight, our boss or the line at the DMV. The moment we can release our resistance, come back to the present moment and simply feel what is really happening—our feet on the floor, cool air, people around, breath moving in and out, sounds and voice—the feeling of stress can decrease dramatically.

I would add to this the concept of pain versus suffering. Buddha was once asked how an enlightened person experiences pain versus a regular person. He answered, "An enlightened person experiences one arrow, the physical experience of pain. A regular person experiences two arrows: the pain, *plus* their reaction to the pain." In life, there will always be pain. There will always be things we don't like and would rather not experience. No one can take that away. That is the first arrow. However, we *do* have the choice to suffer or not. This is related to how we choose to react to what happens.

Suffering is what happens after an initial event. It is what we do with the event, the story we make up about it. Do events happen? Yes. It is like a door slamming once. Often we slam that door over and over in our own head. Did the situation or other person do that? No. Did life do that? No. We do that. It may very well be that someone did something to you, but they did it once. We are the ones who repeat it, relive it and react to it over and over in our own minds. We blame them, but really it is us. This is where we have the choice. It is our self-caused suffering that becomes chronic stress. Think of who you resent, who you blame, the regrets or self-judgments you have. The only person it continues to hurt is you.

Assumption

Closely related to resistance are the stories, assumptions and expectations we create in our own heads. Nothing may be happening, but the mind is quite capable of manufacturing all kinds of stories and making all kinds of assumptions based on its own fears. Someone might not say hello, and we may make the assumption they are upset with us. Before we know it, we find ourselves sleepless, concocting reasons why they are angry, or rehearsing what we will say based on each possible angle the other person might take. We not only rehearse our "lines" but their "lines" as well. We check out everything we plan to say to them *on ourselves first* to make sure it is hurtful enough. Often, we don't end up saying anything to the other person, we just rehearse it on ourselves! The problem is, your body chemistry doesn't know you are rehearsing. It feels everything you say and everything you think. Those are real chemical and hormonal reactions happening in you, and that is real stress you are building into your body. This is another example of the imaginary tigers of the mind. Perhaps it turns out the other person was just pre-occupied. That doesn't take away the damage you did to yourself the night before. Learning to exercise *pratyahara*—the ability to withdraw and not feed the habit of the mind—is key here.

Have you ever had a boss say, "I need to talk to you. It is really important, but I can't talk about it now"? Do you see what your mind can do with that? "Is my boss angry?" "Did I do something wrong?" "Maybe I'm getting a promotion." "Or maybe someone else is getting a promotion and she is letting me down gently." Based on each one of these thoughts, there is a chemical reaction happening in the body. The body does not know the difference between what is real and what we are strongly imagining. If we imagine the boss wants to meet with us to let us down gently, we experience it as truth. It is no wonder the body gets tired living out each and every one of the scenarios the mind can create.

Yoga Nidra helps us *dis-identify* from the mind enough to see the thoughts and assumptions it generates. From there, we have the choice to go with the thoughts and deepen them, or withdraw from them and weaken them. A good practice when we cannot totally withdraw is to "make a deal" with the mind. We can say to it, "You are allowed to be upset and have a reaction, but only when you know the facts and not before." It is natural and human to be upset when things happen. What we want to prevent is being upset when things are *not* happening.

Threat to Self-Image

When stress becomes more psychological than physical, our survival instinct expands to include our self-image. We don't just fight for the Physical body; we use the same survival instinct to fight for the life of our self-image and the images of our loved ones. We don't just fight for the right to live, we fight for the life of our ideas and opinions. Have you ever noticed yourself getting riled up watching television when someone expresses an opinion different from yours? When those opinions are very near and dear to our hearts, we can literally feel the stress response kicking in—our blood pressure and body temperature go up, our heart rate increases, and our muscles tense. The more opinions, thoughts and beliefs we have to defend, the more sensitive our stress response will be. We all know people who "wear a chip on their shoulder." Their whole being is a ball of defensiveness just waiting for someone to say the wrong thing.

Our image also expands to defend what we *do*. Let's say you create a PowerPoint presentation, and someone gives you a suggestion on how to make it better. Notice how it may feel like so much more than just a document on a computer. It may feel like an extension of *who you are*. If someone criticizes the presentation, you might feel *you* are being criticized. This happens when *what we do* has merged with *who we are*. When this happens, our presentation is defended with the same energy designated to protect our life. In this case, it may be helpful to ask yourself, "Is this worth defending with my real life energy?" Keep in mind, the energy you are burning is energy that could be healing and sustaining your body.

Self-image can hit closer to home as well. It has to do with how we appear to others. In the age of social media, some of us know what it feels like to have someone say something not-so-favorable or even untrue about us to colleagues, on Facebook or in the media. It literally burns. We want to set the record straight, to show that what the other said is not true and to show what really is true. Yet, at the same time, we feel powerless. It is natural to feel this way, but in these kinds of circumstances, it is also helpful to realize that nothing real has been taken away other than an *idea* of who we are. We are no different. Nothing from our person has been taken away. We are still alive and our body is not in danger. People have thoughts about everything, including us, all the time and these thoughts change all the time. Yet, we can feel so assaulted by what people think and say, that we literally make ourselves sick.

Our self-image can also expand to include everything to which we are attached, whether it is things or people. Preserving the life of our image can escalate to the point where it is stronger than the will to live. In the 1920s, when people lost their entire fortunes, many leapt to their deaths. Their status in life, standing with peers, money and belongings became the defining element of who they were. When these disappeared overnight, some felt as if they were nothing, because their status defined who they were. They could not conceive of a "self" without those things. It was like losing an essential part of themselves, and many of them took their lives as a result.

Sometimes our image expands to include our family and loved ones. Of course it is completely natural to love our family, to want the best for them and even defend them. One of the most difficult positions we can find ourselves in is to identify with a family member's problems as our own. This is quite a sticky spot because, out of love, we rest our happiness on theirs. When a daughter has a rough marriage, or a son lands in jail for drugs, we feel all these experiences as if they were our own. The problem is now we've gotten ourselves attached to an outcome over which we may have no control. If our son is in jail for drugs, we may worry until his problems are in the past, but he is the only one who can resolve his own problems. See the Catch-22? Out of love, we make a problem our own, but we cannot get out of it until the other person has resolved it. Now we are chained to them and their experiences. *Now, our body is not only at the effect of our own personal experiences, but the experiences of the other person.* This makes us very vulnerable to stress.

Perhaps it is more helpful to love our loved ones, but allow them their own journey. We often try to solve the problems of those we love by jumping into the hole with them out of a misplaced desire to be helpful. Now both of you are stuck! It would be more helpful *not* to jump into the hole to save them. Help them as much as you can, but from a place of realizing they need to work out their own lives and live with their own consequences. Their consequences are not your own. They are theirs. From this position, you are truly in a position to be a helpful, steadying influence. From the edge of the hole, you are in a stable and steady position to be able to reach down and give them a hand to help them get out. They may not be ready for the hand now, but when they are, you will be there.

Control

Another very common stress-producing habit is control. We try to get life to fit our individual picture of what we *think* it should be. This planet was running itself for billions of years before we arrived. It has its own intelligence, yet we have decided what it should look like, and we try with all our might to get life to fit our personal picture. In case you have not noticed, life has no allegiance to your plans. One thing falls into place and another falls out. We are constantly running toward that perfect picture and never quite arriving—at least, not for long. When we *do* arrive at those rare moments when everything fits our picture, what happens? We don't stop to enjoy it. Our tendency is to run to find the next one.

We try to organize our life into submission to manage our fear of painful things to come and our fear of loss of the things we love. We try to make sure things will go our way through the sheer force of our will. In the name of being relaxed, we create even more stress. We do all this to be happy, but when do we actually *allow* ourselves to be happy?

Trying to control reality is like trying to control the weather. The weather will just do what it does. No matter how much you yell and scream and try to organize life to fit your plans, it won't follow your lead. Every once in a while the weather will cooperate, but the truth is you will never own reality. To try to master reality is to pit yourself against an unbeatable opponent. You will exhaust yourself trying to get life under control. That doesn't mean you don't plan. You do your best. *But you also have to be flexible and develop the skill of being happy and relaxed even when things don't go your way.*

Yoga Nidra is a powerful method to develop your capacity to allow all experiences to come and go and to be peaceful in the midst of all of them. The more you know that peace is always present and always available, the less you need to fear or hold onto what comes and goes. You know that no matter what comes, you are okay. This allows you to soften your grip on life. You are more able to abide and flow amidst the natural tides of life. You do your best to make things happen, but you know that even when things don't go your way, your essential being remains intact.

Responsibility

Control and responsibility often work hand in hand to drive us to *do more* and *try harder*. This throws us into excess doing. Many of us operate under the unconscious belief that we *create* everything and therefore are *responsible* for everything. We believe everything is created because of what we *do* or *don't do* well. If things go our way, we attach it to what *we did*. If things don't go our way, we attach it to what *we did wrong*. That means that if things don't go well for us it is our *responsibility* and we just have to *try harder*. This throws us into excessive action-oriented, sympathetic nervous system (*pingala*) activity. Through our doing, we are trying to solve a riddle that cannot be solved. The truth is we are responsible for our part of outcomes, but there are millions of factors over which we have absolutely no control. You can do your best to be successful and make a million dollars. However, there is no guaranteed link between what you do and the results you can expect. There are people who work hard and don't succeed, and there are people who don't work hard at all and stumble into their success. That doesn't mean we won't try our best, but we have to recognize the millions of factors that play into any one thing. Even now, you might think it is solely due to your control and will that you are reading this book. But so many things had to happen for this one moment to occur. Many forces had to come together for the book to be written and published. You had to hear about the book, you had to have the means to acquire it, it had to be available, and so on.

To take full responsibility for outcomes over which we have limited control is setting ourselves up for a never-ending struggle. *We are pitting our "doing" against the forces of life.* Sometimes there is just no more that can be done. It is what it is. Steven Covey, author of *The Seven Habits of Highly Effective People*, describes this beautifully. He recommends taking responsibility for what is *within our circle of influence.* That is all we have control over anyway. Do your best with what you have and let go of the rest. If you don't, it will drag you down.

I find taking responsibility for more than what is realistic is a common habit that throws us out of ha/tha, sympathetic/para-sympathetic balance. Recognizing what is realistically within our circle of influence and stopping when it is time to stop is key to keeping this mental and emotional agent of stress at bay.

Secrets/Holding Stuff Back

Sometimes, out of a desire to preserve our image, we hold secrets—either for ourselves, or others. We may hide something about ourselves, our true desires in life, or something we've done, like an affair, or debts we have. There are things we've done that we know, if shared, would only create pain for the other and would not be helpful except to get it off our own chest. In that case, perhaps it is better to share it with a neutral third party. There are also instances in which we feel fine about keeping our secret to ourselves. If keeping the secret doesn't cause your stomach to clench every time you see that person, or to hate yourself or the other person for reminding you of what happened, it is fine from the point of view of stress. However, if there is a physical effect to keeping the secret, it is important to pay attention. The incidence of heart attacks and illnesses among those who keep stressful secrets is very high. It is important to find a way to let that truth come out in a safe environment.

The more you do a practice like Yoga Nidra, the more you come in contact with your body. Your body will tell you very clearly when something is off. Just like a crooked picture on the wall, it will constantly draw your attention to it until you do something to correct it. Inward practices enhance your sensitivity. They enhance your ability to listen to your body and the signals it is giving you. The more you act in accordance with those signals, the more easily your energy will flow. Your body's energy knows exactly what it needs. You just need to listen to it and honor it.

Fragmentation

Fragmentation is a very subtle mental habit that most of us don't even recognize as a stressor. Up to a certain point, we can be effective with multi-tasking, but over a certain threshold, we are no longer getting more done, we are getting less done. Most of us know when we cross that threshold. When we are effective, we can focus fully on one thing at a time—but do so very quickly. We do each thing with concentration, precision and clarity. However, we know what it feels like when we are running around like a "chicken with its head cut off." We are running around in so many directions, we don't quite know where to begin with all the things we have to do. We are so scattered, we can no longer think clearly.

The most important element of fragmentation is that it can deprive us of the one and only place we can ever experience *Relaxation—now.* We have already discussed how *Relaxation* can only be experienced in the present moment. Yet most of us are married to the "then." We are married to a future point in time when everything will be good, when everything will work. Attention is constantly sliding to the next thing and the next thing as we tell ourselves we will truly let go and enjoy our lives "then."

Let's say you are at work. You can't wait to go on a vacation. The whole time you are at work, all you can think about is the vacation. You are not really present at work, because part of you is divided to where you would rather be. You are not present or fulfilled in the now. Your body is not restoring itself. It is waiting. You are telling yourself when you get "there," to the vacation, *then* you will be able to relax and everything will be good.

Finally, vacation day arrives. You tell yourself when you get on the plane, *then* you will relax. Just getting on the plane will be enough. You sit on the plane, order a glass of champagne and for a moment you relax—until your attention slides to the next thing. Getting to Rome! You tell yourself when the plane flight is over and you are finally in your hotel room, *then* you will relax. Finally, you find yourself in a gorgeous hotel in Rome. You check out the view, the bathroom, try out the bed. Amazing. And for a moment, you relax. Then the mind leapfrogs to the next thing, "Oh I can't wait until I have my first Italian meal— *that* will really do it."

So in pursuit of *Relaxation*, you get dressed up, you walk into town and find yourself a nice restaurant. You have an incredible meal, wine, music, the whole thing. And for a moment, you relax—until the mind comes up with the next thing it needs in order to relax. In the ceaseless jumping of the mind to the next thing and the next thing, we miss *this* thing. Through the fragmented mind, we miss the deep *Relaxation* and restoration that is only ever available in the present moment. Wherever you happen to find yourself, be there. You might find being settled just where you are gives you the peace you are seeking.

Stress Producing Mental Tendencies are Manufactured

The point of the mental tendencies we've just discussed is to realize they are happening *within us*. These are not true threats to our physical life. When we are resisting the everyday events of life, we don't realize *nothing is actually happening to us except in our own mind*. We are not in true physical danger. It is *our own mind* that is assaulting us. Many of the stories we create are not even true, we are simply playing them out *as if* they are real. No one is driving us harder than ourselves to live up to an ideal. And no one deprives us of the simple pleasures of the present moment in favor of a promised future except us. This is self-inflicted stress that plays itself out through our nervous system, and imbalance in our body is the result. We become perpetually trapped in a cycle of hyper-defensiveness and the body no longer even knows what it is to return to a state of parasympathetic balance.

Yoga Nidra works at Two Levels

The beauty of Yoga Nidra is that it works at both the psychological and physiological levels. At the somatic body level, the body has a chance to deeply replenish and rejuvenate itself. Yoga Nidra helps the body reset itself back to natural parasympathetic balance, where doing and relaxation are restored to synergistic harmony. The effects of excess tensions in the body that have already begun to set the stage for ill health can be neutralized and released.

At the psychological level, Yoga Nidra allows you to create a different relationship with the stress-producing habits of the mind. By identifying thoughts as nothing more than thoughts, allowing them to simply move through the space of awareness, and even by redirecting unhelpful thoughts in more helpful ways with *Intention*, we become capable of having thoughts without being owned by them. There are many *Relaxation* techniques out there and, like a massage, they calm the body and allow it to return to a state of equilibrium. However, if you do not address what is causing the imbalance, it will keep coming back. The stressed mind can beat any relaxation technique it wants. You know you can go to the gym or the sauna, even listen to a *Relaxation* CD; but if you cannot tame your anxious mind, it can keep you from relaxing in any one of those environments. If you really want to manage your stress, it is essential to learn how to create a different relationship to the thoughts that are creating it. That is exactly what Yoga Nidra helps you do.

The combined psychological and physical benefits of Yoga Nidra help you reverse the effects of stress that have already taken a toll on your body. In the regenerative state of Yoga Nidra, the body has a chance to heal and restore itself back to vitality and health. It has a chance to reverse the effects of premature aging that stress puts on the body. In the chapter to follow, we will explore the physiological and restorative benefits of Yoga Nidra.

CHAPTER THIRTEEN

The Sixth Tool of Yoga Nidra: *Restoration*
What is Yoga Nidra Doing for Me?

Yoga Nidra powerfully heals and restores the body at a purely physiological level, returning the body to an optimal state of health and vitality while supporting the prevention and reversal of disease.

What is happening during Yoga Nidra to so powerfully restore the body to its natural balance? Every day, throughout the day, we are moving from sympathetic arousal and demand to parasympathetic relaxation (Figure 13).

The moment a demand is made on us, big or small, we experience an immediate *fight or flight* response. The breath becomes shallow. Muscles tense. We become hyper-alert. The pupils dilate to take in all the information needed to tell the brain what to do next. Body temperature increases. All non-essential functions, such as digestion and reproduction, temporarily shut down. This is all in response to the hypothalamus, responsible for the autonomic nervous system, telling the pituitary to release stress hormones such as cortisol from the adrenals. This process takes place through a complex interaction between the hypothalamus, pituitary and adrenals—called the HPA axis.

When all systems are in balance and the demand is over, the parasympathetic response will kick in via the Vagus nerve and the body returns to balance. Calming and balancing substances such as GABA, melatonin and serotonin are released into the system. The heart beat and blood pressure slow down, digestion and reproduction resume function, breath becomes deeper and more diaphragmatic and muscles relax. A feeling of *Relaxation* and well-being overcomes the body and we return to homeostatic balance.

The definition of homeostatic balance is "the ability of the body to maintain the condition of balance, even when faced with external changes." An example often provided for homeostatic balance is the ability of the body to maintain a temperature of 98.6 degrees Fahrenheit, no matter what the temperature is outside.

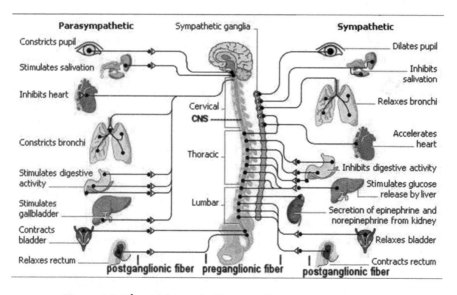

Figure 13: The Autonomic Nervous System

TENSION/SYMPATHETIC RESPONSE

- Hypothalamus, pituitary tell adrenals to release epinephrine, norepinephrine, cortisol
- Heart rate, blood pressure and oxygen consumption increase
- Vessels in lungs dilate, pupils dilate
- Body temperature alters
- Blood flows to limbs and digestion is disrupted
- Reproduction and growth are disrupted
- Large muscles tense

RELAXATION/PARASYMPATHETIC RESPONSE

- Vagus nerve stimulates return to homeostasis
- Heart rate slows, normal blood flow resumes
- Balanced concentration is restored
- Normal digestion is activated
- Reproduction and growth functions are restored
- Increased GABA (the body's tranquilizer)
- Melatonin, serotonin[28]

We know that when we get stuck in sympathetic dominance, the body never fully comes back to homeostatic balance. The heart rate and blood pressure may remain elevated, muscles remain tense, and breath stays more shallow than normal. The experience of full relaxation in the body is not reached. Over days, weeks, months or years, you may not even notice you are missing full relaxation. This is what Yoga Nidra is designed to do—deeply discharge and profoundly release excess tension in the body. Digestion, elimination and reproductive functions normalize. All the organs and systems of the body, including the brain, heart, kidneys and liver, can rest, normalize and rebuild.

The hormones and neurotransmitters released during Yoga Nidra give you a clear mind and an intense feeling of well-being. Inflammation and stress are reduced.[29] A sense of peace and calm floods the system. The tension on the face diminishes, and you immediately appear more youthful and refreshed. The mind is quiet and at rest. The body feels open and pliant. The first time some people do Yoga Nidra, they say they didn't even know they could feel that relaxed.

Meditation and Changes in Body Chemistry

Every time you practice Yoga Nidra meditation, you are giving your body the very best environment in which to experience health, peace and vitality. You are nourishing your body with hormones and neurotransmitters that will make you happier, more relaxed, stronger and younger and it all happens effortlessly by doing something that feels great.

The effects of Yoga Nidra are profound. Yoga Nidra creates a deep restoration state that triggers the brain to release neurotransmitters including GABA, dopamine, serotonin, oxytocin, and endorphins.[30] Melatonin, a hormone, is also released. Each of these chemicals creates greater ease and wellbeing, stronger physical health, mental balance and reduced inflammation. In addition, potentially harmful substances such as cortisol, and norepinephrine are reduced.[31] Most of the facts I will share with you on the benefits of Yoga Nidra are the documented benefits of meditation. *Yoga Nidra is a type of meditation.* The benefits of both Yoga Nidra and other forms of traditional meditation stem from the increase in parasympathetic activity in the body. Yoga Nidra is shown to induce a parasympathetic response in the same way (if not deeper) than other forms of meditation. We'll first examine the general benefits of Yoga Nidra as a form of meditation. Then we will look at further studies specific to Yoga Nidra.

General Benefits of Yoga Nidra as a Form of Meditation

Serotonin

- Yoga Nidra as meditation increases the brain's production of serotonin. Serotonin is a valuable neurotransmitter that profoundly influences both mood and behavior. Serotonin makes us feel good. It brings us to a calm, balanced and focused state of mind along with a relaxed body.[32]

- Low Serotonin can be related to depression, anxiety, bipolar disorder, apathy, low self-esteem, obesity, insomnia, migraine headaches, premenstrual syndrome, and fibromyalgia.[33]

- Drugs such as Prozac, Paxil, and Zoloft are used to treat mood disorders through the restoration of healthy serotonin levels. Though medication is sometimes needed and useful, why not support your own body in creating its own chemical balance through Yoga Nidra as well?

- Serotonin also plays a role in overeating, excess drinking and other compulsive behaviors. Its function is to provide the body with the signal of satiation, letting it know when it has had enough. Thus, having enough serotonin in the system can reduce our tendency to over-indulge in food, sweets or alcohol and instead enjoy them in moderation.

Oxytocin

- Oxytocin, a pleasure hormone, is released during meditation and Yoga Nidra, as well as massage.[34] It initiates a sense of calm, contentment, and security, while reducing anxiety and fear. Oxytocin levels rise during sexual arousal and breastfeeding. It is involved in maternal bonding and the experience of being in love. It generates a sense of bonding, fulfillment and connection within ourselves, our environment and our loved ones.

- Oxytocin affects core structures in the brain including the amygdala, hypothalamus, hippocampus and nucleus accumbens. Oxytocin reduces fear, increases trust and enhances the ability to interact with others in a healthy way. Oxytocin works through oxytocin receptors found in amygdala pathways that mediate fear, trust and social recognition. Strong social networks, being in supportive relationships and social interactions all promote the release of oxytocin as does Yoga Nidra meditation. Some scientists speculate that the release of Oxytocin due to social interaction helps manage stress and anxiety.

- Oxytocin levels are typically low in those with chronic depression, obsessive compulsive disorder and in post traumatic stress disorder. High oxytocin levels reduce the sense of anxiety, increase calm and are related to non-verbal, emotional intelligence.

- Oxytocin is linked to many physiological effects including reduction in cortisol, pain, blood pressure and accelerated wound healing. Both oxytocin and positive experiences can increase the building, growth and restorative aspects of the body's metabolism.[35]

Endorphins

- Endorphins are types of neurotransmitters that have a morphine-like, anti-pain, anti-depressant effect. They positively affect mood and well-being. Endorphins may act as anti-cancer agents in the body and contribute to reduced blood pressure.[36] Endorphins can produce what is commonly known as "runner's high." These same euphoric feelings are also produced through Yoga Nidra meditation.

- In fact, Yoga Nidra as meditation creates the same Endorphin release as running! Research proves that running and meditation *both* release the same amounts of endorphins and endorphin-facilitating substances that keep endorphins circulating in the body. Measurements of mood elevation after both running and meditation were found to be the same.[37]

GABA

- GABA (gamma aminobutyric acid) is known as one of the major inhibitory neurotransmitters in your central nervous system. It plays a central role in the stabilization of mood disorders, reducing muscle tension and cardiac stress.[38] Anxiety, tension, insomnia, and epilepsy are believed to be caused by the lack of adequate production of GABA. *Those who regularly meditate with Yoga Nidra show consistently higher levels of the neurotransmitter GABA.*[39]

- As you will learn, GABA is a very important factor for the prefrontal cortex of the brain. It allows you stay calm under more situations and gain mastery over your reactions. Having enough GABA in your system gives you greater resistance to stress, so that you can handle more pressure before the body initiates a *fight or flight* response.

- Levels of GABA in those suffering from panic disorder are 22% lower than those without panic disorder, concluded a study at Yale University. GABA deficiency is the common denominator in all kinds of addictions including alcohol, drugs, tobacco, caffeine, food, gambling, and even shopping.[40] As you can see, GABA is of vital significance. The cutting edge of treatment for PTSD (Post Traumatic Stress Disorder) includes the administration of GABA.

DHEA

- DHEA sharpens memory, relieves depression, and can cause remarkable improvements in psychological and physical well-being. It is foundational to immune system function—so much so that many scientists are convinced that DHEA hormone deficiency is the major contributor to immune decline as we age.

- Low DHEA levels are extremely common in many individuals who are not even aware of being chronically stressed. In one study of a group of 50 healthy individuals, only 6 DHEA levels were above the laboratory means—suggesting that many who may not appear to be chronically stressed are still experiencing its negative effects.[41] Meditation as Yoga Nidra provides a natural boost to DHEA hormone levels.[42]

- Low levels of DHEA are strongly associated with the risk of heart attack, cancer, osteoporosis, chronic fatigue, obesity, hypertension, immune deficiency, diabetes, and rheumatoid arthritis. Natural enhancement of DHEA has been shown with stress reduction programs, meditation and exercise.[43]

Melatonin

- The pineal gland utilizes the amino acid tryptophan to manufacture the hormone melatonin. Blood melatonin levels peak before bedtime to create a restful sleep. Balanced melatonin levels result in a sound and refreshing sleep.

- Researchers have also demonstrated that melatonin acts as a powerful antioxidant.

- Stress significantly reduces melatonin levels, but *healthy levels of melatonin can be maintained through meditation and stress reduction.*[44]

- Melatonin also sets the biorhythms of the body and our biological clock. It is one of the factors determining the rate at which we age. Perhaps melatonin is the substance Yogis refer to as *amrita*, the nectar of immortality, that

Yoga Nidra: The Art of Transformational Sleep

drips from the pineal gland. Yogis say *amrita* is released during meditation through attention on the *third eye* and keeps one youthful and radiant. If you look at people who meditate with Yoga Nidra or do Yoga consistently, you will notice they appear significantly younger than the average population. Perhaps this is one reason why.

- Low levels of melatonin are associated with higher instances of breast cancer.[45] Studies indicate that women who work late night shifts and are exposed to artificial light have lower melatonin levels which seem to contribute to the incidence of breast cancer.[46]

Human Growth Hormone

- Meditation, as practiced in Yoga Nidra, gives a considerable boost to human growth hormone (HGH), production.[47] HGH is the agent that stimulates growth throughout childhood and then maintains the tissues and organs throughout life. In our 40s, the pituitary gland located at the base of the brain, begins to decrease the amount of HGH it produces (Figure 14).

- The diminished production of HGH is associated with symptoms of aging which can include poor stamina, decreased muscle mass, increased body fat, poor mood, lack of motivation, and decreased bone density.[48] This is why we hear so much about HGH supplements nowadays. Essentially, it slows the aging process. Human growth hormone is *naturally* released at the deepest stages of Yoga Nidra, maintaining youthfulness and allowing for the growth and regeneration of all the organs and tissues of the body.[49]

Cortisol

- When the body is under stress, cortisol is released into the system. Though useful and necessary in small amounts, in excess it can be very damaging to the body.

In the short term and early stages of stress, the cortisol released into the body suppresses the immune system, its resistance, and its inflammatory processes. Controlled inflammation is part of the way the body heals and protects itself. The immune system is suppressed under short-term stress because it is non-essential for survival. If stressed for longer periods of time however, this leads to a chronically suppressed immune system. For many people, cortisol is the one hormone which you want to decrease. Yoga Nidra as a meditation practice is proven to significantly decrease this potentially harmful hormone if needed.[50]

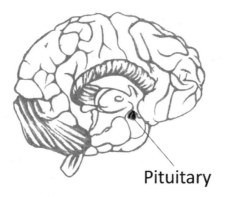

Pituitary

Figure 14: The Pituitary gland secretes human growth hormone during deep meditation, sustaining the organs and tissues of the body.

Artwork by JoElizabeth James

- Higher and more prolonged exposure to cortisol accelerates aging. When actively circulating in the bloodstream, cortisol leads to a host of symptoms. Some of these are: elevated blood pressure, blood sugar imbalances, decreased bone density, compromised thyroid function, weakened memory and problem solving, decrease in muscle tissue, lowered immunity and inflammatory responses in the body, increased abdominal fat (which has its own health risks), heart attacks, strokes, increased levels of "bad" cholesterol (LDL) and decreased levels of "good" cholesterol (HDL).[51] Too much cortisol is destructive. Meditation-based Yoga Nidra takes excess cortisol out of the system and reduces the risks of its many harmful effects.

- When the adrenals secrete cortisol for long periods of time the adrenals can become tired, depleted and unable to produce the hormones that the body needs. Cortisol levels begin to rapidly decline and a chronically stressed person may switch from having *too much* cortisol to *not enough*. This means the anti-inflammatory effect of cortisol is absent. The immune system is left running unchecked. Without sufficient cortisol, there is nothing to prevent severe, widespread and chronic inflammation in numerous bodily pathways. The result is increased vulnerability to inflammatory diseases including auto-immune diseases, chronic fatigue, type 2 diabetes and fibromyalgia. Yoga Nidra can help the adrenals heal and repair so that the body can begin to produce the cortisol it needs. The way to do this is through deep bodily rest so that the adrenals can bounce back from having been overworked.[52]

- The idea is not to have low cortisol or high cortisol, but a good baseline balance. If cortisol levels are normal, then inflammation is neither suppressed nor overly expressed. Whether too high or too low, Yoga Nidra helps restore the proper baseline.

Additional Studies Specific to Yoga Nidra

In addition to the many benefits of Yoga Nidra as a meditation technique, there are other studies which demonstrate benefits specific to Yoga Nidra.

Yoga Nidra and Dopamine

- Studies show that Yoga Nidra techniques increase the endogenous release of dopamine in the system by up to 65%![53]

- Dopamine is a key player in our ability to experience pleasure, feel rewarded, and maintain focus. Dopamine is a critical antidote to depression and amplifies your motivation and positive outlook on the world.

- It helps you take focused, directed and willful action. It helps you be productive.

- Not having enough dopamine in the system is part of the problem that causes Parkinson's disease. Through the natural release of dopamine in the body, Yoga Nidra can be a good aid in the treatment of Parkinson's disease.

- The dramatic boost in the release of the body's own dopamine heightens your ability to manage the impulse to act on unhelpful habits and addictions. In fact it has been scientifically proven that having enough dopamine in your system reduces impulsivity and increases your ability to withstand cravings without acting on them.[54]

Reduced Worry and Depression, Increased Mindfulness

Yoga Nidra practice is associated with reduced stress, worry, and depression, and increased mindfulness in college students. Sixty-six students, ages 18-56, completed an 8-week Yoga Nidra intervention. The results showed significant reduction in perceived stress, worry, and depression. Mindfulness-based skills—the ability to remain calm and centered with neutral attention to the present—also improved pre-to-post-test after 8 weeks of Yoga Nidra.[55]

Reduced Stress, Enhanced Health, Sleep and Immune Response

Yoga Nidra is shown to create a total relaxation effect. It strengthens the parasympathetic (relaxation) response and boosts the immune system. Yoga Nidra increases Alpha brainwave activity, important for relaxation and sleep. In addition, GSR—Galvanic Skin Response tests, measuring the change in the electrical resistance of the skin, show Yoga Nidra reduces the stress and anxiety of the practitioner. Stress leads to a build-up of a cortisol that eventually inhibits the body's ability to fight off bacteria and viruses, while Yoga Nidra is shown to strengthen the immune system.[56]

A key study conducted at the University of Tel Aviv (Israel) found that Yoga Nidra significantly lowers levels of serum cholesterol in cardiac patients.[57] Another study, conducted by Lekh Raj Bali at the Langley Porter Neuropsychiatry Institute in California, demonstrated that Yoga Nidra reduces blood pressure and anxiety levels in hypertensive patients.[58]

A preliminary case study was conducted on the Integrative Amrit Method of Yoga Nidra by Nicola Vague in Melbourne Australia.[59] The four-week program involved a two-hour class per week for nine participants incorporating Yoga Nidra and art based practices in a supportive group setting. Participants were requested to commit to a 30-minute (approximately) guided Yoga Nidra practice each day and were encouraged to keep a journal of their experience. A stress indicator assessment was completed prior to the start of the program, and at the end of the program. This self-assessment covered key indicators of overall stress levels including sleep quality, general health and wellbeing, mental and emotional balance and unhealthy habits, cravings and behaviors. There were nine participants from diverse backgrounds, stages of life and life experience. The group ranged from experienced meditators to those new to meditation. Participants committed to their home recorded Yoga Nidra practice an average of three times between sessions.

Positive changes were experienced across the following metrics: ability to manage stress 43%, sleep quality 43%, mental and emotional balance 57%, reduction of unhealthy habits, cravings and impulsive behaviors 29%.

Volunteer staff and I conducted a similar case study during Amrit Method Yoga Nidra training at the Virginia G. Piper Cancer Center in Scottsdale Arizona.[60] Preliminary findings of the seven participants showed impressive positive results for the Integrative Amrit Method of Yoga Nidra practice across the following metrics: decreased levels of stress 85%, improved mental and emotional balance 83%, improved general health and wellbeing 82%, enhanced sleep quality 57%, greater connection to personal spiritual beliefs 52% and a more positive outlook on life 27%. Additionally, resting heart rates and blood pressures were taken before and after four of the Yoga Nidra sessions. The average drop in resting heart rate after each Yoga Nidra was just under ten beats (8.5 beats) per minute. That is quite a significant drop. Interestingly, those with lower initial resting heart rates dropped the least while those with highest resting heart rates dropped the most. A similar trend was noted with blood pressures. The general trend appeared to indicate that lower-than-normal blood pressures went a little bit higher toward the norm and that higher blood pressures lowered back toward the median average of 120/80. However, more study would be required to verify this.

Decreased Anxiety and Depression

Yoga Nidra consistently improves physical and mental health.[61] A number of studies have repeatedly demonstrated that the practice of Yoga Nidra decreases anxiety and positively increases general well-being. In one study, 80 students reduced stress levels as compared to controls. Several other studies show that Yoga Nidra alleviates anxiety in both men and women.[62] In addition, research shows significant and measurable relief from symptoms of anxiety and depression in those with menstrual disorders.[63]

Reduction in Guilt Levels and Regression to Old Thinking Patterns

Yoga Nidra has been shown to lessen guilty feelings and diminishes the tendency to revert to self-sabotaging patterns of thought and emotion. This effect is consistent among both men and women.[64]

Diabetes

Several studies indicate that Yoga Nidra helps control blood glucose levels of those with diabetes and assists in the management of associated symptoms.[65]

PTSD

Pioneered by Richard Miller and the iRest method of Yoga Nidra, clinical research on Yoga Nidra and PTSD began in 2007 when the Department of Defense approved a study to explore the effect of Yoga Nidra on returning soldiers diagnosed with PTSD. The nine-week study took place at Walter Reed Army Medical Center in Washington DC and found that Yoga Nidra did indeed reduce symptoms of PTSD.[66] In 2010, the War Related Illness and Injury Study Centers conducted a survey of those attending Yoga Nidra classes and found that 85% reported improvements across 13 different symptoms including intrusive memories, headaches, anxiety, depression, insomnia, hypervigilance, irritability and angry outbursts.[67]

Yoga Nidra has been endorsed by the military as a complementary therapy and is being offered in military hospitals and VA centers around the country. Richard Miller's work with Yoga Nidra has extended to a number of underserved populations with a focus on trauma and chronic pain among veterans.

Chronic Pain

In 2010, the US Army Surgeon General endorsed Yoga Nidra as an intervention in treating chronic pain.[68]

Multiple Sclerosis and Cancer

Yoga Nidra is an effective technique for reducing stress for cancer and MS patients. A study utilizing Richard Miller's style of Yoga Nidra examined the effects of a 6-week Yoga Nidra meditation program on perceived stress in multiple sclerosis and cancer patients. Over the course of the program, stress was significantly reduced. While the chronic illness did not go away, the mental and emotional relationship to the illness changed—creating a reduction in the *experience* of stress. Further, it was noted that Yoga Nidra practices are accessible and lend themselves to populations with physical limitations.[69]

Disruptive Behavior

Another study was conducted with boys displaying unruly behaviors. The study showed that boys with disruptive behavior generally display unstable breathing patterns throughout the day. It was demonstrated that Yoga Nidra restored calmer behaviors, reduction of hostility and anxiety along with a corresponding return to stable breathing patterns.[70]

CHAPTER FOURTEEN

Effects of Yoga Nidra and Other Meditation Techniques

Brain Changes during Yoga Nidra

If you are reading this book, you have probably experienced some form of Yoga Nidra. You know how it feels experientially, and now you know what happens with the chemistry of the body. So what is happening in the brain?

The first thing to know is Yoga Nidra is not the same as sleep. It is a distinct state. Researchers have documented physiological and neurological activity that distinguishes Yoga Nidra from relaxation and also makes it a unique form meditation. Parker proposes the following definition: "Yoga Nidra represents a state in which an individual demonstrates all the symptoms of deep, non-REM sleep, including Delta brainwaves, while simultaneously remaining fully conscious."[71]

In a study of Yoga Nidra conducted by H.C. Lou, T.W. Kjaer, L. Friberg, G. Wildschiodtz, S. Holm, and M. Nowak in Scandinavia, an electroencephalograph (EEG), measuring brain activity displayed significant increase in Theta brainwaves (11%) typical of sleep state, while at the same time Alpha waves decreased by 2%. This is not the same as typical sleep in which Alpha brainwave activity also increases. This indicates a state of conscious awareness that is not sleep, but is *sleep-like* due to increased Theta and even Delta brainwave activity. In addition, PET scans show the state of Yoga Nidra is constant and evenly distributed over the entire brain for the full length of the Yoga Nidra session.[72]

Through a series of studies conducted at Cherring Cross Medical School London, Mangalteertham demonstrated that Yoga Nidra is a technique in which one can alter the state of consciousness from Beta to Alpha and then to Delta brainwaves. It was shown that an individual knowingly experiences these different states of consciousness in Yoga Nidra.[73]

Scientists once believed it was impossible to be in these deeply relaxed states, going as deep as the Delta brainwave state, while still conscious. Furthermore it was believed impossible to be able to *direct and manage the brain's activity* in a highly concentrated, consistent, and sequential manner *while in* these deeply relaxed brainwave states. Yet the Scandinavian researchers observing the PET scans of Yoga Nidra practitioners were struck by the degree to which practitioners were able to be deeply relaxed, yet control the brain's activity with a high degree of concentration and precision.

For example, when mentally scanning various parts of the body during Yoga Nidra, especially the face, the corresponding *visual* and *tactile* centers of the brain, were most active, as if these areas of the body were actually being *seen* and *touched* by the practitioner. The same was true in the visualization stage of the Yoga Nidra; the brain was shown to register both *seeing* and *feeling* the image. When in the deepest point of Yoga Nidra—resting in awareness and integration, the temporal lobe (just above the ears) was particularly active, an area of the brain which increases in density with the practice of meditation techniques such as Yoga Nidra and is associated with empathy, compassion and perspective taking. In fact, those who meditate with Yoga Nidra report experiencing changes in their empathy and compassion for others as well as their ability to take a greater, more objective view of events and situations.

Even more remarkable, each practitioner progressing through the various stages of Yoga Nidra demonstrated the *same* sequential changes in the brain *corresponding to the stage of Yoga Nidra* and the technique being utilized. In summary, researchers are seeing that the correlation between the technique and the part of the brain activated is not a matter of chance. As Troels Kjær, Brain Researcher at The Kennedy Institute in Copenhagen, Denmark, said, "We had not expected the meditators to be able to control their consciousness to such an extent."[74]

Another interesting aspect of Yoga Nidra is that the areas of the brain stimulated are virtually symmetrical in both halves of the brain. According to Troels Kjaer and accompanying authors/researchers, "The experience of conscious control of actions is… bilaterally in dorso-lateral orbital and cingulate frontal regions, posterior parietal region, temporal region, and the caudate nucleus, thalamus, pons, and cerebellar vermis and hemispheres."[75]

This is very unusual because most of the time, the brain does not operate in symmetry. From a Yogic perspective, one could speculate that we are seeing what the brain looks like in a state of Oneness. We are no longer internally divided. We are not relying on just the right or left brain, but the whole brain is operating as one. In Yoga Nidra, we physiologically and spiritually *are* One.

How Meditation Can Shape Our Brains

Prefrontal Cortex

One of the most groundbreaking studies in the field of neuroscience and meditation is the work of Sara Lazar from Harvard University. Ms. Lazar had a running injury and discovered Yoga as she was healing. Skeptical of the teachers' claims that Yoga would make her feel better, calm her mind, make her more empathetic and better able to handle difficult situations, she nonetheless began to observe these effects. She noticed she was more able to see things from other people's perspectives and was indeed less reactive. Curious, she embarked on research to discover how meditation changes the brain.

The first study was based on the idea that the brain is *plastic*. That certainly does not mean that the brain is *made of* plastic; it means that the brain has the ability to change. When we repeat something over and over again, the repetition can lead to changes in the brain. This is what is referred to as *neuroplasticity*, which means that neurons can change how they talk to each other through repeated experiences.

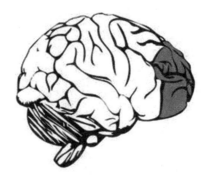

Figure 15: Prefrontal Cortex

Attribution: CC License-Share Alike 3.0 Unported. Link to license: https://creative-commons.org/licenses/by-sa/3.0/legalcode Wikimedia http://commons.wikimedia.org/wiki/

The first study she conducted was done with average individuals who meditated in the Boston area. Not monks, just average people who meditated thirty or forty minutes a day. When compared to people who were demographically matched, but who did not meditate, it was found there were indeed areas of the meditators' brains that had more grey matter as compared to the control group. One of these areas was in the front of the brain, called the prefrontal cortex—the area responsible for executive decision-making and active working memory. This vital region of the brain, located just behind the forehead,

Yoga Nidra: The Art of Transformational Sleep

regulates both short-term and long-term decision making and allows for attuned communication and socialized behavior by modulating our actions or reactions rather than acting upon the base impulses arising from the instinctive regions of the brain. Additionally, the prefrontal cortex, or PFC, (Figure 15) helps one to pay attention, learn, and concentrate on goals. This area is also the part of the brain that allows humans to follow several parallel, yet different lines of thinking when evaluating complex ideas or solutions.

One of the most interesting findings from this first study suggests that meditation slows, or may even prevent, the age-related declines in the prefrontal cortex. Usually, as we age, cortical structure shrinks. This makes it harder for us to do things like work out problems and remember things. However, with the use of Mindfulness techniques like those used in Yoga Nidra, the 50-year-old meditators had the same amount of cortex as the 25-year-old meditators![76]

The prefrontal cortex, the anterior part of the frontal lobe, is like the "parent." It is the one who should be making the final and executive decisions. When operating well, it regulates our behavior and mediates conflicting thoughts, making choices between right and wrong, as well as predicting the probable outcomes of actions or events. This brain area governs management of our emotions, exerts social control, and manages our fears and sexual urges. It is strongly implicated in human qualities like consciousness, general emotional and social intelligence, empathy, insight, intuition, personality, and attuned communication.

The prefrontal cortex primarily develops its strength and resilience to difficulty through caregiver bonding—through feeling safe, secure, loved, and being held. When we experience prolonged neglect or trauma in childhood or as an adult, it affects the physical structure of the brain, especially in the middle prefrontal cortex. Very often, people who have had difficult childhoods or later trauma, have less ability to regulate their emotions, their primal urges, or make good choices for themselves. They have more difficulty attuning to others as well as acting in an appropriate manner in social situations. This can be due to deficiencies in the development of the prefrontal cortex.

Previous thought was that the brain could not heal once a trauma occurred. However it now appears that *meditation can strengthen and even repair areas of the brain affected by childhood difficulties, stress, and later trauma.* This is an amazing breakthrough for those who have suffered trauma and childhood deficiencies. As the physiological counterparts of these experiences are healed, so too can the mental, emotional and behavioral habits that accompany them.[77]

Bigger Hippocampus

A second study by Sara Lazar was done with those who had no meditation experience whatsoever. The participants were put through an eight-week Meditation-Based Stress Reduction Program where they were told to meditate every day for thirty to forty minutes. At the end of the eight weeks, there were significant changes in various regions of the brain. The first was in the hippocampus (Figure 16), associated with emotion regulation, learning and memory. Reduced grey matter in this area is associated with depression and PTSD. However, meditation releases serotonin and acts as fertilizer for the hippocampus, stimulating growth and regeneration. After the eight weeks of meditation techniques like those used in Yoga Nidra, the hippocampus became significantly larger. *Researchers suggest larger volumes in these regions might account for meditators' ability to cultivate positive emotions, retain emotional stability, and engage in a more neutral, responsive stance to daily life events. Studies suggest that these regional alterations in brain structures correlate with long-term meditation regardless of a specific style and practice.*[78]

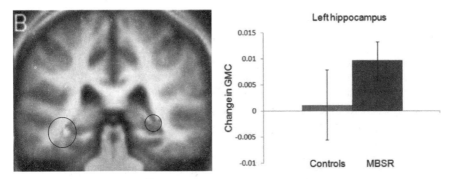

Figure 16: Left Hippocampus grey matter concentration increased after just eight weeks of meditation.

The yellow area (indicated within the circles) on the left side of the brain shows the grey matter concentration (GMC) increases in the left Hippocampus after 8 weeks of Mindfulness Based Stress Reduction training (MBSR). In the graph on the right, you will see the change in grey matter concentration charted in the meditation group (right) versus the control group (left). You can see the change is significant after just eight weeks.

Attribution: Fig. 1. "Left Hippocampus." Hölzel, B.K., J. Carmody, M. Vangel, C. Congleton, S.M. Yerramsetti, T. Gard, and S.W. Lazar. "Mindfulness Practice Leads to Increases in Regional Brain Gray Matter Density. " Psychiatry Research: Neurimaging 191.1 (2011): 36-43. Reprinted with permission.

Temporal Parietal Lobe–Thicker–Perspective Taking, Empathy and Compassion

Another alteration in brain landscape was the temporal parietal junction—located on the side of the brain, approximately above the ear. This part of the brain is important for perspective taking, empathy and compassion.[79] These are all effects practitioners commonly report after consistent practice of Yoga Nidra. "Perspective taking" might be termed as *"witness"* in Yogic terminology. Remember that, according to brain scans, this is the area of the brain stimulated during the deepest stage of Yoga Nidra—the "resting in awareness" phase. This phase is in fact designed to develop the ability to observe and rest as the witnessing space behind the mind. Science appears to verify that we are in fact cultivating the brain's ability to be the witness in the deepest states of Yoga Nidra.

Smaller Amygdala as Less Stressed

Another region that changes as a result of meditation is the amygdala—the part of the brain responsible for threat perception and our instinctual *fight or flight* response (Figure 17). When people have a highly sensitized amygdala, they are more likely to see things through the filters of past experiences. These past experiences may be chemically imprinted in the *fight or flight* pathway. When a new experience occurs, this part of the brain matches new experiences to old ones and determines how to instinctually react as programmed by the past. For example, a child who was left out when playing with other children might perceive and re-experience feeling left out as an adult when there are no chairs at a dinner party. In effect, the amygdala acts as the anatomical counterpart to our *samskaras*—neuronally and chemically recording and storing them as protection from future threats.

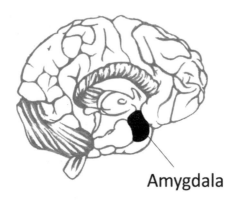

Amygdala

Figure 17: The Amygdala
Artwork by JoElizabeth James

The amygdala causes us to re-experience the stresses of the past over and over through the present moment's experience. Whenever we perceive a potential threat or experience of pain, we react instinctually and pre-mentally. We don't think or consider; we just do. Only *after* doing, do we realize what we did or said. Sometimes, once our consciousness has kicked in, we regret our actions. Keep in mind, however, that the amygdala does not just function to avoid pain. It also records highly pleasurable experiences and gives us the motivation to re-acquire them when they once again move into our field of awareness. In science, the actions of the amygdala are called either "appetitive" (e.g. food) or "aversive" (e.g. electric shock). This seems to correlate with ancient Yogic teachings outlining the process by which the mind works through *raga* and *dvesha* (attraction and aversion).

If needed, meditation can actually decrease grey matter in the amygdala. In the study by Sara Lazar, the change in grey matter was correlated with the amount of stress a person was experiencing.[80] The less stress a person reported, the smaller the amygdala. This is not to say the amygdala becomes abnormally small, but that, if needed, its dominating influence in the brain can be brought to more normalized levels.

As the amygdala normalizes, the prefrontal cortex, responsible for skilled communication and choices, grows in strength. The current understanding is that the stronger the prefrontal cortex becomes, the more fibers grow from it toward the amygdala—part of the limbic system. These fibers release inhibitory peptides, particularly GABA, which help keep the instinctual and reactive patterns of the amygdala under conscious control.

This allows the prefrontal cortex, the "parent," to re-establish its position as the executive decision maker and allows the instinctual center, the amygdala, to come under conscious regulation rather than running the show. For example, instead of instinctively lashing out at someone for hurting you, you will notice you have more ability to step back, consider your actions, and choose what you want to say and how you want to say it. You will observe you have more ability to see the situation from the other person's perspective and are more able to respond consciously rather than react unconsciously. When an old *sams-kara* gets triggered, you will be better able to dis-identify and recognize it as an old tape being replayed. You will have the choice to believe and act on the old tape or set it aside and deal with the current situation independent of the past.

You can see how meditation potentially changes the way you live your life, interact with others and interact with your own thoughts and emotions. Its potential is nothing less than life changing and the effects are scientifically visible in the anatomy of the brain and the biochemistry of the body. You can literally change your brain and your body chemistry to support a happier, healthier and more balanced inner life. In fact, researchers report that *just eleven hours of learning a meditation technique induces positive structural changes in the prefrontal cortex. In other words, if you listen to a 40-minute Yoga Nidra CD 17 times you could begin to observe for yourself some of the positive brain changes we have just discussed.*[81]

Yoga Nidra is Mindfulness and More

A style of meditation that has been exhaustively studied is Mindfulness Meditation. Mindfulness is bringing neutral attention and non-judgmental awareness to body, breath and sensations as well as anything passing through the field of awareness. A Mindfulness practice can involve anything that brings attention to now via body, breath and sensation.

Mindfulness includes the following techniques:

- Entering the Alpha brainwave state

- Concentrating attention on sensations or places in body with neutral awareness

- Tension and relaxation of muscles to help induce deep muscle relaxation

- Paying attention to the flow of breath with neutral attention

- Repeating a simple word, prayer or anything that is personally uplifting

If you look at these techniques, you will notice Yoga Nidra includes ALL of these. Commonly, Mindfulness training involves one technique performed at a time. Yoga Nidra utilizes all the techniques of Mindfulness. What makes Yoga Nidra unique is the *way these techniques are structured to move from the gross to the subtle—easily taking you from active brainwave states to deep slow-wave states.* Mindful body, breath, and awareness techniques are structured in a series to gradually slow the brainwaves at each subsequent stage of Yoga Nidra allowing you to progressively enter deeper states of stillness where the neutral state of awareness naturally arises without any effort whatsoever. In fact, effort only hinders the process. Here, you naturally enter neutral gear about all thoughts, feelings, and sensations. Mindfulness is something that *happens* in Yoga Nidra. It is not something you *do*.

Yoga Nidra is designed to gradually slow the mind by beginning with muscular contraction in the body, then progressing to the more subtle sensation of the breath, then moving into an even subtler level of attention through body rotations and visualizations. We move from the scattered thinking mind, to feeling the body, to consciously placing neutral attention on various locations in the body—but Yoga Nidra goes even further— it eventually even transcends the neutrally observing mind altogether *guiding you to the place where you rest as the space of neutral awareness itself.*

Yoga Nidra can take you to a deeper state than typical Mindfulness practices. Yoga Nidra is guided. The practitioner effortlessly follows the guidance of the facilitator. Mindful meditation requires more effort and keeps you operating at a more active brainwave level.

Eventually, Yoga Nidra transcends both mind and time. Mind and the sense of time co-arise. With mind comes past and future—an awareness of what came before and what is not yet done. In the space beyond mind and time all of this disappears. This is where you go in Yoga Nidra; to the timeless state of being.

Yoga Nidra delivers the benefits of meditation, relaxation, and Mindful meditation, and yet is so much more than any one of them. Given this understanding, let's look at some of the proven benefits of Mindful meditation, relaxation, and also guided imagery as these make up components of a Yoga Nidra experience.

Benefits of Mindfulness Meditation, Relaxation and Guided Imagery

General Health

No matter the type of meditation or relaxation technique, research findings consistently show a reduction in blood pressure, cholesterol and severity of angina attacks with continued practice.

Adult Onset Diabetes

Relaxation and meditation techniques are beneficial for adult onset diabetes. Yoga Nidra has also been proven to improve the body's ability to regulate glucose. In studies, the length of Yoga Nidra varies from 30-40 minutes daily to 20 minutes, five times a week. However, the medical benefits are present even with the latter.

Improves Immune Function

It has been shown multiple times in multiple studies that meditation and the relaxation response it induces can strengthen the immune system.[82] This is important because people who are stressed are three times more likely to suffer from the common cold. They are also more likely to suffer from autoimmune disorders such as asthma and diabetes. Stressed individuals show weaker immune responses to vaccines.[83]

In one study, an eight-week Mindfulness Training Program was carried out in a work environment where healthy employees were vaccinated with the influenza vaccine. Those subjects who meditated showed significant increases in antibody titers to influenza vaccine compared with those in the control group. There was also a significant increase in left-sided anterior brain activation, which is usually associated with positive feeling and behaviors. Interestingly, the magnitude of increase in left-sided activation predicted the magnitude of antibody titer rise due to the vaccine.[84]

Researchers from United Lincolnshire Hospitals and Queen's Medical Centre in the United Kingdom evaluated the effects of relaxation training and guided imagery on breast cancer patients. Eighty patients underwent chemotherapy followed by surgery, radiotherapy, and hormone therapy. Patients were taught relaxation and guided imagery. The number of mature T cells (a type of white blood cell that plays a role in immunity) was significantly higher following chemotherapy and radiotherapy for patients in the relaxation and guided imagery group. In conclusion, relaxation training and guided imagery were shown to beneficially alter anti-cancer host defenses during and after cancer therapies.[85] In other words, practices like Yoga Nidra, which include both relaxation and guided imagery, can help prevent declines in healthy immune function after cancer treatment.

Decreases Pain

At the University of Massachusetts, a study was conducted with people suffering chronic, severe pain from a variety of causes including back pain, migraine headaches, cancer, mishandled surgeries and car accidents. After meditation training, a sharp decrease in pain-related symptoms was reported. Most of the participants were able to lessen or stop pain medications. After four years, people who continued their meditation practice remained free of pain or experienced less discomfort.[86]

In another study, after four days of meditation training, those asked to meditate in the presence of an uncomfortable stimulation reduced their rating of pain unpleasantness by 57% and pain intensity ratings by 40%. The decrease in pain seems to correlate with how a person constructs a pain experience. Meditation can lessen the subjective experience of pain. However, meditation also causes changes to the brain itself to manage how pain is registered.[87]

Decreases Inflammation at the Cellular Level

It has been shown that meditation not only reduces emotional reactivity, but also the inflammatory response that occurs after we are under stress.[88] Inflammation starts the process of healing via the release of a variety of chemicals known as proinflammatory cytokines. One of these is interleukin-6. As an injury or wound heals, it swells as part of the healing response. A simple example is a sprained ankle. Now imagine that the swelling remains and the ankle never returns to its original state. You can see how the ankle would not be able to operate properly and its function would be impaired. This kind of inflammation is not just visible, it is also invisibly happening inside the body. A reaction that was meant to be a temporary healing response to protect the body, becomes a more permanent state that can actually act against the body's normal processes. This is called chronic inflammation. This occurs when a process that is usually closely regulated by the body, gets out of control. Excess inflammation in the body can lead to a host of diseases, such as hay fever, periodontitis, heart disease, rheumatoid arthritis, and even cancer. It has been implicated in the development of Alzheimer's disease, Parkinson's disease, type 2 diabetes, and many more medical conditions.

Many things cause excess inflammation in the body; some of the greatest contributing factors are stress, negative emotions, loneliness and other psychological stressors. In a study of caregivers, the annual rate of increase in serum interleukin-6 levels, an inflammation marker, was four times greater than individuals without caregiving responsibilities.[89] Yoga Nidra as a Mindfulness meditation technique manages excess inflammation.

Improves Memory, Productivity and Focused Attention

One study sought to determine if meditation could improve office workers' abilities to multitask on a computer more effectively and/or with less stress. While overall task time and errors remained the same, the meditation group reported lower levels of stress and showed better memory for the tasks they had performed. They also switched tasks less often and remained focused on tasks longer.[90]

Research has found that even short-term Mindful meditation practice enhances social communication, cognition, mood, and the ability to sustain attention. After just four days of meditation training, participants with *no prior meditation experience* were tested for mood, verbal fluency, visual processing, and working memory. The meditation training not only reduced fatigue and anxiety, but also significantly improved visual and spatial processing, working memory, and executive functioning. Findings suggest that four days of meditation training can enhance the ability to sustain attention—a benefit that was previously only associated with long-term meditators.[91]

Hot Flashes

Researchers from the University of Massachusetts Medical School studied fifteen women with severe hot flashes. After eight weeks of practice, the quality-of-life measures increased significantly and the median severity of hot flashes decreased by 40%.[92]

Other Stress Related Symptoms

SUNY at Albany researchers studied the effects of Relaxation Response Meditation on the symptoms of irritable bowel syndrome (IBS). Sixteen adults either attended a six-week meditation class or were on a six week wait list (control group). Patients in the meditation group practiced relaxation twice a day for 15 minutes. During the three-month follow-up, significant improvements were found in meditation group patients regarding flatulence, belching, bloating and diarrhea. The study tentatively concludes that relaxation response meditation is a viable treatment for IBS.[93]

Researchers from the University of Louisville in Kentucky explored the effects of Mindfulness Based Stress Reduction (MBSR) on sympathetic nervous system activation among 24 women with fibromyalgia. Over-activation of the sympathetic nervous system is thought to be the major factor in the pain and fatigue symptoms associated with this disease. Following meditation training, basal sympathetic nervous system activity was reduced. In addition, fibromyalgia is very often accompanied by depression related to loss of former lifestyle.[94] An earlier study showed that meditation reduces depressive symptoms in patients with fibromyalgia. These gains were still maintained at the two month follow-up.[95]

All these benefits and more are easily gained through the practice of Yoga Nidra. The beauty is that it is not hard. Anyone can do it, and that means anyone can receive these benefits.

CHAPTER FIFTEEN

Yoga Nidra for Health

The mind and body are one unified organism. Our psychology affects our physiology and our physiology affects our psychology. In other words, the way we think and interact with our emotions affects our health. Conversely, the way our body *feels* affects the way we *think*. We all know that a night of too much food and drink can leave us feeling irritated or moody the next day. We also know that incessant worries and fearful thoughts can show up in the body.

Yoga Nidra works at both levels—physiological balance *and* better regulation of our mind and emotions. To me, any comprehensive program for health and well-being *must* include management of our thoughts and emotions. While it is commonly accepted that taking care of our body is an essential part of health, it is less common to take our thoughts and emotions into account. Let's look at how thoughts and emotions affect our health from both Yogic and scientific perspectives. Using the Tools of Yoga Nidra we have learned so far, we will examine how Yoga Nidra can benefit our health at both the psychological and physiological levels.

Intention Applied: Thoughts and Your Health

Yogis, due to their understanding of the *koshas*, have laid out as principle: *the subtle affects the gross*. The *koshas* work in a hierarchical fashion. The subtler *koshas*, like the Bliss, Wisdom and Mental bodies, exert a strong influence on the Energy and Physical sheaths below them. (See Chapter 5, Figure 7). For example, when the mind is irritated and upset, our Energy and Physical bodies, the sheaths below the mind, tangibly experience what originated at a more subtle level.

237

The reverse is also true. It is pretty obvious to us that what we do with the gross Physical body affects our Energy and Mental bodies as well. When we go to the gym, we work with the Physical body to positively affect the subtler Energy and Mental bodies. We work with the gross body to improve our energy and mental state. Well, here's the catch: the subtle will almost always trump the gross. Imagine you leave the gym feeling physically relaxed and energized. As you approach your car, you immediately notice a dent in it that was not there before. In moments, the mind undoes what it took the body to achieve in an hour!

This is because the subtle (in this case, the Mental body) is more powerful than the gross. The gross Physical body is like ice. It takes time, effort and repetition to change it. Your Energy body is like water. All you need to do is give it a direction and energy will take whatever form it is given, causing the Physical body to follow. If the Mental body is in reaction, it is only a matter of seconds before the Energy body fuels the reaction and the Physical body experiences that reaction. This is why a yoga class is most effective when it works with the body, but also works with managing the mind, since the mind is more powerful than the body. Without this element, we may exercise the body daily, but have no control over that which can undo all our hard work: the mind.

The subtle-affects-the-gross principle can work against us, or it can work for us. Used consciously, it is the principle upon which an *Intention* is based. Let's see how this works. Stand up and try to touch your toes by bending forward. You might push yourself just a bit to see how far your Physical body can go. Make a note of how far you go and how it feels in your body. Now close your eyes. Stand up tall without moving. Do not bend forward. In your *mind's eye only*, on an exhaling breath, visualize your Physical body easily and effortlessly bending forward and releasing toward the floor. With each breath out, imagine the hamstrings getting longer, the low back releasing, the head dropping down, the torso heavily dropping toward the floor. *Now do the same exercise with your Physical body.* Take a breath in and as you exhale, bend forward. Make a note of how your body feels and if you are deeper in the pose. *Most people will find they have moved further into the pose.*

This demonstrates the principle that *form follows thought.* The gross is affected by the subtle. The body follows what we see in the mind's eye. Working with the subtle as a means to influence the gross is extremely powerful. You can change what is happening in the body much more quickly and easily by working at the subtler levels beyond it.

It has been proven in many different studies that visualizing the body repairing itself will increase the rate at which it heals.[96] It has also been shown that visualizing a particular gymnastic routine, baskets made, or high jump achieved actually increases real-time performance. Data compiled from 19 published studies, covering 23 interventions, has concluded that relaxation and visualization-based techniques *are* effective for athletes.[97] This further demonstrates the principle that we can increase the body's capacities and potentials by simply working at the subtler levels of being.

Unconscious Intention

However, if not conscious, this same principle can produce unconscious, inadvertent intentions we don't necessarily intend to create.

Any persistent thought patterns coming from the Bliss body are continuously moving from the subtle to the gross to affect the Physical body. What we repeatedly think with conviction and feeling can eventually materialize into the Physical body.

This is not so different from what science tells us. The body is hearing everything we say. Thoughts are translated into their biological equivalent called *neuropeptides*. These thoughts and feelings in the form of neuropeptides are received everywhere in the body: stomach cells, intestines, heart, lungs and kidneys. These neuropeptides fit into the receptors on other cell walls like a lock and key. They tell the cells—brain cells, immune cells, lymphocytes, monocytes, and T cells—how to behave based on the thoughts, moods and emotions we are experiencing. As Indian-American author, medical doctor and Ayurveda advocate Deepak Chopra states, "Your cells literally hear everything you say about yourself in every moment of your existence." Every part of your body is "talking" to other parts of your body.[98]

Interestingly, your heart and gut can also create the same neuropeptides the brain makes—meaning *they are* sensing and speaking to you in some fashion. When we say to ourselves, "My heart is saying I should do this," or, "My gut is telling me something is wrong here," our heart and gut *are* communicating with us!

A study done at UCLA measured immune markers of method actors fully embodying various emotions for an entire day. One group acted out helpful, happy, optimistic emotions, while the other group acted out sad, heavy and pessimistic emotions. Both groups fully embodied and personified the emotions and feelings they were given. At the end of the day, immune markers were again measured. Those who had embodied the oppressive emotions throughout the day showed significant declines in their T-cell production—a critical part of the immune system.[99]

As long as the various thoughts, feelings and emotions related to the human experience are coming and going, there is no problem. It is simply a part of the richness of life played through the body. However, there are certain thoughts, beliefs and events we tend to latch onto over and over. When they come around, we hang on to them. We chew on them and repeat them—not just for an hour or two—but sometimes for days, months and even years. That means we are telling our cells how to behave over and over in a particular way. If the thought and feeling pattern is not helpful, it will be consistently detrimental to the body. *Persistent thoughts will have a persistent effect on the body.*

I am not suggesting the only cause of disease is our thoughts. However, I am suggesting that the thoughts we think and the emotions we consistently revisit *do* have an influence on our health. The way we interact with our thoughts can help or hinder our body's ability to heal. The subtle has enormous power and influence on the health of the body, and this is often overlooked or even dismissed by modern medicine.

In fact, American psychologist Jeanne Achterberg in her published and peer-reviewed article in the *Journal of the American Society for Psychical Research* concluded, after reviewing numerous research studies, that *the mind contributes the greatest variance to the course of health* and that to ignore the role of mental factors in the treatment of disease is a gross oversight.[100]

A Few Studies Demonstrating the Influence of the Subtle *Koshas* on Body and Health

Deepak Chopra in his audio CD *The New Physics of Healing* describes a study conducted at the Health Education and Wellness Program of Massachusetts to determine the greatest risk factors associated with death from coronary heart disease. All the traditional sources of heart disease were on the list: diet, exercise, smoking, heredity, weight and stress. However, the study revealed that the *greatest determining factors* of one's likelihood to die from coronary heart disease were the answer to two simple questions: "Are you happy?" and "Do you enjoy your job?" These had to do with self-happiness and job satisfaction ratings. Take a moment to ponder your response to these questions. Your answers might tell you a little bit about your thoughts and how they may be affecting your health.

The point is that what we think matters. I'm certainly not suggesting we all go out and eat hamburgers, french fries and smoke cigarettes. But it is critical to recognize that *how we think* is the greatest determining factor above *all* the diet and exercise we do or don't do. That is a phenomenal piece of information and something to which we need to pay attention. It once again demonstrates the principle that the subtle affects the gross. It is like going to the gym. We can work out all we want, but if the mind is still creating worry, stress and fear, it can undo much of what we accomplish at the Physical body level. The same is true here. We can diet and exercise, but if we are not attending to the mind, it can be our own undoing.

The study on coronary heart disease cited by Dr. Chopra also examined the day and time most people die of a heart attack. When do you suppose that is? *Monday morning, 9am.* It is almost as if we are saying to ourselves over and over, "I hate my job, I can't do it anymore." Eventually the body takes the order and says, "Yes sir, you can't do it anymore." And we no longer can.[101]

Study after study confirms the same trend: what you think matters. At the University of London, *three 10-year studies* concluded that emotional stress is more predictive of death from cancer and cardiovascular disease than smoking. People who were unable to effectively manage their stress had a 40% higher death rate than individuals who were non-stressed.[102]

According to a Mayo Clinic study of individuals with heart disease, the strongest predictor of future cardiac events, such as cardiac death, cardiac arrest and heart attacks, was psychological stress.[103]

A number of well-controlled studies have linked depressive symptoms with coronary heart disease as the leading cause of death in the United States. For example, a 13-year prospective study suggested that individuals with major depression had a 4.5 times greater risk of a heart attack compared to those with no history of depression. In data from the Normative Aging Study, higher levels of anxiety were associated with almost double the risk of fatal coronary heart disease.[104]

Chronic anger and hostility also negatively impact health. One well-conducted nine-year population-based study found that men with high hostility had more than twice the risk of cardiovascular mortality compared with men low in hostility.[105]

In theory, doing less should be less stressful on the body. However, unemployment has just the opposite effect. The subtle unseen factors of worry, uncertainty and loss of self-esteem all take an enormous toll. Unemployed men and their families show increased death rates, particularly from suicide and lung cancer. They show significant reduction in psychological well-being with a greater incidence of intentional self-harm (parasuicide), depression and anxiety. Studies show that the use of doctor and hospital services increase even for those who previously did not use medical services, and that those who are unemployed use more prescribed medicines.[106]

It is clear that our thoughts and emotions affect our health. The question for us is, "How can we manage our thoughts and *the effects* of our thoughts with Yoga Nidra?"

Yoga Nidra: Influencing Health with *Intention*

The good news is we are all good at manifesting—we can effectively create results from subtle levels. The bad news is we are often manifesting what we don't intend to create. We are unconsciously and inadvertently manifesting what we *don't* want, rather than what we *do* want.

An *Intention* makes *conscious* use of the principle of manifestation. By changing subtle thoughts and feelings consciously, we can change the body quickly and effectively—much faster than working with the density of the Physical body. Working with the Physical body is like working with a block of ice. Working at subtler levels is like working with water. With *Intention* placed at subtle, more malleable levels, we can easily shift what appears dense and difficult to change.

The subtler the level at which an *Intention* is placed, the more powerful it will be. An *Intention* placed at the mind, will always be influenced by what is held above it in the Bliss body. If we can place an *Intention* at the Bliss body itself, the effect on the Mental, Energy and Physical bodies will be the most powerful. This is exactly what Yoga Nidra is designed to do. In Yoga Nidra, the *Intention* is established and rooted in the Bliss body—the most potent and influential of all bodies or *koshas*, including the mind.

In Yoga Nidra, we enter the Bliss body and are completely disengaged and free from other voices that have been affecting the body/mind system. Then, in the absence of conflicting voices, we plant the seed of *Intention* here. While affirmations in the waking state might be effective to some degree, they will not compare to the depth and power of an *Intention* placed in the deepest states of Yoga Nidra.

Yoga Nidra: Influencing Health through *Turiya*

Science now demonstrates that the body is not a static machine. Although it appears to remain the same, as Deepak Chopra puts it, it is more like a perpetually flowing river in which each part of the body is constantly regenerating itself. On the molecular and cellular level, our skin cells are replaced every 30 days, the liver cells turn over every six weeks, the stomach lining every five days. In two years, 90% of the whole body will be replaced, and some say the whole body will be replaced brick by brick, atom by atom, in seven years.[107]

What is keeping the body the same then? If the body is constantly in flux, it must be something outside the body that is constantly directing it into a particular form. In Yoga, this would be considered the effect of *samskaras*. We have all seen people who have literally come to "wear" their lives. The beliefs they hold are evident in the way they hold their bodies and the expressions on their faces. Their physiology has formed itself to match their beliefs or *samskaras* about the world.

Yogis go so far as to say the body is the visible version of our thoughts and beliefs. And that the reason we recreate the same body patterns over and over again is due to the concepts (*samskaras*) we are holding which are directing the body's physiology. Change the concepts and we can change the physiology.

There are of course biological changes that *do* happen with time. It is true that the body ages and will die at a certain point. Nevertheless, how we look, feel and act *as* the body ages is very flexible and subject to our thoughts and emotions.

Breaking the Glass Ceiling of Our Beliefs Frees Our Healing Potential

Perhaps, it is these same beliefs and *samskaras* that limit the true healing capacity of the body. Deepak Chopra, Bernie Siegel and numerous pioneering non-traditional doctors, healers and researchers believe this. If the body is constantly renewing itself and is fully capable of healing itself, they suggest the belief that the body *cannot* change is actually limiting its ability to heal.

In India, elephant trainers train baby elephants by chaining them to a tree. The baby elephant is not only physically hampered, but eventually becomes bound by its own perception that if it is chained, it cannot move. Even when the elephant is fully grown and could easily uproot a tree and go anywhere it chooses, it remains stationary—even if it is not tied to a tree and only has a chain around its neck. In the same way, even though we are free to create any kind of reality we want, we do not know it. *We believe ourselves imprisoned, and therefore we are. In truth, we are not imprisoned except in our own memory and thoughts.*

What if the body is actually much more capable of healing itself than we give it credit? When we see it as a dense block of ice, essentially unmoving and difficult to heal, it becomes just that. Perhaps our own beliefs limit our ability to heal.

Years ago, cancer was almost synonymous with death. Now it is quite normal to have all kinds of cancers and survive. Perhaps the belief that one can survive and heal from cancer is as much a factor as new treatments. In fact, it is now common for doctors to tell patients that their *attitude and will to heal* will be one of the most critical factors in their survival.

When HIV was first diagnosed, people were passing away in great numbers. Then people like the legendary basketball player Magic Johnson began to demonstrate it was possible to be HIV positive and live a healthy, normal life. Twenty years later, Magic Johnson is still going strong. Today, thousands of people are HIV positive and live full lives. Is this just medication? Or is it also that once we *believe* we can live, the body actually does? Even without modern drugs, about one in five hundred HIV-positive individuals have managed to keep their own AIDS at bay for decades without any antiretroviral therapy.[108]

This phenomenon is not just limited to medicine. We see it in high performance sports. Researchers used to say it was physiologically impossible to run a four-minute mile. They said the heart would stop and a person would die. The first time Roger Bannister broke the record, the "limit" of reality was broken. Within 46 days the record was broken again, and in the next year three or four other people achieved the same feat. It is not that these individuals were physically incapable before—now they just *believed* it to be possible. *This was what unlocked the potential of the body.*

What if, in the deepest states of Yoga Nidra—the *turiya* state— the beliefs and limitations that normally shape and bind the body, drop away? Can you see how the body would be free to spontaneously heal itself? This is exactly what Ayurveda, the sister science of Yoga suggests. Spontaneous healing happens in the state of *turiya*. This is because we are temporarily freed from the limitations of our own mind which usually curb the body's true healing potential.

Aligning Behind the Body's Ability to Heal Itself

Intention can help us break free from narrow, outdated concepts and open up the body's greater potential. *Intentions* align the entire body/mind complex behind the body's ability to heal itself. It unfetters the constraints within which we believe the body operates and unleashes its full potential.

This phenomenon is known to modern science as the "placebo effect." The body's ability to heal itself through firm conviction has somehow been seen as suspect. If a medication with all kinds of side effects is curing your illness, that is fine. Yet if you have healed your own body through belief, with no side effects, there must be something wrong with that. What is wrong with your ailments disappearing if they are truly gone? Does it matter if healing was achieved through something other than medication? I believe this distrust of the placebo effect comes from the notion that healing just can't be that simple. It has to be harder, more complicated. *To believe that, is to make it so.*

Yoga Nidra: *Dis-Identification* and Health

These days, there are more and more studies about the health benefits of meditation. Yoga Nidra is a meditation technique. It is designed to help the practitioner *see, versus believe,* the thoughts that are moving through the sky of awareness. This is our Tool of *Dis-identification*. Meditation engenders and gives rise to *Dis-identification*. This effect of meditation and Yoga Nidra is crucial to our health because: *the level of effect of a thought is directly related to our attachment to it.*

The problem is not thoughts, but our relationship to those thoughts. If thoughts are "seen" rather than believed or worn, they will not affect the body chemically. The less attached we are to thoughts, the less effect they will have on us. Thousands of thoughts, feelings, emotions and their chemical counterparts are moving through the body all the time. Yet not all of them are affecting us in the same way. In fact, most of them come and go—creating little or no chemical effect. Like a ticker tape parade, thoughts are constantly moving through with a ceaseless commentary on everything. Thoughts have no power to hurt us unless we believe them and invest energy in them. The thoughts we attach to and invest in are likely to be the same ones we have attached to in the past, reinforcing our world view. These are the ones that can wreak havoc on our health and the ones we need tools to manage.

The beauty of *Dis-identification* is that we don't have to get rid of our thoughts. This is a good thing because the more we fight our thoughts, the more they grow. As Yogi Desai says, "Fighting thoughts is like fighting fire with gasoline. The more you fight, the stronger the thoughts will become."

Meditation is the opposite of fighting. It is simply allowing the thought to move through unobstructed—with no attachment, no fear, no commentary at all. It is the act of noticing a cloud of thought moving through awareness. The beauty of Yoga Nidra is that it takes you to spaces where this happens effortlessly and teaches your body and brain the skill of doing it in everyday life.

If we are not attaching to thoughts, it is as if the thoughts are not there. There is no effect. Even if we *do* engage a thought and react to it, we can still shorten the period between the time we pick it up and put it down again. Each instance in which we succeed in shortening the reaction phase, we are lessening the overall chemical effects on our body, and we are actually building our health.

A study of 5,716 middle-aged people found that those most able to regulate their mind and emotions were over 50 times more likely to be alive and without chronic disease 15 years later as compared to those with the least self-regulation skills.[109] This demonstrates the power of learning to regulate our thoughts and emotions rather than being dragged around by them. Yoga Nidra, a powerful combination of meditation and *Intention*, gives us these Tools of self-regulation.

Yoga Nidra: *Integration* and Your Health

Integration helps manage the *effects* of thoughts to which we have repeatedly and consistently attached. Habituated thinking patterns create biochemical changes in the body. These minute physical changes can eventually manifest as disease in the body. Yoga Nidra clears the effects of these crippling thought patterns, resistances, and blocks from the system, preventing manifestation on a physical level. It helps us release core issues that keep us orbiting around the same concerns over and over. Once the core issue is released with Yoga Nidra and is no longer an issue, the mind no longer circulates around it. For example, the more we release core fears around having enough, feeling safe or feeling worthy, the less the mind will be occupied with those fears and the less the body will have to pay the price for them.

Yoga Nidra: *Relaxation, Restoration* and Your Health

Prana, when free of the mind, accelerates the healing of the body. This is because the same fuel that feeds the body, feeds the mind. *The less energy burned by the mind, the more energy is available to heal the body.* This is why a doctor will tell you to get plenty of rest when you are ill. Mental rest, along with physical rest, will allow the energy normally hijacked by the mind to be reallocated to heal the body. Yoga Nidra provides not only physical, but also deep mental rest with even greater potency and effectiveness than sleep.

Many healing modalities work at the levels we have mentioned above. The beauty of Yoga Nidra is that it includes all of these benefits in one modality. An acupuncture session will increase the body's restorative abilities. A psychotherapy session can help integrate emotions and events that may be related to a current illness. A meditation class may help manage your relationship to thoughts. Yoga Nidra does *all* of this.

Yoga Nidra: *Realization* and Health

The more we rest in *turiya*, the more we are freed from identification with that which is causing disease. Freedom from old thinking patterns provides room for spontaneous healing to occur. In addition, the Tool of *Realization* can also be particularly helpful in the midst of a non-negotiable physical condition that is unlikely to change.

Many report that Yoga Nidra provides respite from doctors, family concerns, worries and treatments which commonly accompany an illness. It is a place where a person in physical distress can retreat and completely let go of everything. Having time each day free of the fear and uncertainty around illness, gives the body time to heal itself if it is going to happen. If it is not going to happen, it allows us to accept the changes of the body with more grace and surrender to the process through the *Realization* that we are more than the body.

If there is no sense of anything beyond the body itself, it is very difficult to watch the body decline from conditions like multiple sclerosis, Parkinson's, Alzheimer's or terminal cancer. If the body is *you*, when the body cannot do what it once did, it can be very hard to accept. Loss of memory, muscle movement, pain—everything that is happening to the body feels like it *is* you. It can feel like you are losing who you are when you lose what the body can do. *The truth is you are more than the body.* Even as the body changes, the Presence beyond it always abides. Yoga Nidra allows you to connect with this part of you and anchors you in the steadiness of the unchanging Self.

Yoga Nidra is a powerful tool for hospice work and terminal illness. When we have identified with the body and mind as the totality of who we are, the fear is that when the body dies, there will be nothing more. For many, this can be the basis of our fear of dying. It can also be the reason we have such a hard time letting go of our loved ones. Yoga Nidra practice allows us to progressively let go of identification with the body. In essence, it is practice for the definitive release of the body—death—which at some point we will all experience. Every time we go into Yoga Nidra we are resting beyond the temporal existence of the body. Consciously recognizing that there is an abiding Self that resides beyond the Physical body gives peace and a greater ability to let go more naturally and effortlessly when the time comes.

CHAPTER SIXTEEN

Yoga Nidra for Depression and Anxiety

In this section, we will apply our knowledge and understanding of Yogic teachings to various common ailments in society today. We will explore the Yogic perspective on the root causes of modern conditions and look at how the Tools of Yoga Nidra can help. The ancient truths of Yoga were designed to solve all core human conflicts. They carry the power and essence of thousands of years of accumulated wisdom. It is not necessary to adapt the teachings, rather we can investigate how their timeless truths are still relevant to every aspect of our lives. Even though we live in a technological age, we still suffer from the human condition—a ceaselessly restless mind and a forgetfulness of our peaceful nature. Today, we call these effects stress, anxiety and depression. We experience insomnia, disease, and addiction. We will see how the core truths and practices of Yoga Nidra can help resolve every one of these conditions and more.

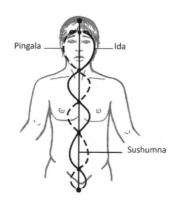

Figure 18: *Ida, pingala,* and *sushumna* imbalances may play a role in depression and anxiety.

Artwork by JoElizabeth James

Earlier, in the chapter on stress, we discussed *pingala* and *ida* as two elemental inner energies that relate to the sympathetic and the parasympathetic nervous systems (Figure 18). *Pingala*, corresponds with the sympathetic nervous system, the right nostril and left brain. Too much *pingala* creates excess tension through overdoing. *Ida* corresponds to the parasympathetic nervous system. It is the resting, recuperative state which relates to the left nostril and right brain. Too much recuperation can also act as a stressor on the body. Too much sleep, lack of activity and movement can set the stage for disease just as much as too much doing.

Yogis believe that the imbalance in these two energies is one of the primary root causes of disease. In science, this imbalance is called stress and is similarly proven to cause disease. According to Yoga, the balance between these energies creates optimal health. Yoga Nidra balances these energies.

One of the measurable effects of Yoga Nidra is balanced activity in both halves of the brain so they work in simultaneous unity. You can also see this effect with the even flow of breath through *both nostrils equally* following Yoga Nidra practice. This indicates right/left brain balance in which both energies are operating in complementary unity. This state of balanced energy allows the body to heal symptoms arising from tension/relaxation imbalances and allows entry into unified states of consciousness.

So far, we know that the imbalance of tension and relaxation, *pingala* and *ida*, creates a state of excess stress in the body on the physical level. What if imbalances in *ida* and *pingala* do not just manifest on a physical level, but on a psychological level as well? What if depression and anxiety could indicate a *subtle* imbalance of *ida* and *pingala*, resulting in corresponding mental and emotional states?

Let's explore this idea and see if it makes sense to you. Whether or not you experience anxiety or depression at the clinical level, we all have certain internal habits and ways of being that manifest on the *ida/pingala* spectrum.

Stress is usually connected to fear. We fear we will fail—that we won't get to work on time, get a project done, will lose our job or our marriage. Fear can cause stress at an even greater level—such as a trauma. Each of us has certain "go-to" behaviors in the presence of fear. These could be strategies we learned in childhood. They could be based on our personality or simply how we have learned to best survive in life.

The strategies fall into one of two major categories which I will call an *ida* strategy or *pingala* strategy. Most of us have a combination of both, or we swing back and forth between the two to some degree. The *ida* strategy in the presence of fear and stress is *collapse*. The *pingala* strategy in the presence of stress is *control*. I suggest that each of these strategies taken to their extreme can result in depression (collapse) or anxiety (control).

Depression: An *Ida* Pattern Under Stress

The state of stress in the body parallels fear in the mind and puts the body into a constant, low-level, *fight or flight* state. Stress generates a chemical condition in the body that can predispose it to certain mental and emotional states, most commonly, depression or anxiety.

Depression often begins under some kind of stress. It could be mental or emotional demands, like pressure at work or the loss of a relationship or the death of a loved one. In the presence of this kind of pressure, excess *ida* will tend to collapse into fear, insecurity and uncertainty. *Ida* is the resting, receptive energy, but taken to an extreme, it can move us toward being passive and listless.

An excess *ida* person will typically feel depleted and hopeless. They tend to experience the world as a victim—weak, paralyzed and helpless. Any effort seems impossible and being in the world feels like moving through molasses.

Excess *Ida* Cycle

- Depletion
- Hopelessness
- Listlessness
- Feel like the victim
- Weak, unable to act
- Paralyzed
- Hopeless thought cycle

We can have a pre-existing tendency to move to the *ida* side. This pre-existing vulnerability can include a genetic pre-disposition or chemical and hormonal conditions such as postpartum depression. These chemical and hormonal states can incline a person toward collapse and feeling overwhelmed by life. Old beliefs and thought patterns resulting from world views learned in childhood can do the same thing. Some examples of *ida* beliefs or *samskaras* could be: "Things never work out for me.", "I might as well not even try.", "Why bother?", "What's the point?" or "I might as well not be here."

This excess *ida* state seems to strongly coincide with what we commonly call depression. Depression is not the same as being sad. Depression can include sadness, but can also include a lack of feeling. It can be experienced as the absence of excitement, hope or happiness about anything. The Webster's Dictionary definition of depression is: "A disorder marked especially by inactivity, difficulty in thinking and concentration, a significant increase or decrease in appetite and time spent sleeping, feelings of dejection and hopelessness, and sometimes *suicidal tendencies.*"

If you read this in the context of excess *ida*, there does seem to be a strong correlation between science and Yoga. Perhaps depression is, at least in part, a mental and emotional state resulting from too much *ida* energy and not enough *pingala energy.*

In fact, in Western treatment models, the antidote to depression is very often to try to help the person bring in more *pingala* energy. The effort is to develop goals, motivation, and hope—to have something to look forward to and feel excited about. A therapist will encourage a depressed person to physically move, to exercise and to *do* things. These are more *pingala* qualities, which trigger *pingala* states in the body.

Which Comes First?

You might ask, "Which comes first, our ways of thinking and behaving, or the chemical states that create the environment for us to think and behave in a certain way?" Current research indicates it is both. The cycle of depression is not merely thoughts, nor is it merely body chemistry. The more we tend to view life situations in a collapsed, hopeless way, the more we create chemical states in the body that perpetuate this mental and emotional cycle.

Conversely, the biological state of the body can predispose us toward certain thought and emotional patterns. Participation in these thoughts and emotional patterns only exacerbates the issue. In short, a chemical state in the body can trigger certain ways of thinking and feeling and certain habitual ways of thinking and feeling can create corresponding chemical states in the body.

The cycle can be triggered at any point. Once triggered, depression is like a revving engine that gains momentum with each added thought and chemical response until we find ourselves being pulled down into a whirlpool of thoughts, sensations and emotions from which it feels like we cannot escape. The beauty of Yoga Nidra is that it not only creates the biological state of chemical balance where we are less likely to drop into habitual mental and emotional patterns, but it *also* helps us disengage from, and redirect those thoughts before they gain a momentum of their own.

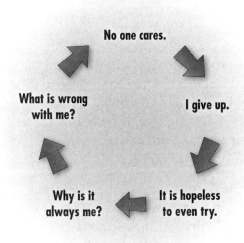

Figure 19: An example of the thought and sensation cycle associated with depression.

In this diagram (Figure 19) are some thoughts that can be triggered in the presence of stress or in the presence of certain body chemistry. If the cycle begins at the level of thoughts, there may be a triggering event. For example, a loved one ending a relationship. The first thought, which could be any, will trigger a cascade of chemical reactions in the body. For example, "No one cares" may trigger a feeling of heaviness in the heart. The way we interpret and label that sensation serves as fodder for the next thought, "I give up."

Believing, attaching to, and participating in this thought only increases the intensity of the sensation in the body, drawing us even further down into the depression spiral. That gives rise to the next thought, "It's hopeless to even try" which creates another sensation, and another story *about* that sensation—with each progressive thought and resulting sensation pulling us even deeper. Once it begins, one thought/sensation adds to another. Within a short time, the feelings and thoughts may no longer be just about this one event, but are magnified to include our whole life. We might say to ourselves, "Why is it *always* me?" or "What is wrong with me?"

It is not one thought, but groups of thoughts, sensations and feelings that trigger one another. Suddenly our whole life is colored by this experience. Not only that, but the accumulation of thoughts and feelings has moved so close to us, it has become all we can see in our field of vision. We have no perspective, no ability to see anything else. It feels as if these thoughts and feelings are the whole of our existence.

The more we engage in the cycle, the deeper the cycle becomes until it may feel like we can't get out. What might have begun as conscious participation in feeding a particular thought or feeling, has gained momentum of its own—pulling us down into its whirlpool. If we have a history of being dragged down into the whirlpool, we will be more disposed to have it retriggered under the right circumstances. Eventually the body can become so accustomed to this biochemical state that it operates here even in the absence of precipitating thoughts.

Depression is a *Samskara*

Let's say that when in the presence of stress, we tend to get into a hopeless mindset. The mind is "set" because this has been repeated before and a chemical pathway has been imprinted to predispose us to think and feel a particular way. In essence, it is a *samskara*. Whether mental or chemically predisposed, the more we repeat and go with the tendency to think and feel a certain way, the deeper its groove becomes. However, just because you may have a predisposition to pessimistic thinking or depression, doesn't mean that is your only choice. It just means that for whatever reason, there are certain impulses that will tend to move you in that direction. This is not something to be afraid of, but something to learn how to manage and work with just as you might a tendency to get a backache. Once you know what they are and where they come from, you can do what is necessary to help head them off or cut them short when you see them coming.

How does Yoga Nidra Help?

Restoration

A consistent practice of Yoga Nidra will help get and keep the body chemistry in the ideal place, in addition to whatever medication or therapy may be necessary. In particular, Yoga Nidra releases serotonin, which is a key factor in many kinds of depression, as well as dopamine, which has to do with focus, motivation, energy, pleasure and the desire to *do*.

We know that meditation significantly increases the size of the hippocampus, which is also related to mood and depression. Serotonin acts as fertilizer for the hippocampus and brain changes in this area can be seen in as little as eight weeks of consistent Yoga Nidra practice.[110]

Sleep Cycles

Abnormal sleep cycles are often associated with depression. Yoga Nidra can help establish a healthy sleep cycle.

Relaxation

Stress hormones in the system create an environment in which depression can be triggered. Yoga Nidra reduces stress hormones.

Dis-identification and Intention

Yoga Nidra helps create a different relationship to the triggering thoughts so it is easier for you to withdraw and redirect them. In fact, this is what cognitive therapy is designed to do for depression; it helps you manage your relationship to thoughts. Yoga Nidra is a way to teach your brain and body how to do this naturally.

Anxiety: A *Pingala* Pattern Under Stress

Pingala is our active, doing, making it happen, energy. It is the gas, while *ida* is the brakes. In balance, *pingala* will give us the fire to do and *ida* will tell us when to stop, let go and relax. When we are under stress, we can easily go to the side of trying to do too much. We try to keep too many balls in the air, doing and doing and doing. We think that we cannot stop doing, because if we do, all the balls will drop. This can lead to a state of excess *pingala* energy, which I believe is comparable to what we now call anxiety. In fact, anxiety is often defined as, "Intense, excessive and persistent worry and fear about everyday situations." The *pingala* (or anxiety) approach is to feel responsible for everything and to try to control everything. Excess *pingala* has us trying to control even the uncontrollable things that are outside our influence.

Out of balance with *ida*, *pingala* will manage stress, fear and uncertainty with *doing*. We become afraid when life gets uncertain. To manage, we tell ourselves to just do more. If we can get everything under control, or just get one more thing done, then everything will be okay. We keep running and running, telling ourselves that one day we will relax, but that day never comes.

The more we do, the more it feels like we have to keep doing. We can't get off the treadmill.

It may only take a small trigger to move from such stress into full blown anxiety. Like the straw that breaks the camel's back, suddenly the amount of stress is no longer manageable. The body gets pushed into a highly overactive condition tipping the nervous system over from stress into a bodily state experienced as pure fear. Eventually this pathway can become so entrenched, we may go there without any apparent trigger at all. Anxiety is actually just the experience of fear. The heart constricts and beats faster. Our breath becomes shallow or constricted, body temperature rises, or we begin to perspire. If the sensation lingers longer than usual, or if it arises unbidden and for no apparent reason, we are likely to become afraid of the sensations themselves. This only makes it worse. We panic about the sensation and instead of passing, it tends to remain and escalate. A full-blown panic attack is an anxiety attack with the added thought, "I must be having a heart attack." The thought fuels the anxiety and can continue until one goes to the emergency room. The more we can stay relaxed amidst those sensations without adding a story to it, the more quickly they will pass.

As with depression, the excessive chemical state of stress in the body can create just the right environment for anxiety to take hold. Stress hormones, already heightened in the body, are more than ready to trigger a strong *fight or flight* response. If we have created a pathway (*samskara*), it will more and more often become the automatic response.

Remember that at the mental and emotional levels, the habit for those with excess *pingala* is to think they are responsible for everything, even things that are outside of individual control. The thought/sensation cycle can go something like this. A stressor, perhaps a job promotion, triggers us to want to do our best. Doing is not just about getting things done. *What we do* is very much connected with *who we are*. If *what we do fails, we see ourselves as a failure.* This creates a tendency to take on more and more things, and it drives us to need to do them all perfectly. Imperfection and mistakes are all seen as a reflection of our essential being. We feel responsible for more and more. We try to keep feeling good about ourselves by making sure we do it all perfectly, but at the same time, we know we cannot ensure the outcomes we are relying on. So along with doing and perfection arise fear and a sense of powerlessness.

Burnout

Tying our sense of self-esteem to what we do and what we achieve can play a significant role in anxiety and burnout. What we do and the outcomes we create are so connected with our sense of self-worth, we *must* succeed at everything. Not only that, we can't stop doing because our achievements are our source of self-esteem. This is often what drives our *over-doing.* We are so focused on proving ourselves to be worthy by what we do, that we are willing to override the body's own well-being. Maybe we don't work twelve hour days because we want to, but because that is what is needed to gain the acknowledgment, appreciation and approval we seek—even from ourselves. Work is often not about work at all. It is used as a medium to remedy our lack of self-worth.

In my experience, it is these unconscious mental and emotional drives that push us to overdo. We think that to *be* more we have to *do* more. This lead to a lack of balance. The body, stuck in doing mode, can overtax the adrenals—leading to a state of complete physical exhaustion. What is needed in addition to restoring the body is to expand our sense of self-worth beyond what we accomplish and develop a true spiritual practice that reinforces our internal wholeness.

- Will

- Make it Happen

- Control

- Perfectionism

- DOING

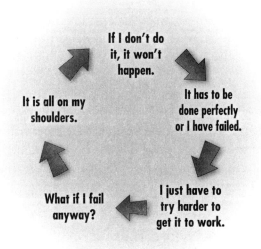

Figure 20: An example of the thought and sensation cycle associated with anxiety.

In anxiety and burnout, the same principle of thoughts and sensations triggering and building upon one another applies. Let's take the example of a job promotion. You are excited, but at the same time anxious. You know you got the promotion over a lot of other people who might be quite happy if you make some mistakes. This circumstance triggers a sensation of tightness in your chest, and the thought cycle begins (Figure 20) with "It's all on my shoulders." You tell yourself you will make it happen. You have to. "If I don't do what needs to be done, nothing will happen." It's all on you now. That thought increases the sensation of pressure in the body. Maybe the stomach tightens, breath shallows, muscles tighten. Perhaps you stay awake at night trying to think of all the details you might have missed. The thought going through your head is, "It has to be done perfectly or I have failed." To keep away the fear, you say to yourself, "I will make it work. I have to. I just have to try harder." You get yourself into even more of a *pingala*/doing state. Then the thoughts come in, "What if I fail? What if I missed something? What if people talk behind my back?" You know that no matter how hard you try, something will eventually go wrong.

You can see how these thoughts and sensations combine into mounting pressure, which at some point will tip the body over into a fear/anxiety response. Once the body becomes habituated to going into this cycle, it can take just a simple thought or sensation to trigger a full blown anxiety attack. Even something as simple as needing to pick up kids at school after work can trigger an episode. Sometimes there is no apparent trigger at all. The body can become so habituated to living in this groove, it wakes up in the anxiety state, or cannot fall asleep because of it.

How Can Yoga Nidra Help?

Relaxation

The stress state easily triggers anxiety. Getting the body out of the stress state significantly reduces the chance of triggering anxiety. The release of GABA, the body's version of valium, calms the system, as does the release of melatonin and serotonin. During Yoga Nidra, the entire body is flooded with the *Relaxation* response and excess stress hormones are removed from the system. The muscles relax, the heart slows down, and the breath deepens. The body remembers what it is to be relaxed, open, soft and at ease. In fact, it is actually difficult to be in an anxious state when the body is physically relaxed.

Restoration

A stronger prefrontal cortex and smaller amygdala allow discrimination and neutral perception to take control of the hair trigger *fight or flight* response that tends to hold us hostage. A widened perspective allows us to relate to worries differently. We see worries not as truths, but simply as thoughts passing through. As such, it is easier to take them less seriously.

Realization

Finally, in Yoga Nidra, we see and experience wholeness independent of what we have achieved. We remember we are more than what we do. This makes it easier to make choices that serve the whole person and our overall health and well-being. You might notice at the end of a Yoga Nidra that everything feels good. Yet nothing has changed. You haven't done more on your "to do" list, but everything still feels okay and peaceful. You recognize that feeling good exists independent of what you achieve. It comes from experiencing *who you are*. It doesn't mean you don't get things done, but that is less and less used as a metric to define who and what you are. When there is less pressure on the results of outside circumstances to bolster your self-esteem, there is less fear and anxiety about them. You can more easily just do your best and then let go.

Most of us Experience *Ida* and *Pingala* Swings Under Stress

Regardless of whether we experience true, clinical depression or anxiety, I believe we can all recognize ourselves in these patterns. Perhaps you have seen yourself go into a collapse pattern under stress. Perhaps feeling sorry for yourself. Or maybe you whip yourself into a frenzy to "get it right," telling yourself to "try harder" and "do more."

Maybe you see yourself doing a combination of *both* at different times. I think most of us do this. We become stressed, and we swing from one pole to the other (Figure 21). We feel like the victim— alone and overwhelmed. Then we try to balance things out by moving to the other extreme. We try to "fix" it by doing more and managing better. We do that for a time until we realize that we will never have things totally under control and managed perfectly. So we swing back to the *ida* side saying to ourselves, "Why bother?", "It's too much.", "It won't work out anyway." "Things never work out for me." In each case, we seek the antidote to what we are feeling in its opposite.

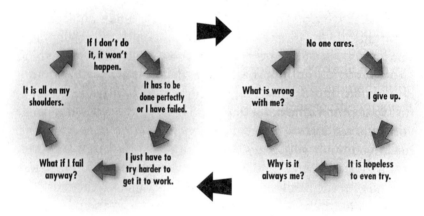

Pingala (I'm Responsible Cycle)   *Ida (Hopeless Cycle)*

Figure 21: In the presence of stress, many of us swing from one polar extreme to the other.

While this may be the right track, the error is in going to the opposite *extreme*, rather than trying to find the *balance* between the two. In a state of too much *ida*, we swing too much the other way. The more healthy place is the central point between *ida* and *pingala*—the state in which we do our best (*pingala*) and let go when we have done all we can (*ida*). This enables us to incorporate the best of both energies and allows us to do and let go in equal measure. Just as the antidote to stress is not endless leisure, the antidote to anxiety is not collapse. It is a healthy balance of *doing and non-doing, exertion and rest, doing your best and letting go*. This is when *ida* and *pingala* come into balance. We are restored to complementary wholeness and a state of health.

Finding the Balance

If you find yourself excessively in one pole, try to find balance by bringing in a *little* of the opposite energy to move back toward center. For example, if you are in too much "hopeless" *ida*, bring in the energies of fire, action, *Intention* and direction. Recognize that no matter what is happening outside, you are not the victim. You have the final say on any experience of your life. Life doesn't determine your experience, YOU do.

I find that people who tend toward depression have suppressed the *pingala*, fire energy. If we are afraid of confrontation, anger, saying "no" or establishing boundaries, we are likely afraid of our inner fire. Sometimes when we are afraid of that fire, we dampen it, suppress it, and put it away. This could be because we have seen what the destructive effects of fire can do, and we are afraid we will act in those same destructive ways.

Also, suppressed anger operates on the hydraulic principle. Suppress it here and it pops up there—often without warning. A significant practice for someone suffering from depression is accepting the energy of anger. This does not mean we dump that anger on other people, but acknowledge it is there and learn to use it and direct it in helpful and meaningful ways. If you learn to express that inner fire in healthy ways—like setting boundaries, saying no when needed, or respectfully contributing your point of view—this energy will begin to manifest in a more steady and balanced way. It will not need to come out in great bursts of unmanageable energy.

If you want to practice this, think of your inner fire as residing in the belly. To communicate it skillfully, it must pass through the heart to the throat *chakra*. Take your inner fire and let it be spoken and expressed through your heart with skill, love, and compassion, yet with truth and inner steadiness. If you recognize this as a practice for you, using it as an *Intention* in Yoga Nidra might be helpful. Maybe something like, "My heart can accept and express my inner fire with love."

If you find yourself with a *pingala* "responsibility" imbalance, you might experiment with consciously letting go and trusting. Rather than hiding your vulnerability or compensating for insecurities and fears with knowledge and achievements, simply *allow them to be*. Experiment with showing a little of your soft side, your imperfections, rather than needing to always have it together.

Here the *Intention* could be about accepting your insecurities, vulnerabilities and imperfections. "I accept my imperfections as a part of who I am." Reinforce that who you are right now is enough. You are not defined by what you do or achieve, but who you *are*. These fears and vulnerabilities about measuring up and having to be perfect are just old stories. They no longer need to run you.

Heart energy, which is your softness and vulnerability, needs space to be felt and allowed. Perhaps it has been dominated and protected by your inner fire. The more you can let the heart lead and be served by the inner fire, the more these two energies will come into balance. Another great intention here is "I do what I can (fire) and let go (heart)."

How Can I Use the Tools of Yoga Nidra Even If I Don't Have Depression or Anxiety?

Realization

Yoga Nidra helps you develop the meditative perspective that contains the tendencies to control and collapse, but can operate beyond either one. It cultivates awareness of the part of you that is already whole and at peace and doesn't need to do more ___ order to feel good about yourself.

Dis-Identification

Yoga Nidra puts the body and brain in the best state to notice thoughts and sensations without needing to add more drama to them. It is this drama that can exacerbate the control and collapse tendencies.

Intention

Use *Intention* to interrupt and redirect the controlling and collapsing conversations in your head and keep the body calm.

Integration

Focus on allowing emotions to move through rather than resisting or suppressing various parts of the human experience. Specifically, allow anger and aggression for depression, and allow vulnerability, fear, and insecurity for anxiety. Feel the physical sensations of worry or anxiety without labeling them.

Relaxation

Yoga Nidra maintains and restores sympathetic and parasympathetic nervous system balance, helping prevent or reverse the tendency to move into mental and emotional swings under stress.

Restoration

In Yoga Nidra, the two halves of the brain begin to operate as one. *Ida* and *pingala* (cooling and heating) come into natural energetic balance. Active and receptive energies return to a state of co-creative harmony where we are not swinging from one to the other, but resting in the sweet spot at the center of

both. Here, we are energetically balanced, centered and resilient to the tendencies of both anxiety and depression.

Related Studies

In fact, science verifies that meditation is most effective for
mood and anxiety disorders such as depression and anxiety.
Of all the benefits of meditation a critical overview of *82 studies, showed that the strongest evidence for the efficacy of meditation
was demonstrated for mood and anxiety disorders.* The studies also
found demonstrable benefit for epilepsy, symptoms of PMS and
menopausal symptoms.[111]

Sleep Cycles

Abnormalities in the circadian rhythm sleep cycle may set the
stage for depression. Longitudinal studies show that disordered
REM sleep appears to precede episodes of depression by about
five weeks. Four or five times a night, we cycle through periods of deep, relaxing sleep, marked by slow brainwaves (low
Theta and Delta). Then we burst into REM dream sleep (high
Theta) marked by dramatic brainwave activity and rapid eye
movements. Depressed individuals enter almost directly into
REM sleep, bypassing the slow-wave sleep cycle and displaying
greater intensity and duration of their REM sleep.

Scientists hypothesize that this disordered brainwave pattern
in sleep affects mood regulation and as a result is creating a
state where negative feelings are not discharged over time.[112]
Given this, Yoga Nidra could very well be of help in "exer-
cising" the natural flow through all brainwave states to help
correct abnormalities and teach the body to enter into a natural
sleep cycle. The release of melatonin may aid in this as well.
Furthermore, the practice of Yoga Nidra itself will move an
individual into deep Theta and Delta brainwave states to help

discharge accumulated mental and emotional detritus that may not have been released through biological sleep.

Anxiety

A study through the Department of Psychology at Stockholm University, Sweden, investigated the efficacy of Applied Relaxation and Cognitive Therapy in the treatment of generalized anxiety disorder. Thirty-six outpatients were randomized and treated individually for 12 weekly sessions. The results showed that both treatments yielded large improvements. Directly after the study, the reduction of anxiety symptoms was 53% for Applied Relaxation, but Cognitive Therapy still came out ahead at 62% effectiveness right after treatment. The most interesting finding, however, was at the follow up 8 weeks later, where a very different picture emerged. The effectiveness of Applied Relaxation *increased* over time, while the effectiveness of Cognitive Therapy decreased! The effectiveness of Applied Relaxation rose to 67%, while Cognitive Therapy had dropped to 56% effectiveness. This implies that relaxation-based treatments such as Yoga Nidra meditation may be more effective in the long term than psychotherapy. At the very least, they could be a powerful adjunct to traditional therapies and could help counteract the decline in effectiveness over time that is sometimes observed with traditional treatments.[113]

CHAPTER SEVENTEEN

Yoga Nidra for Insomnia and Sleep Deprivation

Yoga Nidra is a helpful tool in the resolution of both short-term and long-term insomnia in two ways. First, it helps prepare the proper state for the body and mind to easily fall asleep and sleep deeply. Second, for those who suffer from sleep deprivation, it can help make up for lost sleep and enable the body to rebalance itself.

We all know what it feels like to be lying in bed, eyes wide open, mind racing, waiting for sleep. Maybe our thoughts keep running over what we have to do, appointments we cannot forget, things we have to tell people. Or we're thinking about conversations we had, things that happened, events that could have gone differently. Before we know it, it is midnight, 1:00 am, even 2:00 am, before the mind finally gives up in exhaustion and the body can fall asleep. Or maybe you fall asleep with no problem, but suddenly wake up, unable to fall back asleep.

According to the United States Department of Health and Human Services, approximately 64 million Americans regularly suffer from insomnia. Insomnia is 1.4 times more common in women than in men.[114] A new report from the CDC shows that about 4 in every 100 Americans use prescription sleep aids. This is a concern because long-term use of sleep aids can actually prevent the deep restorative sleep the body needs to regenerate itself. Most doctors frown on long-term use of sleep aids because these "aids" have been linked to negative health effects and dependency as well.[115]

Maybe you don't have any trouble sleeping, but your job requires that you are up for long hours or odd hours. Maybe you are a first responder, a doctor or a nurse. Perhaps you serve in the military or often fly between time zones. Sleep deprivation and deregulated sleep patterns can significantly affect your health and compromise your ability to get restful, restorative sleep. It is important to pay particular attention if your ability to function effectively is diminished or if you feel tired and irritable the next morning.

How much we need to sleep varies from person to person and generally changes as we age. The National Institutes of Health suggests that school-age children need at least 10 hours of sleep daily, teens need 9 to 10 hours, and adults need 7 to 8 hours. According to data from the National Health Interview Survey conducted in 2005-2007, nearly 30% of adults reported an average of less than or equal to 6 hours of sleep per day. In 2009, only 31% of high school students reported getting at least 8 hours of sleep on an average school night. This is important if you consider the following:

If you take an "A" student who is scoring in the top 10% of her class and give her just under 7 hours of sleep on weekdays and 40 minutes more on weekends, she will begin to score in the bottom 9%.[116]

For soldiers responsible for operating complex military hardware, one night's loss of sleep results in 30% loss in overall cognitive skill with accompanying drop in performance. If two nights of sleep are lost, that figure becomes 60%.[117]

Continuous sleep shortages appear to accelerate parts of the aging process. For example, if a healthy 30-year-old is sleep deprived for six days (in this study about four hours per night), parts of the body chemistry soon decline to that of a 60-year-old. If the sleep-deprived person is allowed to recover, it will take almost a week to get back to the 30-year-old system![118]

Sleep Deprivation and Decision Making

We have all experienced what it is like to be sure we've done something right when we are dead tired, only to wake up the next morning and wonder how we made such a mistake. Lack of proper rest severely and measurably affects our ability to think and to make good decisions.

Consider people who need to be awake all night and you will see how important it is that cognitive performance be at its best: emergency room personnel, fire fighters, doctors, nurses and military personnel. Our lives rest in their hands. Performance can be affected and mistakes can easily be made due to lack of sleep.

Investigators ruled that sleep deprivation was a significant factor in the 1979 Three Mile Island nuclear accident, as well as the nuclear meltdown at Chernobyl in 1986. Extreme sleep deprivation played a crucial role in the grounding of the Exxon Valdez oil tanker, as well as the explosion of the Space Shuttle Challenger. In both instances, decision makers were required to make critical judgments while they may have been impaired because of lack of sleep.

The practice of Yoga Nidra shows promising results. In 2010, a study was conducted to assess whether meditation can improve performance and offset the effects of sleep loss. The primary study compared reaction times before and after 40-minute periods of meditation, a nap, or a control activity. *All ten novice meditators showed improved reaction times following meditation.* Sleep deprivation slowed reaction times, as did the nap. These results suggest that *meditation provides at least a short-term performance improvement even in novice meditators.* Now imagine what disasters and mistakes could be averted with a simple 20-minute practice of Yoga Nidra.

A second study was designed to determine whether meditation alters the need for sleep. This study compared sleep times of experienced meditators with non-meditators. It was found that time spent in meditation was associated with a significant decrease in total sleep need as compared to age and sex matched controls who did not meditate.[119] Whether meditation can actually pay off sleep debt is under further investigation. However, the ancient, time-tested teachings of Yoga Nidra already suggest this to be fact.

Sleep and Health

While sleeping well is no guarantee of good health, it does help to maintain the healthy functioning of the body. This is the time when the cells and tissues of the body have the opportunity to recover from the wear and tear of daily life. Functions such as tissue repair, muscle growth, protein synthesis and other critical restorative functions *occur almost exclusively during sleep (or in sleep-like brainwave states)*.[120] Most experts now agree that high-quality sleep is as important to health and well-being as nutrition and exercise. By robbing ourselves of sleep, we actually deprive ourselves of a very simple way to keep ourselves healthy.

<u>Consider the following research:</u>

- People who regularly sleep less than six hours per night tend to have excess body weight, while people who sleep an average of eight hours per night are more likely to have the lower relative body fat.[121]

- Sleeping less than five hours per night greatly increases the risk of having or developing type 2 diabetes while improved sleep can positively influence blood sugar control and reduce the effects of type 2 diabetes.[122] (Yoga Nidra is excellent for type 2 diabetes.)

- Even modestly reduced sleep (six to seven hours per night) is linked with an increased risk of coronary artery calcification.[123]

- Sleep deprivation increases the levels of many inflammatory mediators, which can trigger numerous inflammation-based diseases. While scientists are just beginning to understand these interactions, early work suggests that sleep deprivation may decrease the ability to resist infection.[124]

- Insufficient sleep can influence life expectancy. Compiled data from three different studies indicates that sleeping five or fewer hours per night may increase mortality risk by as much as 15%.[125]

Meditation Prepares Body Chemistry for Sleep

Melatonin

Melatonin plays a vital role in the physiological regulation of sleep. Melatonin is widely used in the management of sleep rhythm disorders due to jetlag, shift work, and insomnia. In addition to its role in sleep, melatonin acts as an antioxidant, immunomodulator, mood regulator and anti-aging agent.

Melatonin secretion tends to reduce and can affect sleep quality as we age, but meditation can counteract this age-related decline. Yoga Nidra as meditation increases the release of melatonin and also slows its breakdown in the body.[126] Melatonin levels were found to be significantly higher in meditators than non-meditating controls. It was also found that meditators experience more sleep cycles during the night indicating quality sleep.[127]

DHEA

Initial research is showing that low DHEA may affect sleep quality and that higher DHEA levels may allow sounder sleep at night. Meditation techniques are known to increase dehydroepiandrosterone (DHEA). High levels of DHEA can reduce the risk of depression, cardiovascular disease and even death in some studies. Some experts suggest DHEA might overcome age-related decline. Meditation can also precipitate the release of growth hormone and thyroid stimulating hormone (TSH) if needed by the body.[128]

Slowing Down the Body

When we enter meditation, the parasympathetic nervous system responds. This state favors sleep. Many people cannot enter sleep because they cannot slow the body down enough to enter the relaxation state (the Alpha brainwave state) that precedes sleep.

Meditation practices regulate the hypothalamic-pituitary-adrenal (HPA) axis and reduce cortisol levels. This reduces the stress state and allows the body to move into relaxation and then sleep.

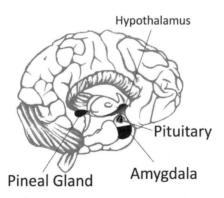

Figure 22: The Hypothalamus, Pituitary and Pineal glands are most often associated with the *third eye*.

Artwork by JoElizabeth James

The Third Eye and Corresponding Glands

In traditional Yogic anatomy, the *third eye* is located in the geometric center of the brain. In some texts, certain sub-points, called *bindu* points, indicate the location of other important areas of the brain. The glands most often associated with the *third eye* and associated *bindu* points are the pineal, pituitary and hypothalamus glands. In the Amrit Method of Yoga Nidra, we bring particular attention to the *third eye* region. (Figure 22). This is one of the key areas area research has shown is regulated by meditation—the (HPA Axis). The HPA Axis controls the body's reaction to stress. Two of the three glands associated with the HPA Axis are here—the hypothalamus and pituitary glands. The third is the pair of adrenal glands located above the kidneys.

The hypothalamus regulates the autonomic nervous system and has the power to create the parasympathetic relaxation response. It directs the function of the immune system and sleep. Also associated with the *third eye* is the pituitary gland, the master of hormones. Directed by the hypothalamus, the pituitary releases hormones telling the adrenal and other endocrine glands how to behave. It makes sense that by bringing attention here and using various Yoga Nidra techniques to stimulate these particular brain centers, we are only enhancing and magnifying our ability to affect the autonomic nervous system (governing both sleep and relaxation) and the endocrine system (governing hormones). This is exactly what ancient texts indicate and brain mapping during the relaxation response shows that the practice of meditation activates neural structures involved in attention and control of the autonomic nervous system.[129]

In addition, research has shown that meditation facilitates the release of melatonin through the pineal gland, also associated with the *third eye* area. The pineal gland produces serotonin in addition to melatonin. Melatonin not only regulates the biorhythms of the body, but also the biological clock that determines the rate at which we age.

Melatonin helps control the timing and release of female reproductive hormones including estrogen which is related to the menstrual cycle and menopause. Several studies have suggested this may be why melatonin levels are associated with breast cancer risk. Others suggest it has to do with exposure to artificial light during normal sleeping hours. Women with breast cancer tend to have lower levels of melatonin. Lab experiments have found that low levels of melatonin stimulate growth of certain types of breast cancer cells, while adding melatonin slows their growth.

Concentrations of melatonin significantly inhibit the proliferation of cancer cells by as much as 60% to 78%. After just four days of exposure to melatonin, breast cancer cells in culture exhibit reduced surface swelling, shedding, and various other types of cell disruption. These results support the hypothesis that melatonin prevents and even reverses the proliferation of breast cancer cells when exposed to the same concentrations of melatonin as are in the body during night hours.[130] Yoga Nidra is a natural and effective way to release melatonin in the body. It could help in the prevention of breast cancer and also serve as an adjunct therapy for those who already have it.

Sleep and Aging

It is a well-recognized fact that sleep medications have a host of side effects and do not offer a lasting, long-term solution. Prescription medications can often be limited in their ability to give you the deep and restorative sleep you need.

Particularly as we age, Yoga Nidra can be important for maintaining a good quality of sleep. Aging can alter the flexibility of the autonomic nervous system to move from stimulation (sympathetic) to relaxation (parasympathetic). In general, as we age, there tends to be an overall *increase* in sympathetic activity along with *reduced* parasympathetic activity. This reduces sleep quality and can make it difficult to fall asleep and stay asleep. Yoga

Nidra meditation helps support the rebalancing and flexibility of the autonomic nervous system. It teaches the body to create a relaxation response in experienced and novice meditators alike.

Continual Resetting Back to a Relaxed Baseline

Many of the positive benefits of meditation are due to its ability to continually reset metabolic functioning back to a relaxation baseline, despite varying levels of stress. Since too much stress is a major cause of insomnia, Yoga Nidra meditation enables practitioners to meet demands and challenges during the day, but then let go, relax and fall into a deep and refreshing sleep at night. The body becomes more resilient and is able to bounce back after stressful episodes rather than getting stuck in a low level stress response. The more consistent the practice, the more this holds true.[131] All these combined factors of Yoga Nidra create global changes in the body and mind which enhance the quality of sleep.

Sleep and Learning

Sleep, learning and memory are very closely interrelated. Although it is not known how sleep enables a person to integrate and access recently formed memories, a number of studies have shown that a reduction in total sleep time or specific sleep stages can dramatically inhibit a person's ability to consolidate memories in this way. Sleep increase has been shown to facilitate overnight learning of a sequenced memory task, while equivalent waking periods produce no such improvement.[132] After sleep, measurements confirm that the brain's "emotional task burden" is decreased. This means we are left feeling lighter, more free and unburdened after a night of sleep. Yoga Nidra does the same thing. Due to evidence of overnight, systems-level changes in motor memory there are important implications for clinical rehabilitation from brain trauma, such as traumatic brain injury or stroke.[133]

The problem is, only 11% of American college students report that they sleep well, and just 40% of those who do sleep well only do so two days per week.[134] The result is that students are often under high pressure to perform while they are not biologically in the best position to access and recall the information they are learning.

Yoga Nidra takes a person into the same brainwave states as in sleep and is shown to improve memory and cognitive performance. One study of a two-week Meditation Training Course improved scores on the GRE, which is the general test one must take for graduate or business school. GRE reading and comprehension scores increased along with working memory capacity. The occurrence of distracting thoughts during completion of the GRE was reduced. *Results suggest that meditation and Yoga Nidra are effective and efficient techniques for improving cognitive function.*[135]

Sleep and Mood

Dr. Lawrence Epstein, Medical Director of Sleep Health Centers and Instructor at Harvard Medical School states, "There's a big relationship between psychiatric and psychological problems and sleep. People who are depressed or have anxiety often have trouble with sleep as part of those disorders." Chronic insomnia can increase an individual's risk of developing depression or anxiety.[136] Studies have found that 15% to 20% of people diagnosed with insomnia will develop major depression. The same study found that people with insomnia are 20 times more at risk for developing panic disorder (a type of anxiety disorder).[137]

Often the first symptom of depression is difficulty sleeping. While sleep research is still exploring the relationship between depression and sleep, studies have shown that depressed people may have abnormal sleep patterns, as discussed in the section on depression. Insomnia two to four weeks before a depressive episode can indicate its onset.

Using Yoga Nidra for Insomnia

Yoga Nidra is a viable option for insomnia. A guided audio experience can help a person suffering from insomnia to naturally fall into sleep. For those who have no trouble falling asleep, but wake up in the middle of the night, Yoga Nidra is a good option to help them get back to sleep or at least give the body the restorative benefits of Yoga Nidra to offset sleep loss. Some people find that doing Yoga Nidra before sleep actually gives them more energy and prevents sleep. In this case, I recommend a practice in the morning or afternoon as the groundwork for a restful sleep at night. Yogis also believe that Yoga Nidra can pay off sleep debt and help the body restore itself from the effects of chronic sleep deprivation.

Summary: How Yoga Nidra Can Help Insomnia

- Yoga Nidra induces the relaxation response which is necessary to be able to fall asleep. Yoga Nidra can "teach" your body to sleep and release worrying thoughts.

- Sleep studies suggest that people who have insomnia with sleep disruption have elevated nighttime levels of circulating cortisol. The relaxation response in Yoga Nidra helps reduce elevated levels of cortisol and initiates the process of sleep.

- Naturally produced melatonin supports sleep without side effects.

CHAPTER EIGHTEEN

Yoga Nidra for Habits and Addictions

In order to understand how Yoga Nidra can be of benefit to habits and addictions, we must first understand how habits and addictions present themselves at different ranges on the same spectrum. As we explore habits and addictions from both a Yogic and scientific perspective, see how this may relate to your own experience.

Consider that every experience we have—failure, heartbreak, joy or conflict—creates a corresponding sensation in the body. We may feel tightness in the belly, lightness in the heart, constriction in the throat or an open, relaxed body. Every experience creates an internal weather pattern, a unique constellation of sensations coming together in a particular way. These patterns of sensation are what we call being angry, sad, frustrated or joyful. However, the common underlying experience is *sensation. Sensation and experience are closely related.* Without sensation, there would be no emotion. There would only be thought. Rejection *without* an accompanying physical experience is a thought; but *with* physical sensation, it is an emotion. There are some emotions and accompanying sensations with which we are comfortable and can allow. Others, we find uncomfortable and have difficulty allowing. Depending on our background, some of us are very comfortable with the sensations that accompany anger. Others of us are not. Maybe we are comfortable with the sensations we feel with sadness, but people we know are not.

Whatever those emotions are that bring you uncomfortable sensations, consider that when they reach a certain level of intensity, you are likely to try to evade or escape them. You might find yourself using all manner of external and internal strategies to keep these sensations at bay. Internally, you might fight the feeling, or tell yourself why you shouldn't feel what you are feeling. Maybe you try to analyze the reasons for the feeling, or blame someone else for the feelings. If you feel bad enough, you might even let off steam by dumping that excess tension on some unsuspecting person who happens to cross your path. It could be your partner, your kids, or the person at the local store. Whatever it may be, notice these are all tactics we use to *manage, but not feel*, emotions and sensations. Unfortunately, these tactics do not bring resolution.

As we have understood with the Tool of *Integration*, emotions are energies which need to be felt fully as a sensation, not a story, and then be allowed to pass through. When allowed, the energy of that sensation will rise to a peak and then return to balance and *Integration*. However, if it is not allowed, and instead is shut down, this energy cannot move through and the emotion will remain as a block.

How do we truly integrate an experience? *We need to be willing to feel the emotions as sensations that we didn't feel before.* When sensations are felt and allowed, apart from the mind's rationalization and justification, the sensations will move through and return to balance. Then, we are able to deal with the situation from a calm, balanced perspective.

Integrating Emotions

When you have an emotional experience, feel the event. Notice what sensation it causes in your body. Then step out of the story that triggered the feeling in your body so you are left with pure sensation: tightness in the throat or tightness in the belly, for example. Now, your only job is *to be* with those sensations in the same way you would be with uncomfortable sensations in a yoga pose. Breathe with the tightness. Let it be there. Don't try to force it away or resist it. Give it space to be. Imagine your body like a tube and keep stepping back, relaxing and making space for that sensation to simply move through the tube. Stay relaxed and open.

When you notice yourself getting back into the story, withdraw from it. Instead, come back to the breath and just breathe with what is there. The mistake most people make is using the breath as a way *to get rid* of the sensation, but that is just a subtle form of managing the discomfort. Instead, use the breath to *be with* the sensation. *Talk* to the sensation as if to say, "It is okay that you are here." You will notice that as you do this, the sensations will literally begin to shift in density and will begin move and flow through different areas of the body. Just follow that energy patiently, continuing to breathe, remaining relaxed and open. At some point, usually after about ten minutes, you will feel that energy take you to a deep, Yoga Nidra state of meditation. This is an indication that the energies are integrating themselves.

Contrary to what we tend to think, *Integration* doesn't happen because we dumped our emotions on someone else. Nor does it happen through suppression. It occurs spontaneously when we allow the sensation to move through the tube. If it is a big event, you may need to do this practice multiple times over a period of weeks or months. If it is a smaller event, it may fully integrate in one round of practice as described above.

If the experiences and accompanying sensations that constitute our life are not fully integrated, we may, instead, manage uncomfortable experiences through avoidance—suppressing what we feel. Avoidance is internal but often includes an external component. We may regularly rely on external substances and distractions to help us avoid the uncomfortable feelings residing within. Food, work, Internet or television can become the habituated ways we ignore and avoid what we don't want to feel inside.

The Yogic Perspective: We are trying to manage the way we feel.

I believe that many of our unhelpful habits stem from wanting to manage the way we feel. This doesn't mean habits are bad. However, if you look at your habits, you may find that you use some of them as ways to take care of everyday discomforts and tensions. Maybe you reward yourself with a drink after work or with junk food after a stressful day. Perhaps you zone out in front of the TV to disconnect from the day. If you go through a breakup and feel down, maybe you engage in a little shopping therapy. These are some of the ways we tend to manage the subtle stressors of our lives.

It is interesting that the more we manage tensions in a particular way, the more frequently we will manage them that way. If we eat cookies to reward ourselves after a hard day of work, that becomes a groove, a *samskara*. The body learns to crave that thing and will want to come back to it over and over. The more we revisit that groove, the deeper it becomes. Eventually, it will become a habit, the automatic way we handle stressors without even realizing it.

At some point, we may not just medicate a hard day with cookies, we may use cookies when we feel any intense emotion, whether up or down. We might eat cookies when we are tense and also when we are tired, sad, angry, bored or even excited. It becomes our "go to" behavior to manage many types of intensity—even the intensity of feeling good. In essence, we might repeat our habit when we feel good, when we feel bad, when we feel bored...whenever! It becomes the thing we just *do,* and we no longer need the intensity to do it. The *samskara* or habit has gained its own self-perpetuating momentum.

Feeling—Not Substance

Notice that the habit is not about the habit. The medicating agent—whether TV, Facebook, shopping, sex or food—is not about *what you are doing. It is about what it helps you feel or not feel.* The agent is helping you do one of two things: it is either giving you *comfort* and making you *feel good* in some way, or it is giving you *relief;* it is *removing some kind of tension.* You might have a drink to give yourself *relief* from a hard day of work. Or, you might buy new shoes to *comfort* yourself. Or it can be a combination of both. The same is true with addiction. Whatever the agent of addiction is—whether a substance, an activity, a person or thing—the addiction is not about the agent itself, but what the agent makes you *feel* or *not feel.*

To use substances as an example, I have a friend who trained in the Amrit Method of Yoga Nidra and is a former heroin addict himself. He subsequently worked as a counselor in an addiction facility and led Yoga Nidra there because of the profound effect it had on him. He once said to me that the first time he took heroin, it took away an essential pain so profoundly and so totally, he knew he would want to go back there again and again. At some point, he no longer wanted to be the person who experienced inner pain. He wanted to be the person who was pain free, who felt good, who felt relaxed, at peace and at ease. Here again, it was not about the substance itself, but about the core pain that the heroin succeeded in taking away—albeit temporarily, and with many more consequences to come.

Eventually, we become so accustomed to the thing that takes away our tension, discomfort or pain, that the lack of it becomes a stressor itself. For example, at the end of a very long work week, we may be really looking forward to our end-of-the-week drink. We can feel our body craving it. If we crave it enough, it can actually become a subtle stress. We want it; we need it.

We can't relax until we get it. *The solution has become a source of stress* itself. This becomes even more of an issue when habits move up the ladder toward addiction.

Habits to Addictions

The problem with repeatedly looking to a habit, like a cookie, to feel better is that it is temporary—it only works for the time we are eating it. Soon, the feeling will come back again. If we want the feeling to stay away, we have to keep eating. Before we know it, we've eaten a whole bag of cookies. The underlying stress will resurface again because it has only been covered up, not dealt with. The same is true of any medicating action—gambling, sex, shopping and the like. As a result, we always need more and more of the "medicating agent or action" and it becomes a vicious cycle.

Habits and addictions operate on the principle of *samskaras*. The more we manage tensions in a particular way, the more we will tend to manage them the same way. Eventually, we may need more and more of the agent to secure the comfort and relief we are seeking and to keep the discomfort we don't want to experience at bay. Furthermore, the more we revisit any kind of substance or activity, the more it moves from the conscious and deliberate to the unconscious and automatic.

Most Addictions Begin Under Stress

Addiction experts suggest that any type of addiction most often begins under some type of stress. These stressors can be biological, like genetics or an underlying chemical imbalance. They can also be mental and emotional stressors like divorce, job loss, or suppressed trauma and abuse. Even compelling negative attitudes and beliefs can set the stage for addictions.

Yogis would say the same thing. Things become habits when we use them to manage circumstances that are uncomfortable—such as pressures or stressors. Habits usually manage a lower level of stress, and there is still at a certain level of conscious ability to withdraw from the habit, if we choose. As we move up the ladder, however, this choice appears to become less and less available as the compulsion to act becomes more and more powerful.

Contributing Factors to Addiction

Overwhelming Circumstances

One of the triggers of addiction is the inability to cope with difficult circumstances. This could be a sudden change in finances, divorce, job loss or the resulting depression, anxiety and loss of self-esteem that can accompany those events. If we did not have healthy social support or experienced undue conflict as children, this can impact our resiliency with struggles later in life. Overwhelmed by feelings and sensations, and not equipped to integrate these feelings in a healthy way, we may turn to a substance or activity to gain temporary relief or comfort from the pain we don't want to feel.

It could even be a recent traumatic event such as rape, abuse or wartime trauma which overwhelm our coping abilities. Ill-equipped to deal with it, we turn to something that takes it away—alcohol, drugs, sex, gambling, and the like. The cutting edge of addiction treatment today is to treat the root trauma that is so often and overwhelmingly present among those who are addicted in one form or another.

Limiting Beliefs and Conclusions about Life

From our environment and experiences, we sometimes adopt limiting conclusions about ourselves and our lives. Distorted attitudes and thinking can drive our behavior in surprisingly destructive ways. I'm sure you know someone who carries the belief, "My life won't amount to anything no matter what I do, so I might as well not try." You can see how it has shaped their choices, their ambition (or lack of it), and their view of the world. You can practically see them foiling every opportunity around them as if on purpose. This belief is the *unconscious intention* guiding their life. Whether it is true or not, it can powerfully thwart happiness, the ability to make self-enhancing decisions, and to find peace.

Now imagine how painful it is to live with such a belief day in and day out. Imagine how good it would feel to have a break from being the person who lives in that negative self-created reality. How nice it would feel not to have to be that person. Imagine that for awhile you get to be someone else. You get to be happy and carefree. Freed from the mental concepts of who you are, you get to choose who you want to be. For a little while, this is what the medicating agent or action can do. It can get you out of your mind. Unfortunately, *it is short-lived and the agent itself soon becomes the problem.*

I will add that Yoga Nidra does something similar, yet altogether different. We don't *temporarily* cover up the belief, nor do we escape from it. Instead, we *neutralize* the beliefs to which we have attached that cause us so much misery. During the Yoga Nidra experience we truly free ourselves of the illusionary grip these beliefs seem to have on us. I say this because the beliefs to which we attach have no power over us, other than the fact that we have held onto them. The moment we truly let them go, we are free.

Yoga masters demonstrate this principle through the example of monkeys and how they are trapped through their own attachment. In order to trap a monkey, a banana is placed in a cage. The only way for the monkey to get the banana is to ease its hand through a hole just big enough for the hand to pass through. The monkey reaches in to get the banana, but the hole is not large enough to pull the banana out. The monkey won't let go of the banana and as a result is "trapped." It is so attached to having the banana, it doesn't realize all it needs to do is let go of the banana and it will be free! The same is true of us. We don't realize the only thing we need to do to be free of the cage is to let go of the banana. The banana is not doing anything to you. The beliefs and experiences you have had are not doing anything to you. *They are holding you captive because you are holding onto them.* Let them go and you are free. This is what the entire practice of Yoga Nidra is designed to do. *It is the true and lasting freedom that no external substance will ever be able to give you.*

Environmental Influences

Another pre-disposing factor toward addiction is how we have been taught by our environment to handle stress. If we grew up in an environment or culture where it was common to manage stress with food or alcohol, we may be more likely to go that route, though this is not always the case. We may do just the opposite. However, our personal history and environmental influences, like an alcoholic parent or our peer group, can be a factor in addiction. We may have seen and learned from a young age or even as an adult, "This is what I do when I'm in pain."

Physiological Stressors: Biochemical Imbalances

External stressors such as job loss or traumatic experiences drive addictive behaviors. Internal, physiological stressors can do the same. It is quite common that those with bipolar disorder, depression, or PTSD don't know how to handle the unstable inner world caused by biochemical imbalances. For those with bipolar disorder, especially when undiagnosed, it can feel as though the only way to stabilize the intense highs and lows is with alcohol or other substances. For those with PTSD, it can feel as if the only way to manage extreme states of stress, hypervigilance and flashbacks is to numb out to make it stop for at least a little while. The same principle applies to depression, anxiety and many other mood disorders. It is actually quite common that people in recovery from an addictive substance have an underlying mood disorder.

Genetics

The role of genetics is a hotly disputed topic in the world of addiction. Some say, "I have an addiction because I was genetically *predisposed* to have an addiction." I believe the evidence proves that genetic predispositions exist, but do not "make" a person addicted. Rather, they increase sensitivity to certain substances. A genetic predisposition can be compared to external *karma*. It is the environment, much like the alcoholic father. However, we always have the choice of *how* we deal with environmental tendencies. We can become just like the alcoholic father, or who we choose to be. We still have the final say. Otherwise, all people who are predisposed to addiction would become addicted and that is simply not true. According to the American Society of Addiction Medicine, environmental factors interact with the person's biology and strongly affect how much these genetic factors will exert their influence. That means that the positive learning and experiences we have as adults, our upbringing as children, our surrounding culture and environment all affect whether a genetic predisposition will actually manifest as an addiction.

So, how *could* genetics fit into the addiction puzzle? Perhaps *heredity can predispose the body to be susceptible to certain ways of medicating intensity.* Perhaps the groove, once set the first time, rapidly deepens. The body learns to crave the medicating substance more quickly and perhaps the substance has a stronger and more powerful effect on the body and mind. From the very first time, the substance takes away something or gives the person something so powerful, they want to go back again and again. In other words, a genetic predisposition accelerates and gives weight to the process by which both the body and mind become habituated and addicted to the medicating agent.

From a Yogic perspective, stress, habits and addictions are very tightly interrelated. Modern addiction science seems to bear out the same conclusion. The less stress we carry, the less we need or want to medicate it. Maybe you can see this with yourself. When you are especially stressed, you might find yourself longing for a glass of wine. But when you are not so stressed, you can easily take it or leave it. This is one of the reasons Yoga Nidra is so valuable for the treatment of habits and addictions. By reducing the underlying stress we experience and integrating the emotions we usually want to cover up, we can prevent the need to use substances to suppress unaddressed stresses and tensions. We can more easily enjoy all kinds of things but not become addicted to them. Of course, I am not referring to highly addictive substances here, though I do find that maintaining a balanced mind, healthy emotions and a relaxed body is one of the best preventative measures for any kind of addiction.

Habits and Addictions from the Yogic and Scientific Perspective

Yoga Nidra speaks to habits and addictions at the *cause* level, while science identifies the net *effect* of the cause. Let's explore this. From the Yogic perspective, addiction is a habituated method of managing the way we feel. From the scientific perspective, addiction occurs when the lack of the medicating agent or action causes such a physical or psychological dependency that its cessation causes severe trauma. Said differently, something is defined as addiction when the person is so enslaved by the habit that they psychologically and/or physically cannot live without it. Unhealthy habits have the potential to move toward becoming addictions. Mapping this process will give us a clearer picture of how the two are related.

We all have habits. If we are human beings, we will have habits. Habits can be equated with *samskaras*. Most habits are good and you don't want to get rid of them. It wouldn't be helpful to have to repeatedly relearn how to dress yourself, drive a car or remember how to get yourself home. These are *useful* habits.

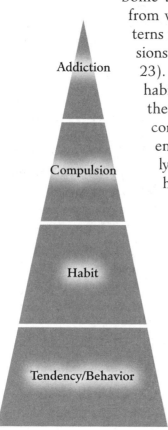

Some *unhelpful* habits become the seed from which deeper, more ingrained patterns form. These can grow into compulsions, obsessions and addiction (Figure 23). The primary differences between habits, compulsions and addictions are the intensity of the habit, how much control we have over the impulses to engage the habit, and how biologically or psychologically entrenched the habit has become.

Understanding your position on this ladder gives you the ability to monitor yourself and your own habits in order to know when you are moving into dangerous territory. You will then be able to use the principles of Yoga Nidra to withdraw and move back down the ladder toward an ordinary habit or tendency.

Figure 23: The ladder moves from light tendencies and behaviors, to deeper habits and compulsions, into potential addiction.

Tendency

Habits begin as tendencies. Tendencies are the first and lightest groove of a *samskara*. The first several times we do something that makes us feel good (comfort) or takes away tension (relief), the initial groove is set. It could be as simple as having a cup of coffee each morning, having an ice cream after work or having a glass of wine with dinner. Once you have done that action and it works, the tendency is set because of all possible choices to feel better, it is just a bit more likely you will choose a strategy that has worked before. With each repetition, momentum builds, tending to move our actions in a particular way.

At first, these just arise as preferences. These are things that you find "nice" to do. They are conscious and deliberate. Your conscious mind is present and consciously chooses to do one thing over another. It consciously chooses coffee over tea, wine over water or jazz over opera. If that preference is not met, little or no inner disturbance arises. You can enjoy the event or substance when it is there, and you can let it go when it is not.

This is the healthiest level of habits. We are all human, and humans are largely unique from each other because of our individual preferences. What makes me unique from you, in part, is that I like pizza and strawberry Häagen Dazs, but you like hamburgers and iced mocha cappuccinos. There is nothing wrong with this. The questions are: When you don't get these things, can you still be happy? Can you enjoy them when they are there, but still be okay when they are not? Or is your happiness and well-being attached to these things?

Tendency/Behavior

> Once we know what makes us feel good, gives us comfort, or relief from discomfort, we will tend to go to that same thing. The groove is set.
>
> Preference: "NICE TO"
>
> • Little or no disturbance.
>
> • *Conscious and deliberate*

Habit

As a tendency is repeated, the groove becomes deeper. Of all possible choices we can make, we begin to unconsciously and automatically choose the things that have historically made us feel good. The choice could be for an activity or a substance. Instead of choosing to have a cup of coffee, it just becomes the thing we do every morning. Maybe we get up and even before being fully awake, that is what we do. We don't think about it anymore. It is automatic.

Obviously, this is not a big issue. However, use the same principle and replace coffee with wine. In the beginning, at the tendency level, you might have a glass of wine with dinner. It is a preference and a nice thing to do. At that level, you can take it or leave it. But let's say that glass of wine gives you a particular feeling, a nice buzz, a little relief from the stress of the day.

At some point, the *preference* for wine can move into a more deeply ingrained *choice* for wine. It's not just something that is "nice" to have, but moves toward something you "want" to have. Of all the beverages you could possibly choose with dinner, wine would probably be the choice. The choice to have it is not even necessarily something you think about; it is just something that becomes nearly automatic. "We always have wine with dinner." Again, not bad, but just understand the principle.

The other difference between a habit and a tendency is that with a habit, wine is missed when omitted. At the tendency level, you can take it or leave it. At the habit level, you will feel a slight tug of missing the agent. It will cause a minor inner disturbance.

Yoga Nidra: The Art of Transformational Sleep

Repeatedly and automatically choosing that which we KNOW will give *comfort or relief* is a habit.

<u>Choice:</u> WANT TO

- The lack of the medicating substance is missed
- Minor Disturbance
- *Unconscious and automatic*

Compulsions

As a *samskara* becomes more deeply ingrained and more automatic, it can become a compulsion, something we don't just *want* to do, but rather something we *need* to do to feel okay. Many of our habits remain at the habit level, but some can move up the ladder toward compulsion.

Now, you might be asking, "Does that mean me driving twenty miles to Starbucks to get a coffee is a compulsion?" By this definition, yes. Now, don't get worried. I seriously doubt the compulsion to have coffee is going to do damage. The principle is important to understand however, because this is where the power differential flips from *you choosing your behaviors to your behaviors driving you*. If you replace this dynamic with alcohol, gambling or some other agent, it can suddenly seem much more concerning.

If you or someone you know has moved from wanting a glass of wine, to feeling its lack intensely enough to go out of the way to get it, this behavior is moving toward a compulsion. The length to which you are willing to go to get it speaks to the degree of the compulsion. If you want wine and drive down to the local grocery store to get it, only to find they are closed, that is one thing. However, if you drive to all the other grocery stores within a 20 mile radius, that is a deeper compulsion indicating a probable cause for concern.

In terms of self-management, it is helpful to be attentive to instances where your habits begin to border on compulsions, moving you into an inverted power relationship with the cravings that drive the body and mind. If you can learn to exercise this principle and manage your simpler, less complex compulsions, you will develop the ability to manage more significant compulsions when they arise.

How do we manage compulsions? *Dis-identification.* The more we withdraw from mechanically acting on our automatic impulses, the weaker they become. In the beginning, when we withdraw from fighting or feeding the impulse and just let it be present, it will burn. It will be uncomfortable. However, over time, the impulse will weaken. It will move down the ladder back toward being a habit. For example, if you see that you are a bit too attached to having a glass of wine after work, experiment with consciously withdrawing for a week or two. In the beginning, it might be uncomfortable, but after a while, you won't give it much thought. It will have reversed momentum from the automatic and unconscious thing you always do, back to something conscious and deliberate.

You will begin to gain personal power as you see these drives do not own you. You have the ability to manage them. Just because a sensation, thought or craving arises in you doesn't mean you are under any obligation to act on it. Once you see this, you will be empowered to more *consciously make choices, rather than having your choices automatically made for you.* This restores the proper power relationship with thoughts and impulses. It is not that you cannot do what the mind thinks or the body wants, but you can *choose it consciously.*

Yoga Nidra is a powerful tool in this regard. As you move into Yoga Nidra, you begin to rest back as the sky-like space of awareness, and the impulses and cravings that seem to be screaming at you in the waking state move further away. The scream is reduced to a conversational tone, then to a whisper. It is like a TV that is playing down the hall versus right in front of your face. The voices may be the same, but because of the distance, it is much easier to disregard what the voices and impulses are saying. A former addict in recovery confided in me that even after completing the addiction program and countless Yoga Nidra sessions, the impulse to use heroin was still present. The difference was the distance between him and the urge was now miles and miles away and Yoga Nidra helped keep it that way. While I'm not suggesting Yoga Nidra as a sole treatment for addiction, it is a powerful adjunct to any addiction treatment. When viewing from a meditative perspective, it is easier to remain removed from compulsive urges.

Compulsions and addictions may become weaker when we withdraw from them and move down the ladder. However, *samskaras*, if deeply ingrained, can be retriggered. For a substance that is potentially dangerous, this is an issue. For example, if a person is an alcoholic and has even one drink, there is a risk of retriggering the *samskara*. It could potentially reopen the groove at the place where it stopped. This is particularly true if the addiction has a strong biological component to it. This can cause the person to binge drink, for example, at the amount they were drinking before, but because the body is no longer accustomed to that amount of alcohol, this can be very dangerous. This is the reason why some substances may require permanent and total withdrawal. It is simply not worth taking the chance. In the addiction world this is called *abstinence*, in Yoga we would call it *pratyahara*: withdrawal of energy and attention, and in this case action.

Compulsion

> The hallmark of compulsion is that our well-being is so contingent upon the medicating action that we are *willing to go out of our way to get it*.

Attachment: NEED TO

- Lack of medicating agent becomes a stressor.

- Significant disturbance: physical sensation/irritation

- We no longer *have* cravings. It feels as if the cravings *have us.*

- *Unconscious automatic and necessary*

Addiction

The final and deepest *samskara* is addiction. Let us come back to the scientific definition: addiction occurs when the lack of the medicating substance or activity creates such physical or psychological dependency that its cessation causes severe trauma. We began with the Yogic principle that habits are often a way to manage the way we feel. We can see that as we move up the ladder, acquiring the substance or action that manages the way we feel becomes increasingly imperative—until not having it becomes, in and of itself, a *stress.* The need to satisfy the craving drives our behavior.

In the beginning, our view of the world is still wide. We have many choices in front of us and directions to focus our attention and energy. As we move up the ladder, our vision becomes increasingly narrowed until, at the addiction level, there is one thing and one thing alone that stands at the center of our attention: returning to the medicating experience. Someone who is at the farthest point of addiction sees no other option except to secure that agent. Children don't matter, jobs don't matter, even clothing, cleanliness or food may not matter. Breaking the law doesn't matter. Anything that needs to be done to get what is needed is fair game.

Of course it doesn't go this far for all people who are addicted, but at its most extreme, it can happen. The reason is that the *need* has moved to *obsession.* We don't just *need* the medicating agent, we feel we *must* have it for our very survival.

In fact, this may be the case in regard to substances. At the addiction level, the *samskara* or groove may no longer be limited to the mental or emotional level, but may move into the biochemistry of the body. The whole body, as well as mind, have adapted and adjusted to the presence of the agent such that taking away the agent could cause the system to collapse. This is the scientific distinction of true substance addiction, the point where the cessation of the medicating agent will cause physical and psychological trauma. The habit has moved from the thing we *like,* to the unconscious and automatic thing we *do,* to the thing we *need,* to the thing we *must have* to survive.

It is important to truly understand that as we become more and more dependent on a medicating agent or action our life constricts around obtaining that one thing. Try a little experiment with me. Take a breath in and hold it. Continue to hold your breath as you read the next couple sentences. Notice that as you continue to hold the breath, your attention automatically withdraws from anything else around you. The longer you hold, the more the pressure builds. The more the pressure builds, the only thing you can think about is taking a breath. Do you feel that? In that state of pressure, nothing else matters but taking a breath. At some point you would be willing to give up everything just to take a breath. Your very survival is at stake. This is how an addicted person feels when in the most intense state of craving. Now take a breath. Notice that as you take a breath, relief floods the whole system. You are back to yourself and you feel okay. That is how it feels when a truly addicted person gets their fix. Unfortunately, after time, more and more of the substance is needed to feel that that sense of relief, with less and less reward actually forthcoming.

Addiction:

The object of addiction is perceived as an absolute need for survival.

Obsession: HAVE TO

- Whole world becomes about getting that thing to the exclusion of everything else.

- *Unconscious, automatic and necessary for survival*

How Can Yoga Nidra Help?

Yoga Nidra can be a very effective method to help disengage from the impulses that drive habits. Depending on the severity and type of compulsion, Yoga Nidra can be used as a stand-alone technique or in conjunction with standard treatment. Here are some of the ways Yoga Nidra can be a benefit in both cases.

Dis-identification and Intention

As we've mentioned, the meditative process of Yoga Nidra increases the distance between us and the medicating agent or behavior, making it easier to make conscious choices versus unconscious and automatic ones. The more we practice seeing these thoughts and impulses without acting on them, the more we realize that *we* hold all the power, not the impulses. However, when we are habituated to acting on the cravings in the body and impulses in the mind, it seems as if we have no choice but to act on them. As we establish the conscious ability to observe cravings and impulses, we gain more mastery over them. Through consciously managing these impulses, we can move our relationship to substances and behaviors down the habit-addiction ladder from the unconscious and automatic and back to the conscious and deliberate.

Yoga Nidra gives us the ability to withdraw from the habits and cravings that don't serve us. We also have the ability to focus and direct that same energy and attention in the direction we want to go.

Yoga Nidra, combined with *Intention,* can consciously and deliberately redirect our attention to areas we want to reinforce. Instead of focusing on our bad self-care habits, overeating or smoking, for example, we can deliberately *redirect* our focus on radiant health and staying vital for ourselves and our family.

Relaxation and Relapse Prevention

We have discussed how stress and life intensity can trigger various habits and compulsions as we attempt to manage that stress. In fact, it is shown that individuals exposed to stress are more likely to abuse alcohol and other drugs. Individuals who already have a history of compulsions and addictions are much more likely to go back to the medicating agent or action in the presence of stress.[138] When you feel good, relaxed and happy, it is usually easier to do good things and avoid bad habits. However, when life gets busy and pressure—at home, at work, or both—builds up, we tend to drop the good habits and pick up the bad ones. The same is true higher up the ladder: the greater the stress, the greater the likelihood of relapse.[139]

Alcoholics Anonymous (AA), one the most known and successful programs for substance addiction has a higher initial relapse rate than one might think. Within the first year success rates are as low as 26%[140] with abstinence rates progressively increasing to 40% after the first year and higher with each year of abstinence, according to AA World Services. In that first year, the biggest contributor to high relapse rates is reconfronting the stressors that cause individuals to seek out the medicating agent in the first place. Helping people manage the stresses that trigger relapse is critical to ongoing success. Yoga Nidra can be a powerful aid to put the body and mind in the best biochemical, mental and emotional state to handle these stressors and prevent relapse.

Research published in the *Journal of Social Work Practice in the Addictions* used Yoga Nidra as the chosen method to research the effect of meditation on relapse prevention. Results demonstrated that Yoga Nidra reduces the rate of relapse and its warning signs— mostly through a decrease in negative mood states. *The data not only provided evidence for the effectiveness of Yoga Nidra to reduce risk for relapse* but also added to the understanding that negative mood states increase the risk for relapse among those in treatment for chemical dependency.[141]

Relapse prevention is quickly gaining ground as a successful adjunct to addiction treatment. At least two studies have demonstrated the effectiveness of relapse prevention for smoking, alcohol, marijuana and cocaine addiction. Both studies include meditation. Research-backed suggestions for relapse prevention include *stress* and temptation coping methods. In 2002, Gordon A. Marlatt, Professor of Psychology and Director of the Addictive Behavior Research Center at the University of Washington proposed a Buddhist-based program called "Skillful Means." In terms of addictive behavior and temptation, it taught observing and accepting the thoughts and urges for the substance or behavior, but not acting on them. This practice was found to significantly weaken addictive behaviors.[142] This is exactly what the Tools of Yoga Nidra, and specifically the Tool of *Dis-identification,* are designed to do. In addition, the Tool of *Relaxation* in Yoga Nidra is a means of discharging the stress that leads us to engage in addictive behaviors and substances.

The last aspect of a suggested relapse prevention program is to redirect from the *motivation to use* to the *motivation to change.* In Yoga Nidra, we accomplish this through the use of *Intention.* Each individual determines the direction toward which they consciously want to move, and with Yoga Nidra, they put more attention and energy on the *Intention* rather than the desire to use. A simple example would be, "No food tastes as good as feeling light feels." The feeling of lightness is the motivation to change. The more attention is devoted to the feeling of "lightness," the more it detracts from the desire to eat.

Lastly, relapse prevention programs also encourage what they call, "positive addiction." Both meditation and exercise have been shown to be effective "positive addictions" that reduce alcohol consumption among male social drinkers.[143]

In another study, authors evaluated the effectiveness of a meditation course on substance use in an incarcerated population. After release from jail, participants in the meditation course showed significant reductions in alcohol, marijuana, and crack cocaine use as compared with those in a treatment-as-usual control condition.[144] Meditation participants showed decreases in psychiatric symptoms as well.

Quality sleep seems to be an important factor in helping prevent relapse. A study of substance-abusing adolescents showed that increased sleep duration was associated with improvements in psychological distress and reduction in relapse. It was found that meditation was a useful component to promote improved sleep.[145] Since Yoga Nidra is a sleep-based meditation, it is likely to be of great use in this regard.

Balanced Body Chemistry Contributes to Moderation

Keeping the system relaxed keeps body chemistry in balance, making it easier to be moderate. Let's understand why. When we are in chronic stress, cortisol is released into the system from the adrenal glands. Cortisol causes a part of the brain's pleasure center, called the nucleus accumbens, to become sensitive to dopamine. That is to say, when we are stressed, the body will crave pleasure and feeling good. If you look into your own experience, you might recognize this. When the body is in this state, and it is given something that creates pleasure, it will easily release high levels of dopamine as a reward.

Dopamine is a neurotransmitter found in the reward pathway of the brain; it is what makes us feel good. It gives us the feeling of reward. It is a motivating force that makes us want more. Low dopamine can make us moody and irritable. When we sleep, dopamine is replenished in the brain. This is why, upon waking from a good night's sleep, we perceive the world from a fresher, lighter and clearer perspective.

Serotonin is a neurotransmitter that balances dopamine. While dopamine makes us want more, serotonin lets us know when we've had enough. It gives us the feeling of contentment, satiation and satisfaction that signals we are done. It takes away the craving. Without serotonin to balance dopamine, the compulsion to act on and acquire substances or experiences to quench our cravings persists. We don't get the message that it is time to stop. Here is the dilemma: *the cortisol released during stress reduces the amount of available serotonin in the system.* In this stress state, *we cannot feel when enough is enough.* This propagates our tendency to over-spend, over-drink, over-eat, over-sex or whatever the habit of choice is, because whatever we are getting never feels like enough.

An example is eating for hunger versus eating from stress. When we are hungry, dopamine will motivate us to get food to reduce our hunger. This is a good and necessary thing. However, if we are eating from stress, we may eat to fulfill our physical hunger, but then keep eating. There is not enough serotonin in the body to tell us we are satisfied and we cannot feel that we have had enough. Without the feeling of satiation, we eat much more than the body actually needs.

The same scenario is true with drinking alcohol. The YouTube video, *The Pathology of Addiction,* uploaded by Janis Dougherty illustrates the theories of Dr. Ronald Ruden in his book *The Craving Brain.* The following example is given. You and a friend go for a beer. The initial craving for the beer is the same. The difference is, when each of you has the beer, one of you is relaxed enough and has enough serotonin in your system. The other is chronically stressed and does not have enough. The person who has enough serotonin will crave one beer, will have one beer, and will feel satisfied. The person who does not have enough serotonin will continue to want more, and likely drink more, because they do not have enough serotonin to give them the signal to stop.[146]

This single understanding of the chemistry of stress is enough of an endorsement of Yoga Nidra in and of itself. Yoga Nidra helps reduce compulsive and addictive sensitivity. The practice not only *reduces the cortisol* in the system, it also *releases serotonin*, allowing the body to reset its own natural dopamine/serotonin balance.

Restoration

In addition to releasing serotonin, Yoga Nidra spontaneously and naturally releases dopamine. Dopamine is associated with focus, concentration and motivation often lacking in those with Attention Deficit Disorder (ADD). Low dopamine is also associated with depression. Having enough dopamine in the system, in balance with serotonin, creates a body that feels good, clear, rewarded, and vitalized. When the body's environment is its own reward, there is less need to get that reward elsewhere.

Impulsivity is a common risk factor associated with substance abuse. If we can control our impulses, we are more able to observe cravings without acting on them. Having enough dopamine in the system *decreases* impulsivity and the tendency to act on cravings. According to a study conducted by researchers at Ernest Gallo Clinic and Research Center at the University of California, San Francisco, *higher* levels of dopamine are found to *decrease* impulsivity in the frontal cortex of the brain.[147] As we have learned, the specific practice of Yoga Nidra (not just meditation, but Yoga Nidra meditation) increases endogenous dopamine release by up to 65%![148]

A good, healthy, prefrontal cortex will help control impulses and cravings while *deficiencies in prefrontal cortex function increase the risk of drug addiction.* This could be part of the reason why people with trauma and PTSD, and adolescents, may be biologically more at risk for addiction. The risks accompanying drug use are increased for teenagers because they do not have a fully developed prefrontal cortex. Their ability to moderate their impulses is already reduced just because of their age. Add in trauma which may further compromise the prefrontal cortex at any age, then add drugs to the mix, and you can see how this can set the stage for addictions to develop quickly in the absence of strong impulse management. Yoga Nidra thickens the prefrontal cortex.

Dopamine levels may be depleted in those who have used certain recreational drugs. Some drugs can release two to ten times the amount of dopamine than a natural reward, reinforcing the feeling that the drug itself is necessary for survival, and making such habits more compelling and difficult to break. The brain responds to the large and rapid surges of dopamine that drugs create by reducing its own dopamine activity. Eventually, the disrupted dopamine system can render the individual less and less able to feel pleasure—even from the drugs that feed their addiction. More of the drug, or a stronger drug, is needed to create the same feeling. When in recovery, the body can be left with very little natural dopamine production due to the over-triggering of this response. *The natural release of dopamine during Yoga Nidra can help correct this imbalance and ease the symptoms of withdrawal.*

This is particularly important for those whose bodies are not producing enough dopamine for other reasons. We've mentioned Parkinson's disease, for example, as a condition where a deficiency of dopamine prevents fluid bodily motion. Yoga Nidra could be an agent to help increase the internal release of dopamine in the body and serve as a natural aid to those with Parkinson's.

Stimulants such as caffeine and medications for Attention Deficit Disorder and Attention Deficit Hyperactivity Disorder (ADD/ADHD) cause dopamine to be pushed into the synapse so that focus is improved. Unfortunately, the consistent artificial stimulation of dopamine can cause a depletion of dopamine over time. Yoga Nidra can help rectify this depletion and may even provide enough dopamine to act as a natural aid for ADD and ADHD.

We've looked at how Yoga Nidra supports the biology of the body to be more resistant to unhelpful habits and addictions. Let's look at how it helps create a different internal and psychological environment.

Integration

Although Yoga Nidra is not a replacement for psychotherapy, the internal clearing of events and associated emotions can help release the underlying issues we may try to cover up with the medicating agent or action. The more we release the underlying issue, the less remains to cover up. For example, if we are sad and finally allow that sadness to be felt and released with the help of Yoga Nidra, the less we will need to bury it in food, drink or other distractions.

Realization

Through the Tool of *Realization*, we rely on a higher power, rather than a substance, to restore our knowledge of wholeness. In AA, two of the most important practices are meditation and prayer.

Establishing a conscious connection with God as we understand it is the Eleventh Step in AA. Yoga Nidra is a powerful, all-inclusive way to do this. It requires no belief in a particular religion or even philosophy for it to work. Meditation is key to AA because once a *samskara* is deeply ingrained, it cannot be managed by the mind or will alone. It needs to be given to a power beyond the mind.

Those who are addicted are often the most spiritual people you will meet. They are seeking wholeness (God), but do not know where to find it. Most of us are never taught how and where to find wholeness. We know something is missing, but we don't know where to look for the solution. So we look for that wholeness in things like money, relationships, and recognition—activities such as work, sex or gambling—or substances like food, alcohol and recreational drugs. The cause is the same, a loss of wholeness. Restoring the *true* experience of wholeness replaces the *false* sense of wholeness the substance or activity temporarily provided. This is the ultimate solution rather than a temporary one.

Studies on Addiction and Meditation

- Analysis of 198 independent treatment outcomes found that meditation produces a significantly larger reduction in tobacco, alcohol, and non-prescribed drug use than standard treatment for substance abuse.

- It was found that the effectiveness of conventional programs declines rapidly within three months, whereas the *effects of meditation increase over time. Total abstinence from tobacco, alcohol, and non-prescribed drugs increased from 51% to 89% over an 18–22 month period.*

- These addiction-inhibiting effects of meditation come from natural improvements in both the psychology of the mind and the biochemistry of the body.[149]

Meditation and Smoking
- A study surveying all available research on smoking cessation published in the *Alcohol Treatment Quarterly* and the *Journal of Health Promotion*, showed meditation to be

twice as effective in helping people to stop smoking as the other treatments, including pharmacological therapy, individual counselling and self-help kits. This result is very significant for the 25-30% of the population who smoke today.[150]

- A study for smoking cessation and abstinence was published in the *Journal of Nursing Scholarship* by Christine Wynd, Professor and Director of the PhD in Nursing Program, University of Akron. This study found that at 24-months after the intervention, smoking abstinence rates were significantly stronger for the *guided health imagery* intervention group over the placebo control group *(26% abstinence rate versus 12%).* The study concluded that guided imagery was an effective intervention for long-term smoking cessation and abstinence in adult smokers.[151] Yoga Nidra includes guided imagery.

CHAPTER NINETEEN

Yoga Nidra for Trauma and PTSD

In the last chapter, we talked about how habits and addictions can begin as a means to manage the way we feel. At times, the present moment is not something we want to experience. There is something other we want to feel—better, happier, more relaxed, rewarded; or something we don't want to feel—tension, stress, pain, fear. We might find that the person we are "under the influence" is more the person we want to be than the person we are when sober.

We want to be the person who is free from fear, worries or concerns. We want to be the person who is free from the inner voices that torment us. The problem is that person and those feelings come back. They are never gone forever—just temporarily forgotten.

Everything Is Related to Everything Else

By now, you are probably beginning to see how everything is related to everything else. Stress is related to sleep. Sleep is related to anxiety and depression. We try to get away from anxiety, depression and other stressors with self-medicating agents or mood-altering activities. The same is true with traumatic experiences. Our unresolved past can cause us to seek agents that will help us get away from the pain, to numb it out, to cover it up, and to escape from it for a little while. We call it self-medicating. Eventually, the medicating substance or action can become a secondary problem arising out of the primary cause of unresolved trauma or pain.

The rate of some kind of trauma or abuse among those who are addicted is phenomenally high. It is no accident that the two tend to co-arise. In fact, among individuals seeking treatment for substance use disorders, approximately 36% to 50% meet criteria for *lifetime* PTSD.[152] Let's look at what trauma is and what PTSD is before we look at how Yoga Nidra can help.

What Is Trauma from the Yogic Point of View?

From a Yogic point of view, *trauma is an undigested, undischarged energy event that continues to affect the body/mind complex at all levels, physical, mental, emotional and perceptual, after the event has actually passed.*

All experiences are expressions of energy. Frustration, loss, grief and happiness are all energy experiences which we feel as varying sensations traveling throughout the body. If allowed to naturally flow through the body/mind complex, these energy-based sensations will be felt, received, and as a result will integrate, returning back to Source—leaving us in a balanced, neutral, baseline state, open and ready for the next experience. This is what we would call an *integrated* energy experience.

However, there are times when an experience coming in from the outside world is too intense and too overwhelming for the body/mind complex to process or digest at the time it is happening. The system simply cannot cope with the enormity of the incoming input through the senses. It could be something that is seen, something we hear, or a bodily experience like a car accident or an assault. Particular smells, tastes and sounds may accompany the experience. These inputs together constitute an energy event, which translates into a kind of electrical "charge" that is felt as sensation in the body. When the charge is simply too great, the body cannot clear the amount of energy or sensation moving through the body and instead of passing through and integrating back to Source, this energy charge remains lodged in the body.

It is as if a thousand-volt experience is moving through a body equipped to handle a five hundred-volt experience. In overload, the nervous system hits the "circuit breaker," and shuts down to survive the experience. This is a healthy protection response. It allows us to live through an overwhelming event by not only keeping us alive, but distancing ourselves from it so that we can come back to it and process it at a later time when we are better equipped to handle it.

Through experience, we know that ordinary energy events, if felt and allowed, will peak, subside and eventually resolve themselves. Experience has shown us that if we are sad and allow the sadness to be felt and experienced, the sadness will pass and will return to zero. We don't have to do anything to resolve it except allow it to be felt and pass through, because energy knows what to do if left alone. However, with bigger events, the enormity of the sensation can be so great, we do not trust that if we feel it, it will safely pass. It feels dangerous to allow the amount of intensity that is present. We don't feel equipped and cannot trust that if we experience the enormity of the sensation, it will restore us back to wholeness. More likely, it feels as if we will be swept away by the sheer immensity of the sensation, drowned in it, and that we will never be able to recover ourselves again. This is what causes us to shut down to what feels like an overwhelming experience.

Essentially we are saying, "I can't feel this." "I don't want to feel this. " "It is too much for me to feel this." This is not bad. It is a survival mechanism. It just means that for this particular experience, we feel unequipped to handle what is moving through. Often quite rightly so. A child may be faced with events far beyond its capacity to manage at that time. In that case, the best strategy may be to put it away and pretend like it never happened because that is what is necessary for mental and emotional survival. As adults the same is true. We may be faced with an event we need to set aside for our own mental and emotional stability until we can come back to it little by little to process it. Or, we may be in a situation where others are relying on us. We have to set our own feelings aside until a later time when we can finally let down. The only issue is that sometimes we never go back. We think that if we simply move on, the past will no longer affect us. Yet, like a hydraulic pump, if you push the experience away it will just pop up somewhere else.

The third law of thermodynamics says that, "Energy is neither created nor destroyed, it simply changes form." This means an event we put away in a closet, doesn't simply disappear, it remains in the closet and will continue to affect us at some level until the original energy of the experience is allowed to move through the system and return to its neutral Source state.

Peter Levine's book, *Waking the Tiger, Healing Trauma: The Innate Capacity to Transform Overwhelming Experiences,* outlines a process by which an incomplete stress response can be the basis of unresolved trauma. When an animal comes out of a *freeze* cycle (known as playing dead), it will discharge the energy associated with the event by running to escape, trembling, shaking, or other kinds of rhythmic muscle contractions. According to Levine's theory, this natural physical discharge of survival energy doesn't always happen in humans. Or, if it does, we often try to suppress that effect when that is exactly what the body needs. An incomplete experience in the body can create residual trauma and prevent the body from returning to its baseline state. Instead of resetting, we are left with a highly activated incomplete motor plan which is left revving the systems of the body indefinitely.[153] This motor plan wants to complete itself and so our unconscious mind may continually resurface memories or flashbacks as part of its mechanism to try to complete and integrate the event. It may replay the event over and over in search of resolution. Or the unconscious may try to reconcile the event through dreams which can feel like recurring nightmares.

315

From the Yogic point of view, this is exactly what a trauma is. It is an overwhelming energetic event that was buried, and because it was never resolved, continues to affect us at the physical, mental and/or emotional level. Imagine the body as a tube and this incomplete event as energy that, like water, is meant to pass through the body/mind tube. Instead, when we shut it down, that energy or water hits a wall of resistance. Like water, the energy simply circles back in on itself, moving into a holding pattern, waiting for the time when the wall of resistance will be removed and the energy of the event will be able to complete its journey through the tube and back to its neutral state. Energy circling in on itself in a continuous feedback loop is called a *granthi,* or energy knot, in Yoga. We all have *granthis* from incomplete experiences.

A trauma is a big *granthi,* or energy knot. This knot remains unresolved in the tube at an unconscious level. When new information and events come into the tube, they can bump up against and retrigger the old event. For someone with trauma or PTSD, for example, a hand placed unexpectedly on a shoulder or a car backfiring is enough to retrigger the old, incomplete energy event—often bringing with it a disproportionate reaction or even memories and flashbacks.

This is simply part of the body's effort to resolve the incomplete event. Flashbacks and triggers are not the enemy. They are part of the healing response of the body. The more we try to suppress the memories and close out the triggers, the more the healing force of the body will try to speak to us, increasing its volume so that we will listen and pay attention. The more afraid we become of the intensity, the more we will try to shut it out, and the stronger it will become. The stronger the suppressed intensity becomes, the more afraid we become and the less we are willing we are to face it. It becomes a vicious escalating circle.

The beauty of Yoga Nidra is that brick by brick, session by session, we are slowly and gently removing the blockage we have put up to the unresolved energy lodged in the body/mind complex. Bit by bit, in titrated doses that the system can handle, this energy moves through the tube and is resolved. Just as the body knows how to heal a physical wound, it knows how to integrate and repair emotional wounds. It is rare for those who practice Yoga Nidra to have flashbacks, and if they do, they are more like passing memories seen before they flow out. Over time, as the original block is released, the triggers also naturally disappear. The beauty is that we are not *revisiting* the event itself. We are *discharging* the energy around the event that continues to affect the nervous system. We will know that the energy around an event is discharged when we can speak about it factually and objectively. We may have a low level of emotion around the event, but talking about it or even thinking about it doesn't put us back into an overwhelmed reactive state.

How Do We Shut down in the Face of Overwhelming Experience?

When we find ourselves in danger, the body goes on high alert. The stress response kicks into full gear and the body prepares itself to survive. In survival circumstances, our attention is not on integrating the experience—our attention is chiefly on survival. The autonomic nervous system operates through the sympathetic and parasympathetic nervous systems. Each system has its own particular survival strategy to protect both the body and the mind. Fighting or running corresponds with the sympathetic nervous system (*fight or flight*) survival response. The parasympathetic nervous system (*rest and digest*) survival response is *freeze*.

Fight Flight or Freeze

When we are faced with an emotionally or physically threatening situation, the nervous system goes into overload and the primal instinctual brain, specifically the amygdala, takes charge. The body goes into high alert, adrenaline is pumped through the body, the heart races, blood flows to the limbs and the senses are heightened to prime the body's abilities to escape or fight. The brain develops a motor plan—a way to survive the situation. The strategy usually involves trying to *fight* the situation or *flee* from it.

In some instances we may feel caught in a dead-end situation where we have no control to do anything. Or our nervous system may be too overwhelmed and we become paralyzed with fear. This is known as the parasympathetic *freeze* strategy, which in animals often manifests as "playing dead." When we *freeze*, we may be unable to move, we feel the whole body go numb, we may go speechless with fear, or we may even feel as if we are watching the situation unfold from a distance. At times we may feel that we are not in our own body, but are watching ourselves from the outside. *Fight, flight or freeze* is not bad. It is a healthy protection response that allows us to survive by mentally, physically and emotionally distancing ourselves from the overwhelming present.

Sometimes, we may experience *fight, flight and freeze* in combination with one another. We may *fight* or *flee*, but feel disembodied at the same time. Whatever the survival response, without resolution, the body can become trapped in a perpetually re-circuiting *fight, flight or freeze* cycle. Instead of returning to a normal baseline, we become stuck in the same instinctual feedback loop *even in the absence of any threat.* This persistent survival-level state locks us into a lingering experience of deep-seated stress which taxes the body's reserves and keeps the mind and emotions in a hyper-vigilant (*fight or flight*) or dissociated (*freeze*) state.

Symptoms that were meant to last for a short time become long-term symptoms. A one-time event initiating a *freeze* response becomes the enduring state in which the body lives—immobilizing us in more subtle ways. Dissociation, a numbed, spaced out or confused response, can be part of the un-integrated *freeze* response. The brain tends to run slowly and inefficiently. It is difficult to focus or concentrate as if operating in slow motion. There is often little or no connection with the body.

Many with PTSD are stuck in the sympathetic *flight* or *flight* response. The mind is still reliving the event and the body is still trying to save them. As a result, the body becomes adapted to living in the *fight or flight* response as the norm. The body, being stuck in this endless feedback loop, lives with a constant hair-trigger response to any reminder of the traumatic event. As far as the nervous system is concerned, the event is still not over and has not reached closure. Until then, the body will continually respond as if it were under imminent threat. Symptoms can include increased startle response, hypervigilance, fearfulness and fear of sleep. Since the body is subsisting in a constant state of threat, sleep is spotty and shallow at best. Many dread sleep in fear of surfacing memories and dreams. Triggers and flashbacks are common. Some take great pains to avoid anything that may trigger the incomplete event, not realizing this is a normal response to a traumatic event. Most people will create this response to a sufficiently severe trauma.

One of the most visible and recognizable signs of being frozen in *fight/flight* is chronic, rapid, shallow chest breathing (hyperventilation), often accompanied by rapid heartbeat, cold, sweaty hands, and neck spasm. This is an indication that the individual is stuck in a threat scenario that seems to have no end. The light switch is stuck on ON, and no matter what they do, where they go, or what they tell themselves, they cannot turn it off. It doesn't turn off with loved ones, it doesn't turn off with sleep. Explosive outbursts resulting from excessive *flight/flight* excitation are also common. The nervous system in extreme stress takes its toll on the entire body and mind which can trigger depression, hopelessness, and meaninglessness. Survivor's guilt, self-blame and depression are often accompanying mental and emotional factors.

In the sympathetic state, our surroundings don't appear as benign or neutral. A possible threat is always around the corner. It is like being stuck in a nightmare and having no way back to the person we used to be. The nervous system is still behaving as if the event never passed and is still in play. There are some, though, for whom the *fight or flight* state is not felt as an unsafe place. It is felt as the *only safe place* to be. These individuals don't want to come out of this state because to be the person they once were is to be vulnerable. For those with wartime trauma, there can be a longing to return to the action—a longing to return to comrades who share common understanding. It is quite likely that the camaraderie of wartime provides the most highly sophisticated anti-stress mechanism we possess as humans—social engagement. Through a highly intricate system of facial expressions and eye contact, the way we interact with each other can actually inhibit the *fight, flight* or *freeze* response. The bonding generated in the military environment may well provide exactly this, and though it may not heal an existing trauma, it might certainly soothe the pain.

A common symptom of PSTD is perception of the world through the lens of survival. This is called *hypervigilance*. Interestingly, Dr. Rajendra Morey, an Assistant Professor of Psychiatry at Duke University and Director of the Neuroimaging Lab at Durham Veterans Administration Medical Center, showed combat pictures along with pictures of everyday people and activities to veterans with PTSD. The amygdala, the *flight or fight* center of the brain, reacted the same to both situations. This study showed exactly what we have described—that even benign situations can be perceived as a threat to someone with PTSD.[154]

Normally, the body should be able to operate in a natural spectrum between *fight* and *flight* (sympathetic) and *rest and digest* (parasympathetic). Even when we become stressed, we should be able to come back to a natural baseline where we feel relaxed and open—available to our environment and able to interact fully with it. According to Peter Levine, with PTSD, it is almost as if the shock to the system throws off this natural rhythm and the nervous system becomes *hyper-responsive*, causing the body to *overreact* both sympathetically and parasympathetically to its environment. Instead of being able to act, focus, concentrate and be directive and determined, we become hyper-vigilant, paranoid, perpetually fearful and explosive. Instead of being able to return to a relaxed and open baseline state, the para-sympathetic nervous system seems to overcompensate—moving into a dissociated, spacey, lethargic, dull and listless state. This may be why many people with PTSD display symptoms of excessive fight, flight and freeze.[155]

The body will heal itself when we are not only able, but also ready, to resolve the stuck energy charge of the event. Only then will the body be able to come out of this mode and back to a neutral baseline state.

Types of PTSD

Even if the body is fixed in a hyperactive threat response, after a time, the body may be able to bounce back and return to normal. For example, after a mugging, we may be in a hyper-vigilant state for a time, but after a while it will pass and we will move on with our lives. Such symptoms of severe stress lasting one month or less are called ASD or Acute Stress Disorder. If the body and mind are stuck in a severe stress response for longer than one month, this is called PTSD or Post Traumatic Stress Disorder. The symptoms are the virtually same as ASD, the main differences are severity and persistence over a longer period of time.

PTSD was first brought to public attention in relation to war veterans, but it can result from a variety of traumatic incidents, such as mugging, rape, car accidents, train wrecks, plane crashes, bombings, or natural disasters such as hurricanes, floods or earthquakes. ASD and PTSD are much more common that one might think. ASD and PTSD occur when an event occurs unexpectedly and is an extreme and overwhelming shock to the system. In natural or other disasters, reality is turned upside down from one moment the next, shattering one's sense of security and safety.

Complex PTSD is a more intricate variation of PTSD that typically results from a prolonged exposure to a threat. Even though the event is shocking and overwhelming, in order to survive, the person learns to adjust to the circumstances in whatever way possible. This could include child abuse, sexual abuse, prison camps and concentration camps, being kidnapped or held captive, and physically or mentally abusive relationships. Not only can Complex PTSD be the result of stress in combat experiences, it can also be the result of growing up in a war torn country, in a dangerous neighborhood or in a violent and unpredictable family.

The main difference between complex PTSD and standard PTSD is that because of long exposure, the person learns to adapt to the environment in order to survive. The symptoms can be subtler, manifesting in the body or in certain self-sabotaging behaviors or thinking patterns. Keep in mind that neglect can be a form of abuse just as much as physical abuse, but may be even more difficult to cope with or even explain because there is nothing tangible to see.

Symptoms of Complex PTSD

Here are symptoms that may present themselves in those who have lived through a long-term, no-win situation:

- Emotional de-regulation which includes difficulty modulating anger, self-destructive and risk-taking behaviors and difficulty modulating sexual involvement.

- Somatization: carrying bodily trauma in the form of various physical symptoms or ailments.

- Alterations in self-perception: guilt, shame, feeling damaged. Trying to rationalize or minimize the importance of the event in one's own mind, or feeling that no one understands.

- Alterations in relations with others: inability to trust and create bonds. Loss of interest in others.

- Loss of beliefs that previously sustained a healthy relationship to life circumstances.

A person with complex PTSD has learned to live with a situation and survive. They can appear to be perfectly normal, yet display erratic behavior, emotions and make poor choices on behalf of themselves. They may feel their world is broken. Their innocence and way of looking at the world is lost. They may try to put aside the event and pretend like it is not important, even though it is. However, this suppressed event often comes out in extremes of emotion, mood and risk-taking behavior. It can lead to addiction as a way to cover up the pain.

Self-destructive, inappropriate or excessive sexual behavior is common. This can occur from a number of different causes. Sex can be a way to feel loved and not be alone for at least a while, and the closeness is a way to keep away the pain. However, at the same time, someone who has been abused, even if not sexually, will tend to dissociate from the act of sex. They will have the closeness they are seeking, but be cut off at the same time.

The other most common difference between complex PTSD and PTSD is somatization. While the mind may not want or be able to remember what happened, the muscles, tissues and cells still remember. Being touched in a particular way, being touched unexpectedly or too quickly will often act as a trigger. Even taking on certain body positions can trigger a traumatic response. For example, I had a client who was sexually molested as a child. In yoga class, she would go into a stress response just by assuming certain yoga poses that involved opening the inner thighs or lying on her back. Just the position itself was enough to trigger her back into a *freeze*, dissociated stress response.

How Yoga Nidra Can Help

Integration

Yoga Nidra is particularly helpful for treating symptoms of PTSD and other forms of trauma. For one thing it enables people to relate differently to their thoughts and emotions. For someone with a history of trauma, emotions and memories can be so intense and unpleasant that unhealthy behaviors, such as substance use, become the means to escape from them. This may work temporarily, but these suppressed emotions quickly come back with even more force.

The skills practiced in Yoga Nidra lead to increased tolerance and acceptance of uncomfortable emotional experiences. Yoga Nidra is a safe, gentle method that allows the unresolved energy of an overwhelming event to slowly begin to unwind and be released. Yoga Nidra does not dig into the past nor make it necessary to relive the event. This is what those working with PTSD and trauma like most about the practice of Yoga Nidra. The body is allowed to discharge what it is ready for in a safe, relaxed state. Residual thoughts and emotions gradually pass like clouds through a clear blue sky. The less these feelings are feared, as in Yoga Nidra, the more easily they can flow through and be released, leaving us more and more whole, relaxed and at peace.

Very often during Yoga Nidra, old fragments of trauma are released outside of conscious awareness. Without even knowing what has been released, individuals report feeling lighter, different, as if some unspoken burden has been lifted. It happens in deep states of relaxation where the body can simply let go of what it no longer needs in the amount and timing that is uniquely appropriate to each individual.

In the meditative state, we are resting in a safe place. Here, life events can be observed as if watching a movie. We become less afraid to face anything that might surface. We dare to face these events because they don't feel like outside uncontrollable forces anymore. They feel like emotions—scared and terrified ones—but emotions nonetheless.

Relaxation

Another significant benefit of Yoga Nidra is that it re-teaches the body how to turn the light switch OFF and return to a balanced interplay between the sympathetic and parasympathetic nervous systems. The nervous system can reset itself to operate within the norm, rather than the hyper-tense (excess sympathetic) or dissociated (excess parasympathetic) state. Step by step, Yoga Nidra teaches the body how to return to a calm, relaxed, neutral state.

In Yoga Nidra, we do the opposite of hyperventilation which is associated with the stress response. We are deliberately slowing and deepening the breath to induce a deep relaxation response. Respiration is the only major system in the body which can be involuntarily affected by stress, but can voluntarily be controlled to return to baseline levels. Somewhat like the flywheel in a car engine, the breath regulates all the other autonomic systems, including brain function.

Yogis have known for thousands of years that controlling and changing the way we breathe can counteract the debilitating effects of nervous system overload. If we want to teach the body how to return to its baseline state, breath is an important key.

Most of us need to change the chronic habit of shallow breathing to diaphragmatic (belly) breathing, which is natural in animals, newborns, and relaxed individuals. Breathing is one of the key practices of the Amrit Method of Yoga Nidra. If you are working with trauma it is advisable to spend extra time and attention on breath.

The Anatomy of PTSD

In the diagram below (Figure 24), you can see the differences between a normal brain and a brain with PTSD. The differences are shocking and dramatic. It literally looks as if the brain has been eaten away by high levels of cortisol in the system resulting from chronic stress. In fact, chronic stress and cortisol can cause the entire brain to shrink in size, including the pre-frontal cortex which affects concentration, decision making, judgment and social interaction. Too much cortisol results in the loss of synaptic connections between neurons.[156] However, this is not all bad news. The body can heal and recover if we provide the proper environment. The key to reversing this process is to remove

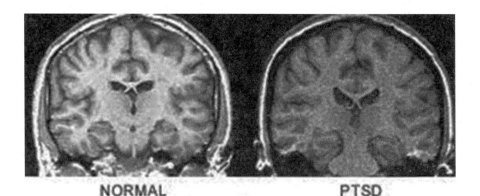

NORMAL   PTSD

Figure 24: A Normal brain compared with a brain suffering from PTSD. The difference is astonishing.

*Attribution: "Figure 4.2", from **Does Stress Damage the Brain? Understanding Trauma-Related Disorders from a Mind-Body Perspective** by Douglas J. Bremner. Copyright © 2002 by Douglas J. Bremner, M.D. Used by permissions of W.W. Norton & Company, Inc.*

excess cortisol from the system, breaking the biochemical momentum of the *fight or flight* response and affording the body an opportunity to heal.

There are three areas of the brain playing a role in PTSD that Yoga Nidra can affect (Figure 24). Yoga Nidra meditation is shown to alter each of them in different ways.

Amygdala

One of the major areas affected by PTSD is the amygdala, the area of the brain responsible for threat perception and fear responses. When a shocking event happens, massive amounts of cortisol are released into the system, which dramatically affect the landscape of the brain. Scientists have found that excessive long-term exposure to cortisol can cause the amygdala to become hyper-reactive.[157] In fact, being under the chronic stress associated with PTSD actually *increases* the activity level and number of neural connections in the amygdala or fear center.[158] This may cause the unnecessary fear responses and hypervigilant threat perception.

As we have learned, Yoga Nidra calms the body and brain by removing excess cortisol from the system. Studies on Mindful relaxation techniques such as Yoga Nidra have demonstrated that the more normal the size of the amygdala, the less stressed people feel. Through these practices, the amygdala actually shrinks back to a more normal size as stress is reduced.

Prefrontal Cortex

The second area PTSD influences is the size and structure of the prefrontal cortex, the area just behind the forehead. This area is responsible for executive function, emotional intelligence, making well-thought-out choices, social and emotional connection, and our ability to feel love. While the amygdala appears to be active in fear acquisition (learning to fear an event), the prefrontal cortex can dampen the original fear response. Different areas of the prefrontal cortex play slightly different roles. The medial prefrontal cortex suppresses the amygdala and controls the stress response. Data supports the involvement of this same area (the medial prefrontal cortex) in the pathophysiology of PTSD, and its role in possibly mediating some of its symptoms.[159] Other parts of the prefrontal cortex help sustain long-term dampening of fearful memories. The size of the prefrontal cortex appears to be related to its ability to inhibit the fear response.[160]

The prefrontal cortex is associated with self-regulation, the ability to manage instinctual reactions, fears and emotions coming from the amygdala. If the amygdala is an unrestrained child, the prefrontal cortex is the parent who can keep the child calm and manage and direct the child in helpful ways. When the weakened "parent" can no longer control the "child" in the way it was meant to, the child is more prone to run amok. Fearful memories and hyper-reactive responses take control without anything to manage them. If weak, the "parent" cannot do its job of both dampening short-term reactive responses and extinguishing the overriding effect of long-term fearful memories.

The experience of love, security and emotional bonding promotes the growth of fibers in the prefrontal cortex. Strong emotional bonds and attachments formed as a child with parent figures strengthen this area of the brain. In addition, studies show that how a mother rat cares for its newborn baby plays a role in how that baby will respond to stress later in life. The pups of nurturing moms are more resistant to stress. Their brains have more cortisol receptors which stick to cortisol and dampen the stress response.[161]

The prefrontal cortex is also developed through meditation and Yoga Nidra practices. As we have learned, just 11 hours of practicing a meditation technique induces positive structural changes in the prefrontal cortex. This enables the prefrontal

Yoga Nidra: The Art of Transformational Sleep

cortex to reclaim its parental role and once again establish its calming, dampening and inhibiting effect on the over-reactive amygdala. A healthy prefrontal cortex allows a person to develop resilience. Such a person will possess a greater resistance to traumatic events and will have an outlook that aids their recovery.

Interestingly, the prefrontal cortex is not fully developed until age 22 to 26. Consider the age of those entering the military. Physiologically, they are not equipped to handle what they may see or experience in war. If there is a history of an unstable youth or background in which strong emotional bonds were not created, that puts them at an even higher risk for PTSD, and this is exactly what we are seeing. Research bears this out. Environmental factors, such as childhood trauma, head injury, or a history of mental illness, may further increase a person's risk by affecting the early growth of the brain.[162]

How helpful would it be to train our troops in a method like Yoga Nidra to put their brain physiology in the best possible position BEFORE a traumatic event occurs? Such resiliency training is slowly being adopted by the U.S. Military Special Forces. Not everyone who returns from war is affected by what they see in the same way. Yoga Nidra gives a person more wartime resilience and resilience to any other life experiences they may have.

Hippocampus

The third area of the brain affected by PTSD and other types of trauma is the hippocampus. As levels of cortisol rise, the hippocampus, the part of the brain associated with mood, learning, memory and stress control deteriorates. Stress profoundly affects the hippocampus and can lead to fewer new brain cells being manufactured in the hippocampus. Severe trauma can trigger a massive release of cortisol into the brain which, in extreme conditions, can even kill cells of the hippocampus.[163] The hippocampus also inhibits the activity of the HPA (hypothalamus, pituitary, adrenal) axis which controls the body's stress response—so when it weakens, our ability to control our stress is diminished.[164] A compromised hippocampus affects the ability to learn and remember things. It can set the stage for more serious conditions such as depression and even Alzheimer's disease.[165]

The common link between stress and depression is likely the hippocampus. Severe stress affects our mood severely, potentially creating serious bouts of depression. Depression is common among those with PTSD. Those who suffer from depression tend to have a smaller hippocampus. Research has shown that Mindful relaxation techniques such as those in Yoga Nidra are associated with an increase in the size of the hippocampus in as little as eight weeks.[166] The practice of Yoga Nidra releases serotonin into the system. Serotonin is like fertilizer for the neurons of the hippocampus. It stimulates the growth of new neurons in the hippocampus. It is also shown that such regeneration of the hippocampus positively restores mood and memory.[167]

In fact, in addition to traditional medications for depression and anxiety symptoms of PTSD, researchers are currently using serotonin-targeted approaches. They are also looking at melatonin because it appears to contribute an anti-depressant effect—though scientists are unsure why. GABA is also on the cutting edge of treatment protocols for its use in mediating anxiety. Do you remember which of these healing agents Yoga Nidra releases naturally in your body? All of them! The body releases a cornucopia of healing agents which are capable of restoring, stabilizing and healing the body both psychologically and physiologically.

Metabolic Syndrome and PTSD

Those with PTSD are stuck in a perpetual stress response, which predisposes them to many stress-related illnesses and most commonly, metabolic syndrome. Metabolic syndrome is a cluster of clinical signs associated with chronic stress including obesity, high blood pressure, insulin resistance and cardiovascular disease. According to a study led by Pia Heppner, PhD, a psychologist with the University of California, San Diego School of Medicine and Veterans Affairs of San Diego, VA Center of Excellence for Stress and Mental Health (CESAMH), veterans with post-traumatic stress disorder (PTSD) are more likely to have metabolic syndrome than veterans without PTSD.[168] Since all the techniques of Yoga Nidra have been shown to produce a relaxation response, it is an ideal aid in reversing the effects of metabolic syndrome.

Related Studies

Veterans

The clinical benefits of Yoga Nidra for PTSD are well documented.[169] A published, peer-reviewed study on PTSD was conducted with returning Vietnam and Iraq war veterans who participated in eight weeks of Yoga Nidra. The results showed:

- Reduced rage, anxiety, and emotional reactivity
- Increased feelings of peace and self-awareness
- Relaxation despite ongoing challenges to mentally focus and intrusive traumatic memories
- Better sleep
- Mood improvement

Clinical research on Yoga Nidra began in 2007 when the Department of Defense funded a study to explore the impact of iRest Yoga Nidra on soldiers returning from Iraq and Afghanistan who had been diagnosed with PTSD. As a result of the study, Yoga Nidra has since been endorsed by the military as a complementary therapy and is being offered in military hospitals and VA centers around the country (33 is the often quoted number of locations offering Yoga Nidra).[170]

In 2010, the War Related Illness and Injury Study Centers found that of 164 veterans attending Yoga Nidra classes, 85% reported improvements across 13 different symptoms including disturbing memories, headaches, anxiety, depression, insomnia, hypervigilance, irritability and angry outbursts.[171] Yoga Nidra has also been studied for the management of chronic pain in veterans with Traumatic Brain Injuries. Conclusions show significant and demonstrable health benefits for those with chronic pain.[172]

Research has shown that meditation is beneficial to people with a history of trauma exposure—including veterans, civilians with war-related trauma, and adults with a history of childhood sexual abuse. Meditation exercises included movement and stretching, focusing on breath, and paying neutral attention to sensations, images and thoughts. We use these same techniques in Yoga Nidra. In one study, veterans who used the meditation skills they learned over the course of treatment had lower levels of clinician-rated PTSD and depression at post treatment.[173]

Another study on meditation showed 47.7% of veterans had clinically significant improvements in PTSD symptoms including: depression, capacity to function and interact normally and the ability to accept versus avoid triggering experiences.[174]

After just eight weeks of practicing meditation, veterans of the Iraq/Afghanistan wars showed a 50 percent reduction in symptoms of post-traumatic stress disorder (PTSD). The study evaluated five veterans, ages 25-40, who had served for 10 months to two years in moderate or heavy combat. The meditation practice significantly reduced stress and depression, and participants showed marked improvements in relation-ships and overall quality of life. The paper's senior research-er, Norman Rosenthal, M.D., is Clinical Professor of Psychiatry at Georgetown University Medical School. "Even though the number of veterans in this study was small, the results were very impressive," Rosenthal said. "These young men were in extreme distress as a direct result of trauma suffered during combat, and the simple and effortless meditation technique literally transformed their lives."[175]

Urban Firefighters

A study among urban firefighters showed fewer PTSD symp-toms, depressive symptoms, physical symptoms, and alcohol problems with the use of meditation. Reduction in symptoms was related to stress reduction and greater mastery of mind and emotions. It was concluded that meditation should be included in models of stress, coping, and resilience in firefighters.[176]

Children

Researchers from the University of Bielefeld in Germany compared the efficacy of two different treatments for children with severe PTSD in a Sri Lankan refugee camp, in the acute aftermath of the Tsunami of 2004. Thirty-one children were randomly assigned to one of two short-term interventions: ei-ther six sessions of Narrative Exposure Therapy for children (KIDNET), where children draw and tell the story of what they experienced, or six sessions of meditation-relaxation (MED-RELAX), without talking about the event at all.[177]

At six months follow-up, recovery rates were 81% for the chil-dren in the KIDNET group, where the event was discussed. The recovery rates for the MED-RELAX group, was an impressive 71% without talking about the event at all. Both techniques showed PTSD symptoms and impairment in functioning were significantly reduced at one month post-test and both showed the effects remaining stable over time. Recovery rates in both treatment groups exceeded the expected rates of natural recovery. I find it remarkable that a technique as simple as meditation and relaxation, without revisiting the traumatic event at all, could be almost as effective as a directed type of therapy. It stands to reason that combining the two could enhance the effectiveness of both techniques.

Intentions for Recovering from Trauma

Personality and life attitudes, a tendency to view challenges in a positive way, as well as availability and use of social support, result in quicker recovery from trauma. Planting *Intentions* in Yoga Nidra based around these factors help strengthen the body/mind complex with the kinds of attitudes that will assist in moving through trauma.

Social Support

Studies demonstrate that those who have even one source of support are more likely to survive and recover from trauma. It can be appropriate to choose *Intentions* that support seeking out social support like: "I ask for help when I need it.", "It is safe to share my inner world.", "I reach out to the support around me." or "The more I share the less I carry."

Even Traumatic Events are Manageable

It is very common for negative thought patterns to creep in after a traumatic event. There is often a loss of belief in God or goodness in the world. The more these negative feelings and thoughts are repeated, the more entrenched they become, leading to pessimistic, cynical, hopeless, disempowered or depressive cycles of thinking and feeling. The underlying cause is seeing oneself as a victim of the event—believing the event has the power to determine how we think and feel.

In fact, *we* have the power to determine how we think and feel. We *choose* our response to life events. Life events do not decide how we feel about them. That is up to us. Understanding that control lies in oneself and how we choose to respond to events, re-establishes this inner power. *Intentions* that support this can have very positive effects. Appropriate *Intentions* could be: "I am free and clear of all that has happened in the past.", "I have the power to choose my response to all life's experiences.", "I release all those who I hold responsible for my happiness.", or "I am light, unburdened and free."

Letting go of the past doesn't mean suppressing it or pretending it didn't happen. It means allowing for the fact that it did happen, allowing for the feelings and sensations that are there as a part of the event, and then realizing at a certain point that we have the choice to hold on to and relive the event over and over in our own mind, or put down the past and leave it where it belongs. You already lived through it, you already survived. It is over. You made it. Now you have the choice to move on, changed but wiser—enriched, but not broken, for having known and experienced what you did. This perspective is one you choose to take, not one that is automatically given. Which perspective on life you choose, will ultimately determine your experience of life.

Understanding and Conscious Meaning

Eventually we may be able to see the event as a meaningful one, allowing us to understand and choose what we want to make of the event rather than the one we automatically adopted at the time. I once experienced a traumatic episode in my own life. My whole family suffered from the aftermath. For many years, my conclusion from this event was that people were not to be trusted and that if only the event had not happened, everything would have been fine.

After some time and distance, I realized I could view that event in a completely different light *if* I chose. I recognized that people act and respond according to what has happened to them in *their* past. They could not help their reactions and feelings any more than I could help mine, and that didn't make them bad people.

With time came understanding. The cost of my believing people were not to be trusted was great; my own health, well-being and happiness suffered. I held the pain in my heart against those people, but it never touched them—it only poisoned me. When I finally admitted to myself that no matter what, these were individuals about whom I cared, I freed myself. The situation hadn't changed, but my heart was free to move on to trust again.

Events don't have meaning. We give meaning to events and the meaning we give, determines how we feel about them and what we do with them. One interpretation of this event left me with a closed and bitter heart, the other helped me open it. *I realized the choice was mine and that that choice would determine the course of my life.*

Since every event is just what it is, we can use *Intention* to help us shift and see events differently, in ways that are more beneficial and helpful for us. The only caveat is that we need to be sure we are not just covering up an old interpretation with a new one, but truly rewriting it, genuinely seeing and experiencing the situation in a different way.

In the episode referred to, I could have looked to the past and tried to tell myself, "Well, everything is as it should be. That is what all the spiritual books say." I could have tried to pretend that is what I felt and kept repeating positive thoughts and affirmations. In that case I would only be using one thought to cover up an older, deeper one. However, if I could feel in every cell of my being that, "Everything is as it should be," I would *know* this truth; I would *feel* it and begin to live from this place. Then I would have rewritten it.

Yoga Nidra is a powerful tool to rewrite underlying beliefs, to truly experience your past and the whole world in a different light. In fact, this is exactly what I did with this event. What I saw deep in a Yoga Nidra experience was that this event was actually the most spiritual event of my life. While painful on one level, it shifted the course of my entire family's life and made each of us grow in ways we never would have if the situation had stayed the same. We were forced to grow, to learn and evolve. And it was this situation, the most painful of my life, that shaped who I am today. *Most people find their greatness in the midst of their greatest pain.* Without that pain, they rarely go as far or as deep in life. *The pain is also the door to freedom.*

From Lock to Key

In the case of trauma, the most important shift in our world-view is from lock to key. Often, the tendency is to see the trauma as the prison that obstructs us from an old life—the person we knew ourselves to be. We might believe the trauma stops us from ever living a normal life again. We feel life is something that will no longer be available to us in the same way. If that is how we choose to focus on it and see the event, then that is what will be experienced.

However the traumatic event can also be perceived as a *key*— not as a lock. It is a key to a new kind of life, different from what came before. It is a life that includes, is informed by and even enriched by the event, but is not a victim of it. Appreciating your life in its entirety for what it has given you and what it has shaped you to be is the key that unlocks the rest of your life. If you want to find an *Intention* for yourself here, you might ask yourself: "Regardless of what happened in the past—who do I want to be now? How can I see that event as having shaped me to be a greater person? How have all the experiences of my past brought me perfectly to this moment where I get to be this person I was meant to be?"

For example, you might feel that a past physically abusive relationship is keeping you from feeling safe enough to move into another relationship. You could feel locked into the fear, "What if I choose the wrong person again," and be limited by it. Or you could see your past experience as wisdom gained, allowing you to move in the direction you *do* want to go. In that case your *Intention* could be something like, "I have the wisdom to make the choices that serve me."

We often believe that because of the bumps, bruises and cuts we have accumulated along the road of life, we are somehow disqualified from the rest of life. I would say it is precisely *because* of those experiences that you are uniquely qualified to make choices that better serve you the next time around. Recognizing this and appreciating your life in its entirety for what it has given you, is the key that unlocks the rest of your life. *Intentions* here could include, "I accept the path that has brought me here.", "I trust that my life is shaping who I'm meant to become."

To quote the Greek philosopher Aeschylus, "Wisdom comes alone through suffering." In the case of more intense or acute trauma, appreciating even one thing you gained from the event is crucial. For example, appreciating the enormity of what you experienced and survived. You made it through and are here to tell the story. That is an amazing feat. The fact that you lived through it reveals some qualities you possess that you may never have acknowledged or recognized. These are qualities you want to put into your *Intentions* to help them grow. Some examples are: "Life has revealed my inner power.", "I face all situations with equanimity and dignity.", "My life has shown me the inner strength I didn't know I had.", "My life is showing me how to face pain with an open heart.", "The setbacks in my life have shown me inner fortitude and courage." or "I have everything I need to be with my life as it is."

Once we become more empowered, it is natural and very healthy to take concrete steps to do something with what we have learned. We may give back and help others who are on the same road. We may have found meaning or purpose from that event and if so, it is important to follow it. It is what will keep you going. It is what will make you feel the event was worth it because it will have made you into a greater version of yourself.

Recommendations for Practice

During Yoga Nidra, the body/mind gently clears itself outside your conscious awareness. Sometimes this clearing results in feeling moody or out of sorts for no apparent reason. It's okay. Let it happen.

If it is more comfortable to practice with the eyes open, you may do so—maintaining a soft, unfocused gaze. You may even prefer to sit up with your back to the wall.

If, at any time during or after the Yoga Nidra, you feel uncomfortable memories or emotions surfacing, let them pass through as if you were watching a movie playing out on a screen. Simply watch them. If you find yourself resisting the movie, becoming afraid or getting drawn into it, ground yourself in the Now as these feelings or memories continue to pass across the screen. You can ground by bringing your attention to the soles of your feet, or by bringing your thumb and index finger together. You can repeat an *Intention* such as, "I am safe and secure right now." You can even observe yourself as the movie watcher watching whatever moves across the screen. You, as the movie watcher, are safe.

Stay in the present by focusing on your breath and remember that whatever it is, it is no longer present. Make the present your safe place, because NOW YOU ARE SAFE! When you are really present, there is no fear because the cause of the fear *is not* here anymore. The fear only comes back when you drift from the present and get caught in the memories, or if you react to the fear and let it pull you away from Now. Use the present as your anchor point. Let all the old stuff pass across the screen you are watching unencumbered, keeping in mind phrases such as: "I am willing to let it arise as it does.", "I allow it to be just as it is.", "It just wants to be acknowledged, allowed and felt as it is so it can pass through." The more you do this, the lighter and freer you will feel with each progressive practice.

SECTION THREE

Practicing The
Ancient Secrets of
Yoga Nidra

How to Practice Yoga Nidra

Now that we've understood how beneficial the practice of Integrative Amrit Method of Yoga Nidra is, let's look at when and how to practice for the most benefit.

When to Practice

Of course the best time to practice is whenever you can. You might find you have a few moments to practice Yoga Nidra while waiting in the car for your kids, on your lunch break, in a waiting room or even while on an airplane. Any time you have extra time is a great time to practice Yoga Nidra.

There are three general times that are ideal. The first is in the morning as soon as you get up. This is a wonderful way to set the course of your day. A Yoga Nidra in the morning helps you remember you are more than the thoughts, events and emotions that will be passing through during the course of the day. It will keep you steady and grounded. You can use *Intention* to help you remain present, calm and focused no matter what happens.

Another good time to practice is in the evening, just before you fall asleep. This is a great way to release thoughts, impressions, reactions and events of the day that tend to occupy the mind and keep us from falling asleep. This is especially helpful if you tend to get stuck in events of the day. Yoga Nidra will help you disengage from and integrate these events in a restful way—dropping you down into the Alpha brainwave state, then allowing you to enter a deep, restful and rejuvenating sleep.

A third time to practice is in the late afternoon when we start to feel tired. This is when our blood sugar is drops. We tend to lose focus and seek out coffee, sugar, snacks or other stimulants to stay awake. The Amrit Method of Yoga Nidra is a great alternative. Yoga Nidra is shown to balance blood sugar and will naturally restore energy, focus and concentration, allowing you to be productive throughout the rest of your day.

Where to Practice

Incorporate your practice into a place where it is easy and doesn't add a lot of extra steps to your day. If you have a Yoga Nidra recording on your iPod, you can just tuck in your earbuds as soon as you awaken, before you fall asleep, or whenever you decide to practice. You can practice seated or lying down. Whatever is most convenient and comfortable for you is best. The most important thing is that you *do* it.

Some people find it useful and helpful to have a meditation space or yoga mat set up to practice. This is wonderful because just entering the space tells the body it is time to move inward. It creates a sacred space in your house for you. However, if you are the type of person who, on the way to your sacred space, will be distracted by emails, coffee, breakfast and the newspaper—and will likely never make it there—you might opt to remain in bed and practice. For those whose lives are packed with things to do, waking up, rolling on your back, putting on your iPod for a Yoga Nidra before you get out of bed can be an ideal way to begin the day without adding a lot of extra effort. If you have back or other body issues, practicing in bed may be a better option. If in bed, practice Yoga Nidra lying on your back when possible. If needed use height under the knees and only as much height under the head as needed to keep the chin parallel to the floor. A very thick pillow that props the head up too high sends an "awake" signal to the brain. If you suffer from chronic pain or other injuries, and cannot lie on your back, any other position where your body is most likely to be still is best.

What to Practice With

Yoga Nidra is about a complete release of doing and effort. For this reason it is most effective when led by a person or a CD. You don't want to have to think about what to do next. Having to remember, anticipate and guide yourself takes away from the effect of Yoga Nidra. However, there are certain techniques which can be effectively used on their own. For example, "61 Points" or breathing techniques are very beneficial to boost energy, make up for sleep deprivation or manage reaction.

Eventually, with consistent practice of Yoga Nidra, you will be able to close your eyes and in one breath, you will be in the depths of meditation. You will be able to take yourself to a Yoga Nidra state without the techniques. Even so, I still suggest a consistent guided practice. This is because the various techniques of Yoga Nidra provide unique therapeutic benefits which are excellent for your overall health and well-being.

How Long?

If you notice you cannot settle down during a Yoga Nidra, try the option of beginning with some yoga poses or stretches. For those who are mentally active, dynamic yoga poses or gentle stretches before the Yoga Nidra practice assist with turning attention inward.

Beginners typically start with a shorter 20 minute Yoga Nidra. As you become more advanced, you will find you can naturally rest in the depths of Yoga Nidra for longer periods of time. The longest Yoga Nidra is usually 45 minutes; it is only body comfort that prevents people from longer Yoga Nidra sessions. However, if this happens spontaneously, there is no problem with it. In fact advanced Yogis remain in states of Yoga Nidra for many hours at a time in various stages of *Samadhi* (the experience of merging into oneness with the whole).

After you become a consistent practitioner of Yoga Nidra, your body will know when it is complete. Sometimes you will only need to go down into Yoga Nidra for twenty minutes (or even less) and then your awareness will naturally rise to the surface. Nothing is wrong. You have touched stillness and that is all you need. You have the option to remain in the Yoga Nidra and may find yourself dropping back down, or, if you feel complete, you may take your time and come out when you are ready.

This is not to be confused with a more common "surfing" experience in Yoga Nidra where you may feel as if you are "surfing" up, down, through and between various brainwave states. It feels as if you are conscious and hearing clearly for a time, then dropping out, then rising back to hearing, then dropping out again. This can be accompanied by a sinking or dropping feeling. Allow this to happen and follow the process. After consistent practice, you will clearly be able to tell the difference between "surfing" the brainwaves versus a true completion in which the body feels clear, refreshed and ready to go.

Position and Propping

An Integrative Amrit Method Yoga Nidra experience will run anywhere from 20 to 45 minutes. Sometimes a Yoga Nidra experience will be shortened to fit the end of a yoga class (12-15 minutes), but ideally, take at least 20 minutes to get down into the deepest states of Yoga Nidra, rest there, and return refreshed. For the time you are in Yoga Nidra, eliminate bodily distractions and discomfort as much as possible.

If accessible, lying on the back is ideal for optimal energy flow through the body. If the low back is sensitive, place more height than you think is needed under the knees. You may use several rolled blankets, pillows, or even place your lower legs on a chair. Sometimes an additional blanket on the chair is needed for extra padding. If you find the legs falling asleep, be sure that the padding is directly behind the knees and not unduly compressing the whole area under the legs.

Yogis state that Yoga Nidra is even deeper than sleep. Once you experience Yoga Nidra for the first time, you may notice certain body parts become super sensitive due to the deep relaxation and heaviness induced in the body and also due to increased energy flow. These areas can include the back of the head, the heels, or even the wrists and sacrum. Placing a folded blanket over the whole yoga mat or any other type of padding will generally help the whole body rest. Additional padding, such as a folded blanket can be placed under any sensitive areas such as the back of the head. Ideally, height under the head should only bring the chin parallel to the floor and no higher than the body. If having a higher pillow is absolutely necessary for comfort, then use it.

If pain or other conditions make lying on the back difficult, any position where the body is most comfortable and least likely to need to move is best. For pregnancy, after three months, or at the first sign of discomfort, side-lying on the left side is recommended to increase the amount of blood and nutrients that are reaching the placenta and baby. Otherwise, side-lying on the right stimulates the *ida*, or calming *nadi*, which is ideal for Yoga Nidra. The yoga mat should be well padded with blankets under the head and between the legs as well. Yoga Nidra in bed is a good option here as well.

Take care that the body is not touching anything, such as a foot touching the wall or a water bottle. While we may think it doesn't matter, stimulating sensory signals are being sent to the brain and this is counterproductive to the aim of Yoga Nidra.

Keep in mind that body temperature drops during Yoga Nidra, so it is usually advisable to cover the body with a light blanket. If you begin with stretches or poses, have it neatly draped at the end of your mat so you can simply pull it over you when the time comes.

If lying down is not an option for you, sitting against a wall or in a chair are both good options. Make sure you are sitting with the spine as straight as possible. If you are in a chair, the feet should be on the floor or on blocks if that is more comfortable. Placing the chair against a wall can be a nice option so that the head can lightly rest on the wall to prevent the head from bobbing forward.

When you become deeply relaxed in Yoga Nidra, the tongue may slip back toward the throat causing snoring, even if you don't normally snore. The letting go that happens in Yoga Nidra can be deeper than in sleep even though the practitioner is still conscious. I have had numerous amusing incidents where I will gently squeeze the toe of someone who was snoring. After, they will ask why I squeezed their toe. They will indignantly say to me, "I wasn't asleep, I heard everything you were saying!" Yet, they were, in fact, snoring. This is not a concern as long as you are not in a group and disturbing others. If you are in a group and have trouble with either falling asleep or snoring, you can try keeping one hand lifted. When you begin to fall asleep the arm will drop slightly and thus will keep you in a state of relaxed awareness. You can also elevate the upper body using stair-stepped blankets, bolsters, a body wedge or reversed Back Jack™ Floor Chair with blankets on it.

If you have extreme low blood pressure or feel dizzy after Yoga Nidra, experiment with upper body elevation. This will often take care of the issue.

Falling Asleep

Over time we are training the body to stay awake in deeper brainwave states. However, in the beginning, it is natural that you may fall asleep as this is what the body is accustomed to doing in deeper brainwave states. Over time you will naturally find a level of conscious awareness remaining even though you are in a deep state of meditative relaxation.

Also keep in mind that if your body is exhausted or sleep deprived, it will take care of its survival needs before spiritual practices. Your body needs to restore itself first. Don't fight it. If you are falling asleep, it is not disturbing anyone, and you know that is what your body needs, then let it happen. Once you feel ready to train yourself to be restfully aware in deeper brainwave states, set an *Intention* beforehand such as, "I resolve to remain awake." Repeat it to yourself three times before you enter the Yoga Nidra. If that doesn't work, try the lifted hand method. Or go to two hands. If none of these work, elevating the upper body or sitting against a wall or in a chair until the body learns this skill is a good option.

Many times people will be in the state of Yoga Nidra but think they fell asleep. This is because in the deepest states of Yoga Nidra, there are gaps of nothingness. We stop hearing what is being said as we drop into the silence behind the words. However, the cells of the body are still registering everything that is said. If you come back at the end of a Yoga Nidra when you are asked to, you were not asleep. You were in a deep state of Yoga Nidra.

Sometimes people will feel they were completely alert during the Yoga Nidra, yet the body was relaxed at the same time. This is also Yoga Nidra. The state can be experienced in different ways at different times. The key is to do the practice and let go of attachment to a particular experience as being the one you want. Rather, let each experience be as it is, trusting that when you let go, the higher intelligence can move through you in the way it needs to. Even if you fall asleep during a Yoga Nidra, you are gaining benefits. Your body is still hearing everything that is said on some level.

Motionless

The purpose of Yoga Nidra is to move into a state of complete non-doing. Any motion activates the sympathetic nervous system. We want to quiet this as much as possible so the body can regenerate itself. However, if the need to move is so great that it becomes a distraction, make the adjustment slowly and consciously and return to stillness as soon as you are able.

Listening

Listening is not intended to be a mental process in Yoga Nidra. It is meant to be an energetic, bodily and cellular listening. When we listen with the mind, we take in the directions, process them through the mind, make sure we understand them, and then "do" them. Listening in Yoga Nidra is a more direct and non-mental process. You don't need to consciously take in every single word. Instead, simply allow the body to receive the words and respond to them directly and non-mentally.

Even if you cannot hear, or if you are listening to Yoga Nidra in another language, you will still get the energetic benefits and transmission of Yoga Nidra. A Yoga Nidra facilitator I trained has a mother who is going deaf. She invited her to class. At the end, she said she couldn't hear anything, but felt very relaxed. She said, "It was really strange though. I felt these different points in my body lighting up one after the other." Her daughter had been guiding the "61 Points" of Yoga Nidra! The body hears even if the ears don't.

Of course, if you do have hearing difficulties, it is always nicer to hear if you can. Try to be as close to the guide as possible. Turn your head to face them for the Yoga Nidra, and let them know you have hearing difficulties. Sometimes those with hearing difficulties prefer to practice seated or elevated with their eyes softly open so they can read the lips of the instructor. This is also an option.

Release of Doing

Everywhere in life, we are learning to do things. Yoga Nidra is just the opposite. It is not about doing anything. It is a release of all doing, all effort to make anything happen. Typically, when someone asks about Yoga Nidra, they ask how to do it right. That is like asking how to do floating. Floating is not something you *do*, it is something that happens when you *let go of any doing*.

In some styles of Yoga Nidra, the purpose is concentration. The techniques are used as a point of concentration, and the intent is to use your will to keep your focus and attention on the technique at hand throughout the entire practice. In the Amrit Method, the purpose is to quiet the mind to a single point of concentration, until even that is surrendered to the ocean of stillness. Here, concentration is seen as a stepping stone to resting as oneness: it is not an end it itself. We are not striving and struggling to stay with the technique. *The technique is designed to take you beyond the technique itself. It is a jumping off point.*

The purpose is to release all doing and to rest, to float, in your true nature, where all effort to be or to do anything is released. The technique serves as a platform from which you can dive into a state of complete non-doing.

Follow the guidance of the technique until you feel yourself dropping away into the ocean of silence. *Let yourself fall away.* When the mind comes back, simply pick up and follow the guidance at that stage of the Yoga Nidra.

Disturbances

Disturbances are a part of life. Even Yoga Nidra experiences, as a part of life, will include disturbances. There are two ways to practice Yoga Nidra. You can practice Yoga Nidra because the environment allows you to notice the profound peace and silence present. Or, you can practice Yoga Nidra as a way to rest in profound peace and silence *despite* the fact that disturbance is present. Both are valuable. One aspect of the practice effortlessly drops you into a state of silence. The other makes you practice it under pressure. The beauty of the former is it trains you to rest as peace. The beauty of the latter is you are training yourself to rest in that peace even when life is disturbing.

In Yoga Nidra, students often notice that the same noises that felt assaulting and irritating at the beginning of the session become less so as they progress through the practice. The volume of the disturbance has not changed. What has changed is their resistance to it. The more you let go, the less things disturb you. The same is true in life. The less you push against disturbances, they less they will be disturbing to you. It is the act of pushing them away that makes them appear more assaulting than they really are. In the midst of environmental distractions, simply affirm that these will only serve to draw you more deeply into the Yoga Nidra. It is amazing to see how effective this technique is.

The same applies to internal disturbances. Maybe you have an internal reaction to someone who is snoring. Or maybe you have a judgment about how the Yoga Nidra is being led. Or perhaps you are judging yourself for your thoughts. These are internal disturbances. The more you engage them or even try to change them, the more they will pull you into them. Instead, do not engage. Simply allow for the fact that this "internal noise" is present and allow that internal disturbance to simply draw you more deeply within. The intention you can use is, "Any disturbances, external or internal, only draw me deeper within."

The Yoga Nidra Script

What follows is one complete Integrative Amrit Method of Yoga Nidra script for Health and Healing. These are just a few of the techniques that can comprise a Yoga Nidra experience. This script is intended as a means for you to dip your toe into an Amrit Method Yoga Nidra practice.

As discussed, when you practice Yoga Nidra it is best to be guided so that you can fully receive its benefits and effects. You can use this script as a personal tool to record and listen to yourself in the Yoga Nidra experience. Or, you can use it to guide others. When guiding someone else, it is important to drop yourself into a meditative space. Take your time, remember to breathe. Feel what you are speaking and let the energy of the words be felt. Use the pauses indicated to allow the *energetic impact* of the technique to be received.

An experienced Integrative Amrit Method Yoga Nidra facilitator is skilled in all the techniques of Yoga Nidra and can tailor experiences for specific populations, needs and conditions. To truly share this powerful modality in the way it was intended and bring transformational shifts to yourself and others in a responsible way, further training is recommended for those who want to go deeper. More information is provided at the end of this book.

The following Amrit Method Yoga Nidra experience is written and created by Yogi Amrit Desai. You will see that many of the points touched on in this book are built into the Yoga Nidra experience. This is your opportunity to *experience* what you have just learned. Enjoy.

The Integrative Amrit Method of Yoga Nidra for Health and Healing

Closing the Eyes and Being Present

Close your eyes and quiet your mind.
Be still.
Let go of all thoughts, worry and tension.
Give yourself fully to a higher power. Relax, trust and let go...
Breathe in fully and exhale with a deep sigh...
And again, breathe in fully and exhale with a deep sigh... And let go even more....
Feel a deep sense of contentment and peace in your heart.
(pause...)

Deliberate Tension and Relaxation

We will move our attention into the body to release trapped energy and move deeper into total relaxation.

Those with cardiac disease, hypertension, or glaucoma should use caution. If you cannot have undue pressure in the head for any reason, it is important that you breathe normally and only lightly tense the body.

Upper Body:

As you inhale, make fists and deliberately induce stiffness and tension throughout your shoulders, arms and fists.
Tighten...tighten...even more.
Now let go completely. Relax.
On your next exhalation, relax even more. Let go.

Observe and feel the flood of energy in your arms...
(pause...)

Lower Body:

This time as you inhale, deliberately induce stiffness and tension in hips, legs and feet. Tighten...tighten...hold..hold.

Let go. Let go completely. Relax.

Observe the flood of energy in your legs...
(pause...)

Whole Body:

This time tighten and tense the entire body as you inhale: arms, hands, shoulders, feet, legs, face....

Tighten...tighten...

Now let go completely. Relax.

On your next exhalation let go even more.

Observe and feel the energy extending to all the muscles, nerves and cells of your entire body.

Release any holding...anywhere.

(pause...)

Bumblebee Breath

I will guide you in the next phase to enter into deeper and subtler levels of relaxation through the bumblebee sound and breath.

Use your thumbs to gently close your ears, just tight enough so that you can still hear me. Rest the remaining fingers on either side of the forehead.

In a moment, we will take a deep breath in and with closed lips, we will begin to hum the sound of the bumble bee. Change the pitch of the buzzing sound to maximize the vibratory sensation felt in your skull.

Now, take a breath in and follow me......Mmmmmmmmm *(Allow up to 7 breaths.)*

Now stop...bring your arms by your sides...and be still.

Bring your total undivided attention to your whole body.

Feel the stimulating impact of the vibrations extending throughout your whole body.

Observe your energy field expand and grow, extending everywhere and filling every nerve and cell of your body...

Now bring your attention to the eyebrow center...

And empty your mind into the flood of energy.

Drop into complete silence and deep stillness.

(pause....)

Universal Instructions

As we enter this next phase of Yoga Nidra, remain as motionless as possible. If you need to move or make an adjustment do so mindfully, returning to stillness as soon as you are able.

Resolve to remain awake staying in touch with the sound of my voice.

Allow your entire body to respond directly and non-mentally to my words.

Allow any disturbances, external or internal to draw you more deeply within.

Now shift from thinking and doing to feeling and being (pause...)

Do absolutely nothing from now on. (pause...)

Drop into the deepest state of tranquility, stillness and peace in the third eye.

Now your consciousness is in direct communion with your energy body.

(pause...)

Complete Yogic Breath

Now follow my guidance as we begin the relaxation breath...

Breathing in deeply fill your lungs from the bottom to the top as if you are filling a water bottle.

As you breathe out empty your lungs from the top to the bottom...

Let your breath be slow and steady.

Observe the movement of your abdomen and chest.

Stay connected to the wonderful feeling of the release of tension and the deep feeling of relaxation.

Let this feeling extend to every part of your body.

Let this entire process of breathing be the vehicle for deepening your relaxation.

(pause...)

Now redirect your full attention to your breath.

Bring your undivided attention to the movement of your abdomen and chest as you breathe in and out.

Create no struggle around breathing; use the breath to release any tensions.

Let the flow of your breath be steady and uniform as much as possible.

(pause....)

With each breath out, release any tension held in your body and anticipations in your mind......let go...

With each breath in, fill every nerve and cell with pulsating, healing energy.

Now breathe normally and be still...

(pause....)

Bring your total attention to the energy field felt in the form of sensations in your body.

Let all the tension simply melt, drain away and dissolve in the expanding energy field.

Bring your attention to your eyebrow center....

Empty your body and mind and enter deeper levels of stillness and silence.

(pause....)

Integrate

Do absolutely nothing from now on.

Settle into the silent Source of your being.

(pause...)

Heavy and Light

Heavy:

As I name the body part bring your total attention accompanied by a feeling of heaviness... sinking....like a stone in water...

Both feet...heavy...like stones...

Calves and knees...heavy...sinking...deeper

Thighs and hips...very heavy...like lead...

Abdomen, chest and back...gravity pulling you down...

deeper...

Shoulders, arms and palms...Very...very heavy

Feel your entire head...heavy like a stone

Give your body completely and totally to the omnipresent field of gravity

(pause....)

Now experience your whole body heavy like a rock.

Feel your whole body sinking...deeper and deeper....

Totally let go...into the pull of gravity...

Sinking deeper into stillness and silent awareness...

(pause...)

Light:

Now shift your attention and as I name the part of the body, let all the heaviness drain away...

Let your body be buoyant and light...like a fluffy cloud...

Both feet...limp and light...

Calves and knees...empty and free...feel it

Thighs and hips...hollow, weightless

Abdomen, chest and back...light and empty

Shoulders and arms and palms...floating...

Head...hollow...empty

Feel your whole body; empty...light and hollow

Sense the emptiness of your body, and silence of your mind

(pause...)

Energy Body: (optional)

Be free of all inhibitions and boundaries of your body and mind, past and future.

Feel the feathery lightness of your Energy body.

Enter the power of Presence and protection of your Energy body.

Feel completely safe and secure.

Give yourself permission and freedom to float out of your Physical body and drift.

Feel yourself getting lighter and lighter until you begin to float in the air.

Release your Energy body from your Physical body.

Let it freely float like a cloud in the sky.

Enter and experience the freedom of this new dimension.

Experience being released and freed from identification with your body and mind.

Witness your body completely at peace resting in stillness.

Recognize you are the Spirit separate from the Physical body.

Enjoy the Spirit freed from all limitations.

Experience your entire body and being, freed from fear of pain, hurt and suffering.

Feel the innate healing wisdom of the body, liberated and functioning optimally.

(pause…)

Now relax back into your physical experience as you remain deeply established in your connection with Spirit in faith and trust.

(pause…)

Integration Resting in Awareness/Third Eye

(Note: Incorporate a few breaths of silence between each line or two, with a space of 8-10 breaths at the deepest point of your integration. You do not need to read all lines.)

Bring your attention to the center between your eyebrows and drop into the deepest level of relaxation. *(pause...)*

Here, there remains nothing to do or achieve, you have entered the domain of grace.

Allow yourself to merge into this space and be empty...

(pause...)

In this domain of integration, you are witness of all that is happening but doing nothing to make it happen...

(pause...)

All that can never be done by your doing can happen only in the non-doing Presence of your being...

(pause...)

Feel completely safe and comfortable as you hand yourself over to the power and protection of the Presence...

Feel it.... experience it....be it....

(pause...)

Hand over all fear, apprehension and anxiety about all that you want to change control and manage...let go of all doing...

(pause...)

Feel yourself as time-transcendent Presence, right now... *(pause 8 breaths....)*

Intention

Here your *Intentions* and affirmations are actualized and fulfilled with effortless ease.

If you have self-defeating patterns or habits that are holding you back that you want to be freed from, make that your *Intention* now.

Repeat your *Intention* now silently three times *(pause...)*

Allow it to go to the deepest levels of recognition with no hesitation.

Know that your higher Self recognizes, honors and accepts your *intention*.

Have faith and trust that it has been heard and is being acted upon by a higher power of the Source within.

There is no need for you to do anything about it...

(pause...)

Affirmations

(Note: You can combine categories, however use up to three affirmations in total or repeat one affirmation three times. Give time to let each affirmation be absorbed.)

Allow your entire Self to respond spontaneously and effortlessly to what I say....

General Affirmations:

I am released from my self-image to experience the infinite potential unfolding from within me.

My Source is silent stillness. I rest in peace.

I am the non-participative observer, separate from my thoughts and emotions that come and go.

I hold no one responsible for all that has happened in the past. I am free and clear of all that has happened in the past.

I go to the Source within that heals all conflicts and restores my health and peace of mind.

I am at peace with myself as I am, and the world as it is.

Health and Healing Affirmations:

I return to the innate wisdom of my body to heal itself. I remain in restful awareness.

I relax so completely and let go so fully that the inner healing blueprint of my body functions freely and optimally.

I have entered a complete state of synergy and balance.

I let the radiant light of love melt and disperse the blocks in my body and mind.

I replace resentment and regret with total acceptance and forgiveness.

(pause...)

Higher Self and Spiritual Guide

Establish yourself firmly in faith and trust to receive the grace, protection and guidance of the higher Self within you.

The more often you go to your Source, the easier it will be to return there and longer you can stay there.

Feel the presence of your own spiritual guides, family members or mentors surrounding you and blessing you...

Accept their blessing and grace...embody it and spread it wherever you go...

Now you have prepared the base from where you can carry out interactions with life and interpersonal relationships with the integrative power of love and the Source within.

You are the emissary of light and love.

Carry it everywhere you go and to everyone you meet.

If you have an area that you feel needs healing, physical, mental or emotional allow this light and love to flow into that area now.

(pause...)

Externalize

Now, begin to become aware of the rising and falling of the breath. *(pause...)*

Slowly...feel yourself beginning to rise to the surface of awareness. *(pause...)*

Sense the body resting on the floor. The quality of the air as it touches the skin. *(pause…)*

Gradually, you can move, as if you are waking from a restful sleep.

Bend your knees and pull them closer to your chest, rock sideways gently,

Take your time; do not hurry.

Then just turn onto your right side and curl into a fetal position.....feel the safety, comfort and protection of the womb of existence.

Bring your *Intention* into your awareness again. Change nothing.

Every time you find yourself in reaction, you are empowered to replace it with your *Intention*.

Now you can gradually move and begin to sit up with your eyes closed.

Continue to stay deep in this deep inner experience.

Regardless of what you consciously recognize that has or has not changed, know that something deep within has shifted to connect you with your *Intention*.

Become aware of your body…and bring a deep sense of peace and contentment with you as you bring attention back to the body…

Notice:

How relaxed the body is…

How soft the breath is…

How silent the mind is…

How quiet the heartbeat is…

Be still…and be grateful.

Know that you can easily enter here again and again.

Now, you may gradually open your eyes.

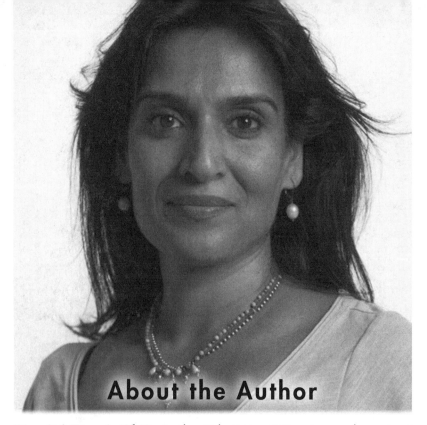

About the Author

Kamini Desai, PhD, is the Education Director and curriculum developer of one of the premier schools of Yoga Nidra in the West, the Amrit Yoga Institute. Considered an expert in the inner sciences of Yoga Nidra, Relaxation and Artful Living, she is author of the acclaimed book, *Life Lessons Love Lessons,* and is a frequent guest speaker and teacher at various institutions for higher learning throughout the United States and Europe.

Kamini's corporate clients have included: Upjohn Pharmaceuticals, Sony, Kellogg's, KEDS, Mars Confectionary, and KPN Telecom in addition to the Netherlands Ministry of Defense and Ministry of Finance. Her guided Yoga Nidra experiences have been used in various United States government facilities.

Trained at the Kripalu Center for Yoga & Health, Kamini also earned university degrees in Anthropology and Psychology, and is daughter of one of the original masters who brought Yoga to the West. Kamini served as Director of Wellness at Yarrow, an executive retreat center in Michigan, and was on faculty of the Foxhollow Leadership Center, Lenox, Massachusetts. She is one of three Founding Directors of the International University of Yoga and Ayurveda with Vijay K. Jain, MD, and Shekhar Annambhotla, MD.

Kamini is a member the Editorial Board of the *Light on Ayurveda Journal*, associated with the University of Massachusetts, Dartmouth. In 2012, she was awarded the title of *Yogeshwari* (a woman of yogic mastery) for her keen ability to bring ancient illumination to the genuine challenges of the human experience. She was featured on the cover of *Natural Awakenings (2015) in celebration of National Yoga Month,* in Dutch *Cosmopolitan, Fit and Healthy Magazine*, and has published numerous articles and videos in the United States and Europe. For more information visit: *www.kaminidesai.com, www.amrityoga.org.*

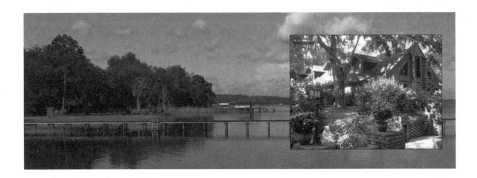

Located in Salt Springs Florida on the tranquil shores of Lake Kerr, The Amrit Yoga Institute is an educational institute devoted to engaging others in the science and system of personal transformation as outlined by the original and authentic teachings of Yoga. Headed by Yogi Amrit Desai one of the original pioneers of Yoga in the West, and through the educational curriculum developed by Kamini Desai, PhD, we offer a unique learning opportunity that will not just change you, but transform you. All of the Amrit Method teachers have been directly trained by Yogi Amrit Desai, Founder of the Amrit and Kripalu Methods of Yoga and Kamini Desai, PhD Director of Education.

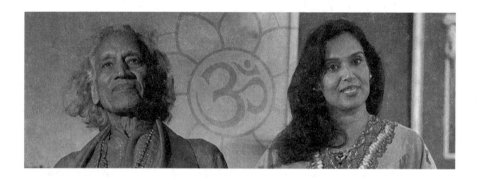

To find out more about Yoga Nidra Programs, or to find an Amrit Method Yoga Nidra facilitator near you, or to become a professionally trained Amrit Method Yoga Nidra Facilitator visit: *www.amrityoga.org*. For more information on worldwide programs given by Kamini Desai visit: *www.kaminidesai.com*. Free Yoga Nidra experiences and teachings are available on the Amrit Yoga Institute YouTube channel: *https://www.youtube. com/user/AmritYogaInstitute* Educational materials and resources may be purchased at: *www.iam.yoga*.

Endnotes

1-----Lutz A., Grieschar L. L., Rawlings N. B., Ricard M., Davidson R. J. (2004). Long-term meditators self-induce high-amplitude gamma synchrony during mental practice. Proc. Natl. Acad. Sci U.S.A. 101, 16369-1637310.1073/pnas.0407401101

2-----Hammond, D.C. "What is Neurofeedback?" *Journal of Neurotherapy* 10.4 (2007): 25-36

3-----Klimesch, W. "EEG Alpha and Theta Oscillations Reflect Cognitive and Memory Performance: A Review and Analysis." *Brain Research Reviews* 29.2-3 (1999): 169-95.

4-----Walker, Matthew P., and Robert Stickgold. "Sleep-dependent learning and memory consolidation." *Neuron* 44.1 (2004): 121-133.

5-----Barnes, D. C., and D. A. Wilson. "Slow-Wave Sleep-Imposed Replay Modulates Both Strength and Precision of Memory." Journal of Neuroscience 34.15 (2014): 5134-142. Web. 23 Mar. 2016.

6-----Strecker, Robert, and David Uygun. "Faculty of 1000 Evaluation for Sleep Modulation Alleviates Axonal Damage and Cognitive Decline after Rodent Traumatic Brain Injury." F1000 - Post-publication Peer Review of the Biomedical Literature. Web. 23 Mar. 2016.

7-----Nishida, M., J. Pearsall, R. L. Buckner, and M. P. Walker. "REM Sleep, Prefrontal Theta, And The Consolidation Of Human Emotional Memory." *Cerebral Cortex* 19.5 (2009): 1158-66.

8----- Lagopoulos, J., J. Xu, I. Rasmussen, A. Vik, G.S. Malhi, C.F. Eliassen, I.E. Arntsen, J.G. Sæther, S. Hollup, A. Holen, S. Davanger, and Ø. Ellingsen. "Increased Theta And Alpha EEG Activity During Nondirective Meditation." *The Journal of Alternative and Complementary Medicine* 15.11 (2009): 1187-92.

9----- Tang, Y.Y., Q. Lu, X. Geng, E.A. Stein, Y. Yang, and M.I. Posner. "Short-term Meditation Induces White Matter Changes In The Anterior Cingulate." *Proceedings of the National Academy of Sciences* 107.35 (2010): 15649-652.

10 --- Lagopoulos, J., J. Xu, I. Rasmussen, A. Vik, G.S. Malhi, C.F. Eliassen, I.E. Arntsen, J.G. Sæther, S. Hollup, A. Holen, S. Davanger, and Ø. Ellingsen. "Increased Theta And Alpha EEG Activity During Nondirective Meditation." *The Journal of Alternative and Complementary Medicine* 15.11 (2009): 1187-92.

11 --- Muzet, A., and G. Brandenberger. "A Quantitative Evaluation of the Relationships Between Growth Hormone Secretion and Delta Wave Electroencephalographic Activity During Normal Sleep and After Enrichment in Delta Waves." Sleep 19.10 (1996): 817-824.

12 --- Arpita. "Science and Service: The Yoga of Swami Rama." Yoga Journal May-June 1983: 34-35. Print.

13 --- Frawley, David. *Ayurveda and the Mind: The Healing of Consciousness.* Twin Lakes, WI: Lotus, 1997. Print.

14 --- Frawley, David. *Ayurveda and the Mind: The Healing of Consciousness.* Twin Lakes, WI: Lotus, 1997. Print.

15 --- Frawley, David. *Ayurveda and the Mind: The Healing of Consciousness.* Twin Lakes, WI: Lotus, 1997. Print.

16 --- Desai, Amrit C., Yogi. *Amrit Method of Yoga Nidra Immersion Manual.* 2015. MS. Amrit Yoga Institute, Salt Springs, FL. p. 78

17 --- Desai, Amrit C., Yogi. *Amrit Method of Yoga Nidra Immersion Manual*. 2015. MS. Amrit Yoga Institute, Salt Springs, FL. p. 78

18 --- Gruzelier, J. "A Working Model of the Neurophysiology of Hypnosis: A Review of Evidence." *Contemporary Hypnosis* 15.1 (1998): 3-21.

19 --- Desai, Amrit C., Yogi. *Amrit Method of Yoga Nidra Immersion Manual*. 2015. MS. Amrit Yoga Institute, Salt Springs, FL. p. 52-53

20 --- Desai, Amrit C., Yogi. *Amrit Method of Yoga Nidra Immersion Manual*. 2015. MS. Amrit Yoga Institute, Salt Springs, FL. p. 52

21 --- Nelson, Portia. There's a Hole in My Sidewalk: The Romance of Self-discovery. Hillsboro, OR: Beyond Words Pub., 1993. Print.

22 --- Robinson, Joe. "Three-Quarters of Your Doctor Bills Are Because of This." *Huffpost* 22 May 2013, Healthy Living sec. Web. 22 July 2105. <http://www.huffingtonpost.com/joe-robin-son/stress-and-health_b_3313606.html.

23 --- Boone, Jeffrey L., and Jeffrey P. Anthony. "Evaluating the impact of stress on systemic disease: the MOST protocol in primary care." *JOURNAL-AMERICAN OSTEOPATHIC ASSOCIATION* 103.5 (2003): 239-246.

24 --- Gazzaniga, Michael S. *The Cognitive Neurosciences*. 3rd ed. Cambridge, Mass.: MIT, 2004. Print.

25 --- Medina, John. *Brain Rules: 12 Principles for Surviving and Thriving at Work, Home, and School*. Seattle, WA: Pear, 2008. 184-185. Print.

26 --- Elder, C., S. Nidich, R. Cobert, J. Hageline, L. Grayshield, D. Oviedo-Lim, R. Nidich, M. Rainforth, C. Jones, and D. Gerace. "Reduced Psychological Distress in Racial and Ethnic

Minority Students Practicing the Transcendental Meditation Program." *Journal of Instructional Psychology* 38.2 (2011): 109-116. Print

27 --- Tafet, G.E., and R. Bernardini. "Psychoneuro-endocrinological Links Between Chronic Stress and Depression." Progress in Neuro-Psychopharmacology and Biological Psychiatry 27.6 (2003): 893-903. Print.

28 --- Carlson, Neil R. *Physiology of Behavior.* 9th ed. Boston: Pearson Allyn & Bacon, 2007. 601-606. Print.

29 --- Rosenkranz, Melissa A., et al. "A comparison of mindful-ness-based stress reduction and an active control in modulation of neurogenic inflammation." *Brain, behavior, and immunity* 27 (2013): 174-184.

30 --- Kasala, Eshvendar Reddy, et al. "Effect of meditation on neurophysiological changes in stress mediated depression." *Complementary therapies in clinical practice* 20.1 (2014): 74-80.

31 --- Newberg, A., and J. Iversen. "The Neural Basis Of The Complex Mental Task Of Meditation: Neurotransmitter And Neurochemical Considerations." *Medical Hypotheses* 61.2 (2003): 282-91.

32 --- Newberg, A., and J. Iversen. "The Neural Basis Of The Complex Mental Task Of Meditation: Neurotransmitter And Neurochemical Considerations." *Medical Hypotheses* 61.2 (2003): 282-91.

33 --- Walton, K.G., N.D.C. Pugh, P. Gelderloos, and P. Macrae. "Stress Reduction and Preventing Hypertension: Preliminary Support for a Psychoneuroendocrine Mechanism." *The Journal of Alternative and Complementary Medicine* 1.3 (2007): 263-83.

34 --- IsHak, Waguih William, Maria Kahloon, and Hala Fakhry. "Oxytocin role in enhancing well-being: a literature review." *Journal of Affective Disorders* 130.1 (2011): 1-9.

35 ---Uvnäs-Moberg, Kerstin. "Oxytocin may mediate the benefits of positive social interaction and emotions." *Psychoneuroendocrinology* 23.8 (1998): 819-835.

36 ---Dhayal, Parveen. "Effect of Meditation on Hormone Creation and Sporting Performance." International Journal of Applied Research 1.4 (2015): 123-26.Www.allresearchjournal. com. Web. 19 Apr. 2016. <http://www.allresearchjournal.com/ archives/2015/vol1issue4/PartC/82.1.pdf>.

37 ---Harte, Jane L., Georg H. Eifert, and Roger Smith. "The effects of running and meditation on beta-endorphin, corticotropin-releasing hormone and cortisol in plasma, and on mood." *Biological psychology* 40.3 (1995): 251-265.

38 ---Dhayal, Parveen. "Effect of Meditation on Hormone Creation and Sporting Performance." International Journal of Applied Research 1.4 (2015): 123-26.www.allresearchjournal. com. Web. 19 Apr. 2016. <http://www.allresearchjournal.com/ archives/2015/vol1issue4/PartC/82.1.pdf>.

39 ---Elias, A.N., S. Guich, and A.F. Wilson. "Ketosis with Enhanced GABAergic Tone Promotes Physiological Changes in Transcendental Meditation." *Medical Hypotheses* 54.4 (2000): 660-62.

40 ---Dhayal, Parveen. "Effect of Meditation on Hormone Creation and Sporting Performance." International Journal of Applied Research 1.4 (2015): 123-26.www.allresearchjournal. com. Web. 19 Apr. 2016. <http://www.allresearchjournal.com/ archives/2015/vol1issue4/PartC/82.1.pdf>.

41 ---Shealy, C. Norman. "A review of dehydroepiandrosterone (DHEA)." *Integrative Physiological and Behavioral Science* 30.4 (1995): 308-313.

42 ---Glaser, Jay L., et al. "Elevated serum dehydroepiandrosterone sulfate levels in practitioners of the Transcendental

Meditation (TM) and TM-Sidhi programs." *Journal of Behavioral Medicine* 15.4 (1992): 327-341.

43 --- Shealy, C. Norman. "A review of dehydroepiandrosterone (DHEA)." *Integrative Physiological and Behavioral Science* 30.4 (1995): 308-313.

44 --- Tooley, G.A., S.M. Armstrong, T.R. Norman, and A. Sali. "Acute Increases in Night-time Plasma Melatonin Levels following a Period of Meditation." Biological Psychology 53.1 (2000): 69-78.

45 --- Blask, David E., Robert T. Dauchy, and Leonard A. Sauer. "Putting cancer to sleep at night." *Endocrine* 27.2 (2005): 179-188.

46 --- Hansen, Johnni. "Increased breast cancer risk among women who work predominantly at night." *Epidemiology* 12.1 (2001): 74-77.

47 --- Jevning, Ron, A. F. Wilson, and Eileen F. VanderLaan. "Plasma prolactin and growth hormone during meditation." *Psychosomatic Medicine* 40.4 (1978): 329-333.

MacLean, Christopher RK, et al. "Effects of the transcendental meditation program on adaptive mechanisms: changes in hormone levels and responses to stress after 4 months of practice." *Psychoneuroendocrinology* 22.4 (1997): 277-295.

48 --- Dhayal, Parveen. "Effect of Meditation on Hormone Creation and Sporting Performance." International Journal of Applied Research 1.4 (2015): 123-26.www.allresearchjournal. com. Web. 19 Apr. 2016. <http://www.allresearchjournal.com/ archives/2015/vol1issue4/PartC/82.1.pdf>.

49 --- Travis, Fred, and Jonathan Shear. "Focused attention, open monitoring and automatic self-transcending: categories to organize meditations from Vedic, Buddhist and Chinese traditions." *Consciousness and cognition* 19.4 (2010): 1110-1118.

50 --- Walton, K.G., N.D.C. Pugh, P. Gelderloos, and P. Macrae. "Stress Reduction and Preventing Hypertension: Preliminary Support for a Psychoneuroendocrine Mechanism." *The Journal of Alternative and Complementary Medicine* 1.3 (2007): 263-83.

Sudsuang, R., V. Chentanez, and K. Veluvan. "Effect Of Buddhist Meditation On Serum Cortisol And Total Protein Levels, Blood Pressure, Pulse Rate, Lung Volume And Reaction Time." *Physiology & Behavior* 50.3 (1991): 543-48.

51 --- Dhayal, Parveen. "Effect of Meditation on Hormone Creation and Sporting Performance." International Journal of Applied Research 1.4 (2015): 123-26.www.allresearchjournal. com. Web. 19 Apr. 2016. <http://www.allresearchjournal.com/ archives/2015/vol1issue4/PartC/82.1.pdf>.

52 --- Dhayal, Parveen. "Effect of Meditation on Hormone Creation and Sporting Performance." International Journal of Applied Research 1.4 (2015): 123-26.www.allresearchjournal. com. Web. 19 Apr. 2016. <http://www.allresearchjournal.com/ archives/2015/vol1issue4/PartC/82.1.pdf>.

53 --- Kjaer, T.W., C. Bertelsen, P. Piccini, D. Brooks, J. Alving, and H.C. Lou. "Increased Dopamine Tone During Meditation-Induced Change of Consciousness." *Cognitive Brain Research* 13.2 (2002): 255-60.

54 --- Kayser, A.S., D.C. Allen, A. Navarro-Cebrian, J.M. Mitchell, and H.L. Fields. "Dopamine, Corticostriatal Connectivity, and Intertemporal Choice." *Journal of Neuroscience* 32.27 (2012): 9402-09.

55 --- Eastman-Mueller, Heather, et al. "iRest yoga-nidra on the college campus: Changes in stress, depression, worry, and mindfulness." *International journal of yoga therapy* 23.2 (2013): 15-24.

56 --- Kamakhya, Kumar. "Effect of Yoga nidra on hypertension and other psychological co-relates; Yoga the Science." *Yoga Publications* 3.7 (2005): 26-38.

Pranav, Pandya, and Kumar Kamakhya. "Yoga Nidra and its Impact on Human Physiology." *Yoga Vijnana* 1.1 (2007): 1-8.

57 --- Cooper, M.J. & Aygen, M.M., Dec(1979). A relaxation technique in the management of hypercholesterolemia. J. Hum. Stress, pp. 24-27.

58 --- Lekh Raj Bali, (1979). Long term effect of relaxation on blood pressure and anxiety levels of essential hypertensive males: a controlled study. Psychosom. Med.,41(8).

59 --- Vague, Nicola. Managing Stress with Yoga Nidra. Working paper no. 1. Victoria, Australia: Evolving Leaders, 2016. Print.

60 --- Desai, Kamini A. Yoga Nidra Case Study. 29 Mar. 2016. Raw data. Virginia G. Piper Cancer Center, Scottsdale, AZ.

61 --- Kumar, K. "A Study of the Improvement of Physical and Mental Health Through Yoga Nidra." *Dev Sanskriti Journal* 4 (2006).

Kumar, K., and B. Joshi. "Study on the Effect of *Pranakarshan Pranayama* and *Yoga Nidra* on Alpha EEG and GSR Levels" *Indian Journal of Traditional Knowledge* 8.3 (2009): 453-54.

62 --- Kumar, K. "Yoga Nidra and Its Impact on Student's Well Being." *Yoga Mimamsha, Kaivalyadhama, Lonavla* 36.1 (2004): 31-35.

63 --- Srivastava, N., K. Rani, U. Singh, S. Tiwari, and I. Singh. "Yoga Nidra as a Complementary Treatment of Anxiety and Depressive Symptoms in Patients with Menstrual Disorder." *International Journal of Yoga* 5.1 (2012): 52-56.

64 --- Praktikui, P. "Psychological changes as related to Yoga Nidra." (2006).

65 --- Amita, S., S. Prabhakar, I. Manoj, S. Harminder, and T. Pavan. "Effect of Yoga-Nidra on Blood Glucose Level in Diabetic Patients." *Indian Journal of Physiology and Pharmacology* 53.1 (2009): 97-101.

66 --- Brogan, Jan. "Ancient Form of Yoga Used to Cure Yuletide Stress." *Boston Globe* 17 Dec. 2013, Health and Wellness sec. Web. 10 Dec. 2017.

67 --- "IHeal." - Bethesda Magazine. Web. 15 Apr. 2016.

68 --- Brogan, Jan. "Ancient Form of Yoga Used to Cure Yuletide Stress." *Boston Globe* 17 Dec. 2013, Health and Wellness sec. Web. 10 Dec. 2017.

69 --- Pritchard, Mary, Patt Elison-Bowers, and Bobbie Birdsall. "Impact of Integrative Restoration (iRest) Meditation on Perceived Stress Levels in Multiple Sclerosis and Cancer Outpatients." Stress and Health 26.3 (2009): 233-37. Web

70 --- Jensen, P.S., P.J. Stevens, and D.T. Kenny. "Respiratory Patterns in Students Enrolled in Schools for Disruptive Behaviour Before, During, and After Yoga Nidra Relaxation." *Journal of Child and Family Studies* 21.4 (2012): 667-81.

71 --- Parker, Stephen, Veda Bharati, Swami, Fernandez, Manuel. (2013). Defining Yoga-Nidra: Traditional Accounts, Physiological Research, and Future Directions. International Journal of Yoga Therapy — No. 23 (1).

72 --- Lou, H.C., T.W. Kjaer, L. Friberg, G. Wildschiodtz, S. Holm, and M. Nowak. "A 15O-H2O PET study of meditation and the resting state of normal consciousness." *Human Brain Mapping* 7.2 (1999): 98-105.

73 --- Mangalteertham, Sannyasi (Dr A.K. Gosh), (1998). Yoga Nidra - Altered State of Consciousness. In Swami Satyananda's Yoga Nidra. Bihar School of Yoga, Munger, 6th edition.

74 --- Nilsson, Robert. "Pictures of the Brain's Activity during Yoga Nidra." / *Bindu 11* / *Issues of Bindu* / *Articles*. Scandinavian Yoga and Meditation School, 7 July 2013. Web. 11 Dec. 2015. <http://www.yogameditation.com/Articles/Issues-of-Bindu/Bindu-11/Pictures-of-the-brain-s-activity-during-Yoga-Nidra>.

75 --- Lou, H.C., T.W. Kjaer, L. Friberg, G. Wildschiodtz, S. Holm, and M. Nowak. "A 15O-H2O PET study of meditation and the resting state of normal consciousness." *Human Brain Mapping* 7.2 (1999): 98-105.

76 --- Lazar, S.W., C.E. Kerr, R.H. Wasserman, J.R. Gray, D.N. Greve, M.T. Treadway, M. McGarvey, B.T. Quinn, J.A. Dusek, H. Benson, S.L. Rauch, C.I. Moore, and B. Fischl. "Meditation Experience Is Associated With Increased Cortical Thickness." *Neuroreport* 16.17 (2005): 1893-97.

77 --- Siegel, Daniel J. *The Mindful Brain: Reflection and Attunement in the Cultivation of Well-Being (Norton Series on Interpersonal Neurobiology)*. New York: WW Norton & Company, 2007. 25, 172. Print.

78 --- Hölzel, B.K., J. Carmody, M. Vangel, C. Congleton, S.M. Yerramsetti, T. Gard, and S.W. Lazar. "Mindfulness Practice Leads to Increases in Regional Brain Gray Matter Density." Psychiatry Research: Neuroimaging 191.1 (2011): 36-43.

79 --- Hölzel, B.K., J. Carmody, M. Vangel, C. Congleton, S.M. Yerramsetti, T. Gard, and S.W. Lazar. "Mindfulness Practice Leads to Increases in Regional Brain Gray Matter Density." *Psychiatry Research: Neuroimaging* 191.1 (2011): 36-43.

80 --- Holzel, B.K., J. Carmody, K.C. Evans, E. A. Hoge, J.A. Dusek, L. Morgan, R.K. Pitman, and S.W. Lazar. "Stress

Reduction Correlates with Structural Changes in the Amygdala." *Social Cognitive and Affective Neuroscience* 5 (2011): 11-17.

81 ---Tang, Y.Y., Q. Lu, X. Geng, E. A. Stein, Y. Yang, and M. I. Posner. "Short-term Meditation Induces White Matter Changes In The Anterior Cingulate." *Proceedings of the National Academy of Sciences* 107.35 (2010): 15649-652.

82 ---Goleman, Daniel. "Relaxation: Surprising Benefits Detected." *The New York Times* 13 May 1986: n. pag. *The New York Times Company*. Web. 8 Feb. 2015.

83 ---Medina, John. *Brain Rules: 12 Principles for Surviving and Thriving at Work, Home, and School*. Seattle, WA: Pear, 2008. 176-178. Print.

84 ---Davidson, Richard J., et al. "Alterations in brain and immune function produced by mindfulness meditation." *Psychosomatic medicine* 65.4 (2003): 564-570.

85 ---Eremin, O., M.B. Walker, E. Simpson, S.D. Heys, A.K. Ah-See, A.W. Hutcheon, K.N. Ogston, T.K. Sarkar, A. Segar, and L.G. Walker. "Immuno-modulatory Effects Of Relaxation Training And Guided Imagery In Women With Locally Advanced Breast Cancer Undergoing Multimodality Therapy: A Randomised Controlled Trial." *The Breast* 18.1 (2009): 17-25.

86 ---Goleman, Daniel. "Relaxation: Surprising Benefits Detected." *The New York Times* 13 May 1986: n. pag. *The New York Times Company*. Web. 8 Feb. 2015.

87 ---Zeidan, Fadel, et al. "Brain mechanisms supporting the modulation of pain by mindfulness meditation." *The Journal of Neuroscience* 31.14 (2011): 5540-5548.

88 ---Rosenkranz, Melissa A., et al. "A comparison of mindfulness-based stress reduction and an active control in modulation of neurogenic inflammation." *Brain, behavior, and immunity* 27 (2013): 174-184.

89 --- Kiecolt-Glaser, Janice K. "Psychoneuroimmunology: Psychology's gateway to the biomedical future." *Perspectives on Psychological Science* 4.4 (2009): 367-369.

90 --- Levy, David M., et al. "Initial results from a study of the effects of meditation on multitasking performance." *CHI'11 Extended Abstracts on Human Factors in Computing Systems.* ACM, 2011.

91 --- Zeidan, Fadel, et al. "Mindfulness meditation improves cognition: evidence of brief mental training." *Consciousness and cognition* 19.2 (2010): 597-605.

92 --- Carmody, J., S. Crawford, and L. Churchill. "A Pilot Study of Mindfulness-based Stress Reduction for Hot Flashes." *Menopause* 13.5 (2006): 760-69.

93 --- Keefer, L., and E.B. Blanchard. "The Effects of Relaxation Response Meditation on the Symptoms of Irritable Bowel Syndrome: Results of a Controlled Treatment Study." *Behaviour Research* and Therapy 39.7 (2001): 801-11.

94 --- Lush, E., P. Salmon, A. Floyd, J.L. Studts, I. Weissbecker, and S.E. Sephton. "Mindfulness Meditation For Symptom Reduction In Fibromyalgia: Psychophysiological Correlates." *Journal of Clinical Psychology in Medical Settings* 16.2 (2009): 200-07.

95 --- Sephton, Sandra E., et al. "Mindfulness meditation alleviates depressive symptoms in women with fibromyalgia: results of a randomized clinical trial." *Arthritis Care & Research* 57.1 (2007): 77-85.

96 --- Cupal, Deborah D., and Britton W. Brewer. "Effects of relaxation and guided imagery on knee strength, reinjury anxiety, and pain following anterior cruciate ligament reconstruction." Rehabilitation Psychology 46.1 (2001): 28.

97 ---Greenspan, Michael J., and Deborah L. Feltz. "Psychological interventions with athletes in competitive situations: A review." *The Sport Psychologist* 3.3 (1989): 219-236.

98 ---Chopra, Deepak. *The New Physics of Healing with Deepak Chopra*. Sounds True Recordings, 2002.

99 ---Futterman, A.D., M.E. Kemeny, D. Shapiro, and J.L. Fahey. "Immunological and Physiological Changes Associated with Induced Positive and Negative Mood." *Psychosomatic Medicine* 56.6 (1994): 499-511.

100--Achterberg, Jeanne. "Mind and medicine: The role of imagery in healing." *Journal of the American Society for Psychical Research* (1989).

101--Chopra, Deepak. *The New Physics of Healing with Deepak Chopra*. Sounds True Recordings, 2002.

102--Eysenck, H.J. "Personality, Stress and Cancer: Prediction and Prophylaxis." *The British Journal of Medical Psychology* 61 (1988): 57-75.

103--Allison, T.G., D.E. Williams, T.D. Miller, C.A. Patten, K.R. Bailey, R.W. Squires, and G.T. Gau. "Medical and Economic Costs of Psychologic Distress in Patients with Coronary Artery Disease." *Mayo Clinic Proceedings* 70.8 (1995): 734-42.

104--Kiecolt-Glaser, Janice K., et al. "Emotions, morbidity, and mortality: new perspectives from psychoneuroimmunology." *Annual review of psychology* 53.1 (2002): 83-107.

105--Kiecolt-Glaser, Janice K., et al. "Emotions, morbidity, and mortality: new perspectives from psychoneuroimmunology." *Annual review of psychology* 53.1 (2002): 83-107.

106--Wilson, Sarah H., and G. M. Walker. "Unemployment and health: a review." *Public health* 107.3 (1993): 153-162.

107--Chopra, Deepak. *The New Physics of Healing with Deepak Chopra.* Sounds True Recordings, 2002.

108--Hadhazy, By. "How Has Magic Johnson Survived 20 Years with HIV?" *LiveScience.* TechMedia Network, 7 Nov. 2011. Web. 15 Dec. 2015.

109--Grossarth-Maticek, R., and H.J. Eysenck. "Self-regulation and Mortality from Cancer, Coronary Heart Disease, and Other Causes: A Prospective Study." *Personality and Individual Differences* 19.6 (1995): 781-95.

110--Hölzel, B.K., J. Carmody, M. Vangel, C. Congleton, S.M. Yerramsetti, T. Gard, and S.W. Lazar. "Mindfulness Practice Leads to Increases in Regional Brain Gray Matter Density." *Psychiatry Research: Neuroimaging* 191.1 (2011): 36-43.

111--Arias, Albert J., et al. "Systematic review of the efficacy of meditation techniques as treatments for medical illness." *Journal of Alternative & Complementary Medicine* 12.8 (2006): 817-832.

112--Marano, Hara Estroff. "Bedfellows: insomnia and depression." *Psychology today magazine* (2005).

113--Ost, L.G., and E. Breitholtz. "Applied Relaxation vs. Cognitive Therapy in the Treatment of Generalized Anxiety Disorder." *Behaviour Research & Therapy* 38.8 (2000): 777-90.

114--Olpin, Michael Nelson. "Perceived Stress Levels and Sources of Stress among College Students: Methods, Frequency, and Effectiveness of Managing Stress by College Students." Diss. Weber, 1996. Abstract. Print.

115--Staff, By Live Science. "Sleep, Anxiety Drugs Linked to Dementia." LiveScience. TechMedia Network, 2012. Web. 16 Apr. 2016.

116--Passer, Michael W., and Ronald Edward Smith. Psychology: *Frontiers and Applications*. 1st ed. Boston: McGraw-Hill, 2001. 193-94.

117--Angus, R.G., and R.J. Heslegrave. "Effects of Sleep Loss on Sustained Cognitive Performance During a Command and Control Simulation." *Behavior Research Methods, Instruments, & Computers* 17.1 (1985): 55-67.

118--Van Dongen, H.P., and G. Maislin. "Investigator: Van Dongen HP, Mullington JM, Dinges DF.–The Cumulative Cost of Additional Wakefulness: Dose-response Effects on Neurobehavioral Functions and Sleep Physiology From Chronic Sleep Restriction and Total Sleep Deprivation." Sleep 26 (2003): 117-26.

119--Kaul, Prashant, et al. "Meditation acutely improves psychomotor vigilance, and may decrease sleep need." *Behav Brain Funct* 6 (2010): 47.

120--"Sleep and Health." Healthy Sleep. Web. 19 Apr. 2016

121--Kohatsu, Neal D., et al. "Sleep duration and body mass index in a rural population." *Archives of Internal Medicine* 166.16 (2006): 1701-1705.

122--Knutson, Kristen L., et al. "Role of sleep duration and quality in the risk and severity of type 2 diabetes mellitus." *Archives of internal medicine* 166.16 (2006): 1768-1774.

123--King, Christopher Ryan, et al. "Short sleep duration and incident coronary artery calcification." *Jama* 300.24 (2008): 2859-2866.

124--Meier-Ewert, Hans K., et al. "Effect of sleep loss on C-reactive protein, an inflammatory marker of cardiovascular risk." *Journal of the American College of Cardiology* 43.4 (2004): 678-683.

125--Altevogt, Bruce M., and Harvey R. Colten, eds. *Sleep Disorders and Sleep Deprivation:: An Unmet Public Health Problem*. National Academies Press, 2006.

Nguyen, June, and Kenneth P. Wright Jr. "Influence of weeks of circadian misalignment on leptin levels." *Nature and science of sleep* 2010.2 (2009): 9.

126--Nagendra, Ravindra P., Nirmala Maruthai, and Bindu M. Kutty. "Meditation and its regulatory role on sleep." *Frontiers in neurology* 3.54 (2012): 1-4.

127--Nagendra, Ravindra P., Nirmala Maruthai, and Bindu M. Kutty. "Meditation and its regulatory role on sleep." *Frontiers in neurology* 3.54 (2012): 1-4.

128--Nagendra, Ravindra P., Nirmala Maruthai, and Bindu M. Kutty. "Meditation and its regulatory role on sleep." *Frontiers in neurology* 3.54 (2012): 1-4.

129--Lazar, Sara W., et al. "Functional brain mapping of the relaxation response and meditation." *Neuroreport* 11.7 (2000): 1581-1585.

130--Hill, Steven M., and David E. Blask. "Effects of the pineal hormone melatonin on the proliferation and morphological characteristics of human breast cancer cells (MCF-7) in culture." *Cancer research* 48.21 (1988): 6121-6126.

131--Nagendra, Ravindra P., Nirmala Maruthai, and Bindu M. Kutty. "Meditation and its regulatory role on sleep." *Frontiers in neurology* 3 (2012).

132--Walker, Matthew P., and Robert Stickgold. "Sleep-dependent learning and memory consolidation." *Neuron* 44.1 (2004): 121-133.

133--Walker, M. P., et al. "Sleep-dependent motor memory plasticity in the human brain." *Neuroscience* 133.4 (2005): 911-917.

134--Buboltz, W.C., F. Brown, and B. Soper. "Sleep Habits and Patterns of College Students: A Preliminary Study." *Journal of American College Health* 50.3 (2001): 131-35.

135--Mrazek, Michael D., et al. "Mindfulness training improves working memory capacity and GRE performance while reducing mind wandering." *Psychological Science* (2013): 0956797612459659.

136--"Sleep and Health." Healthy Sleep. Web. 19 Apr. 2016

137--Neckelmann, Dag, Amstein Mykletun, and Alv A. Dahl. "Chronic insomnia as a risk factor for developing anxiety and depression." *Sleep* 30.7 (2007): 873.

138--Sinha, Rajita, et al. "Psychological stress, drug-related cues and cocaine craving." *Psychopharmacology* 152.2 (2000): 140-148.

139--Kosten, Thomas R., Bruce J. Rounsaville, and Herbert D. Kleber. "A 2.5-year follow-up of depression, life crises, and treatment effects on abstinence among opioid addicts." *Archives of general psychiatry* 43.8 (1986): 733-738.

140--Dodes, Lance M., and Zachary Dodes. *The Sober Truth: Debunking the Bad Science behind 12-step Programs and the Rehab Industry.* Print.

141--Temme, Leslie J., Judy Fenster, and Geoffrey L. Ream. "Evaluation of Meditation (Integrative Restoration – iRest) in the Treatment of Chemical Dependency." Journal of Social Work Practice in the Addictions 12.3 (2012): 264-81. Web.

142--Witkiewitz, Katie, G. Alan Marlatt, and Denise Walker. "Mindfulness-based relapse prevention for alcohol and substance use disorders." *Journal of Cognitive Psychotherapy* 19.3 (2005): 211-228.

143--Marlatt, G. A., et al. "Effects of meditation and relaxation training upon alcohol use in male social drinkers." *Meditation: Classic and contemporary perspectives* (1984): 105-120.

144--Bowen, Sarah, et al. "Mindfulness meditation and substance use in an incarcerated population." *Psychology of addictive behaviors* 20.3 (2006): 343.

145--Britton, Willoughby B., et al. "The contribution of mindfulness practice to a multicomponent behavioral sleep intervention following substance abuse treatment in adolescents: a treatment-development study." *Substance Abuse* 31.2 (2010): 86-97.

146--Dougherty, Janis. "The Pathology of Addiction." Online video clip. YouTube. You Tube, 6 Jul 2010. Web. 17 Apr. 2016. http://www.youtube.com/watch?v=KegfzfqEre0.

147--Kayser, A.S., D.C. Allen, A. Navarro-Cebrian, J.M. Mitchell, and H.L. Fields. "Dopamine, Corticostriatal Connectivity, and Intertemporal Choice." *Journal of Neuroscience* 32.27 (2012): 9402-09.

148--Kjaer, T.W., C. Bertelsen, P. Piccini, D. Brooks, J. Alving, and H.C. Lou. "Increased Dopamine Tone During Meditation-Induced Change of Consciousness." *Cognitive Brain Research* 13.2 (2002): 255-60.

149--Alexander, C.N., P. Robinson, OTR, and M. Rainforth. "Treating and Preventing Alcohol, Nicotine, and Drug Abuse Through Transcendental Meditation: A Review and Statistical Meta-Analysis." *Alcoholism Treatment Quarterly* 11 (1994): 13-87.

Gelderloos, P., K.G. Walton, D.W. Orme-Johnson, and C.N. Alexander. "Effectiveness of the Transcendental Meditation Program in Preventing and Treating Substance Misuse: A Review." *International Journal of the Addictions* 26.3 (1991): 293-325.

Benson, H., and R.K. Wallace. "Decreased drug abuse with Transcendental Meditation: A study of 1,862 subjects." *Drug abuse: Proceedings of the international conference.* Philadelphia: Lee and Febiger, 1972.

150--Alexander, C.N., P. Robinson, OTR, and M. Rainforth. "Treating and Preventing Alcohol, Nicotine, and Drug Abuse Through Transcendental Meditation: A Review and Statistical Meta-Analysis." *Alcoholism Treatment Quarterly* 11 (1994): 13-87.

151--Wynd, Christine A. "Guided Health Imagery for Smoking Cessation and Long-Term Abstinence." *Journal of Nursing Scholarship* 37.3 (2005): 245-50.

152--Brady, Kathleen T., Sudie E. Back, and Scott F. Coffey. "Substance abuse and posttraumatic stress disorder." *Current Directions in Psychological Science* 13.5 (2004): 206-209.

153--Levine, Peter A. Waking the Tiger: Healing Trauma: The Innate Capacity to Transform Overwhelming Experiences. Berkeley, CA: North Atlantic, 1997. Print.

154--Morey, R.A., F. Dolcos, C.M. Petty, D.A. Cooper, J.P. Hayes, K.S. Labar, and G. Mccarthy. "The Role of Trauma-related Distractors on Neural Systems for Working Memory and Emotion Processing in Posttraumatic Stress Disorder." *Journal of Psychiatric Research* 43.8 (2009): 809-17.

155--Levine, Peter A. Waking the Tiger: Healing Trauma: The Innate Capacity to Transform Overwhelming Experiences. Berkeley, CA: North Atlantic, 1997. Print.

156--Murgia, Madhumita. "How Stress Affects Your Brain - Madhumita Murgia." TED-Ed. Animation. Andrew Zimbelman. 9 Nov. 2015. Web. 06 Apr. 2016.

157--Sapolsky, R.M., L.C. Krey, and B.S. McEwen. "Prolonged Glucocorticoid Exposure Reduces Hippocampal Neuron

Number: Implications for Aging." *The Journal of Neuroscience* 5.5 (1985): 1222-227. Print.

158--Murgia, Madhumita. "How Stress Affects Your Brain - Madhumita Murgia." TED-Ed. Ed. Andrew Zimbelman. 9 Nov. 2015. Web. 06 Apr. 2016.

159--Zubieta, Jon-Kar, et al. "Medial frontal cortex involvement in PTSD symptoms: a SPECT study." *Journal of psychiatric research* 33.3 (1999): 259-264.

160--Murgia, Madhumita. "How Stress Affects Your Brain - Madhumita Murgia." TED-Ed. Ed. Andrew Zimbelman. 9 Nov. 2015. Web. 06 Apr. 2016.

161--Murgia, Madhumita. "How Stress Affects Your Brain - Madhumita Murgia." TED-Ed. Ed. Andrew Zimbelman. 9 Nov. 2015. Web. 06 Apr. 2016.

162--Brewin, Chris R., Bernice Andrews, and John D. Valentine. "Meta-analysis of Risk Factors for Posttraumatic Stress Disorder in Trauma-exposed Adults." Journal of Consulting and Clinical Psychology 68.5 (2000): 748-66. Web. 20 Apr. 2016.

163--Sapolsky, R.M., L.C. Krey, and B.S. McEwen. "Prolonged Glucocorticoid Exposure Reduces Hippocampal Neuron Number: Implications for Aging." *The Journal of Neuroscience* 5.5 (1985): 1222-227. Print.

164--Murgia, Madhumita. "How Stress Affects Your Brain - Madhumita Murgia." TED-Ed. Ed. Andrew Zimbelman. 9 Nov. 2015. Web. 06 Apr. 2016.

165--Gross, Gail, Dr. "Effects of Stress on the Hippo-campus." www. drgailgross.com. 19 Mar. 2013. Web. 6 Apr. 2016. http:// drgailgross.com/academia/effects-of-stress-on-the-hippocampus/

166--Hölzel, B.K., J. Carmody, M. Vangel, C. Congleton, S.M. Yerramsetti, T. Gard, and S.W. Lazar. "Mindfulness Practice Leads to Increases in Regional Brain Gray Matter Density." *Psychiatry Research: Neuroimaging* 191.1 (2011): 36-43.

167--Mahar, Ian, et al. "Stress, serotonin, and hippocampal neurogenesis in relation to depression and antidepressant effects." *Neuroscience & Biobehavioral Reviews* 38 (2014): 173-192.

168--Heppner, P.S., E.F. Crawford, U.A. Haji, N. Afari, R.L. Hauger, B.A. Dashevsky, P.S. Horn, S.E. Nunnink, and D.G. Baker. "The Association of Posttraumatic Stress Disorder and Metabolic Syndrome: A Study of Increased Health Risk in Veterans." *BMC Medicine* 7 (2009): 1.

169--Stankovic, L. "Transforming trauma: a qualitative feasibility study of integrative restoration (iRest) yoga Nidra on combat-related post-traumatic stress disorder." *International journal of yoga therapy* 21.1 (2011): 23-37.

170--Engel, C., Goertz, C., Cockfield, D., Armstrong, D., Jonas, W., Walter, J., Fritts, M., Greene, R., Carnes, R., Gore, K., and Miller, R. "Yoga Nidra as an Adjunctive Therapy for Post-Traumatic Stress Disorder: A Feasibility Study."(2007). Samueli Institute and Walter Reed Army Medical Center

171--"IHeal." - Bethesda Magazine. Web. 18 Apr. 2016.

172--Nassif, T., D. Norris, K. Soltes, F. Sandbrink, M. Blackman, and J. Chapman. "Using Mindfulness Meditation to Improve Pain Management in Combat Veterans with Traumatic Brain Injury." (2015). VA Healthcare.

173--Owens, Gina P., et al. "Changes in mindfulness skills and treatment response among veterans in residential PTSD treatment." *Psychological Trauma: Theory, Research, Practice, and Policy* 4.2 (2012): 221.

174--Kearney, David J., et al. "Association of participation in a mindfulness program with measures of PTSD, depression and quality of life in a veteran sample." *Journal of clinical psychology* 68.1 (2012): 101-116.

175--Rosenthal, Joshua Z., et al. "Effects of transcendental meditation in veterans of Operation Enduring Freedom and Operation Iraqi Freedom with posttraumatic stress disorder: a pilot study." Military medicine 176.6 (2011): 626-630.

176--Smith, Bruce W., et al. "Mindfulness is associated with fewer PTSD symptoms, depressive symptoms, physical symptoms, and alcohol problems in urban firefighters." *Journal of Consulting and Clinical Psychology* 79.5 (2011): 613.

177--Catani, C., M. Kohiladevy, M. Ruf, E. Schauer, T. Elbert, and F. Neuner. "Treating Children Traumatized by War and Tsunami: A Comparison between Exposure Therapy and Meditation-relaxation in North-East Sri Lanka." *BMC Psychiatry* 9.1 (2009): 22.

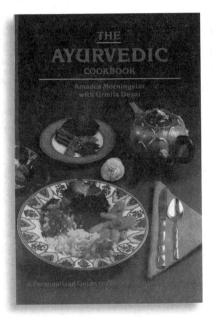

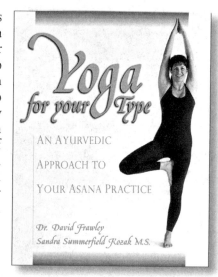